DIABETES

DIABETES

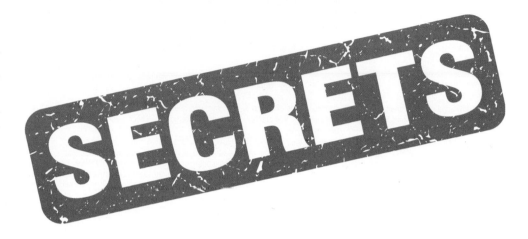

SECRETS

MICHAEL T. MCDERMOTT, MD
Professor of Medicine and Clinical Pharmacy
Department of Medicine
Division of Endocrinology
University of Colorado Denver School of Medicine
Aurora, CO

JENNIFER M. TRUJILLO, PHARMD, BCPS, CDCES, BC-ADM
Professor
Department of Clinical Pharmacy
University of Colorado
University of Colorado Skaggs School of Pharmacy and Pharmaceutical Sciences
Aurora, CO

ELSEVIER

Elsevier
1600 John F. Kennedy Blvd.
Ste 1800
Philadelphia, PA 19103-2899

DIABETES SECRETS

ISBN: 978-0-323-79262-2

Notices

Knowledge and best practice in this field are constantly changing. As new research and experience broaden our understanding, changes in research methods, professional practices, or medical treatment may become necessary.

Practitioners and researchers must always rely on their own experience and knowledge in evaluating and using any information, methods, compounds or experiments described herein. Because of rapid advances in the medical sciences, in particular, independent verification of diagnoses and drug dosages should be made. To the fullest extent of the law, no responsibility is assumed by Elsevier, authors, editors or contributors for any injury and/or damage to persons or property as a matter of products liability, negligence or otherwise, or from any use or operation of any methods, products, instructions, or ideas contained in the material herein.

Library of Congress Control Number: 2021946911

Content Strategist: Marybeth Thiel
Content Development Manager: Meghan Andress
Content Development Specialist: Nicole Congleton
Publishing Services Manager: Deepthi Unni
Project Manager: Janish Ashwin Paul
Design Direction: Bridget Hoette

Printed in India

Last digit is the print number: 9 8 7 6 5 4 3 2

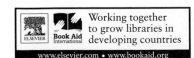

We dedicate this book to our patients, who work so hard to control and overcome diabetes; to our colleagues, who join us in this battle; to our students, whose curiosity and eagerness to learn continually challenge us; and to our families, who support us and keep us focused on the priorities of life.

FOREWORD

Approximately 34.2 million Americans and 463 million people worldwide are living with diabetes. It is the leading cause of kidney failure, acquired blindness, and nontraumatic amputations in the United States. Although the numbers of patients affected with this chronic disease continue to grow in this country and around the globe, we have seen a decline in the chronic complications of diabetes in the United States. Although diabetes can cause significant damage throughout the body, it cannot defeat the human spirit. We see and know of countless people affected with diabetes who daily face this disease head-on with determination and courage. They modify their diets. They count their calories and their carbohydrates. They often take multiple oral and/or injectable medications daily to control their glucose levels. And they monitor their blood glucose levels meticulously with painful fingersticks or with emerging technology. Although we have not found a cure for diabetes, these brave individuals defeat diabetes daily in a most inspiring way.

Knowledge is power. We have gained a great deal of knowledge about diabetes pathophysiology, diagnosis, and monitoring, along with measures to control blood glucose levels and the other metabolic features of diabetes. The purpose of this book is to empower providers, fellows, residents, students, and even patients to overcome this formidable adversary through knowledge of the foe. Although every basic and clinical aspect of diabetes could not be covered in this short book, we hope to have provided our readers with the most up-to-date information available regarding the classification, pathophysiology, diagnosis, complications, monitoring, medications, technology, and overall management of diabetes, with the hope that this will improve the lives of people suffering from diabetes and will inspire some individuals to pursue critical research to strengthen our armamentarium in the fight against diabetes mellitus.

Diabetes has different demographics and clinical features in different parts of the world, and management practices vary greatly across the globe. To supplement the information in our book, which is based mainly on data from the United States and Europe, we have invited colleagues from Ethiopia and New Zealand to write chapters about diabetes as it presents, progresses, and is managed in their parts of the world. We found their chapters to be intriguing and compelling, and we greatly appreciate their generosity in sharing their stories with us.

CONTENTS

TOP 100 SECRETS

Michael T. McDermott, MD, and Jennifer M. Trujillo, PharmD

1. Type 1 diabetes (T1D) is an autoimmune disease characterized by pancreatic beta-cell destruction resulting in absolute insulin deficiency. It is best diagnosed by finding a low or undetectable serum C-peptide and one or more positive islet-cell antibodies: glutamine acid decarboxylase (GAD) antibodies, insulin antibodies, islet antigen-2 (IA-2) antibodies, and zinc transporter 8 (ZnT8) antibodies.
2. Type 2 diabetes (T2D) is a heterogeneous metabolic disorder characterized by the pathophysiologic triad of excessive hepatic glucose production, peripheral insulin resistance, and progressive beta-cell failure; other contributing features include increased lipolysis, excessive glucagon secretion, deficient incretin hormone secretion, increased renal glucose reabsorption, and insulin resistance in the brain.
3. Less common types of diabetes include posttransplant diabetes, diabetes resulting from pancreatic insufficiency or pancreatectomy, cystic fibrosis–related diabetes, maturity-onset diabetes of the young (MODY), and medication-induced diabetes.
4. A complete medical evaluation should be performed at the initial diabetes visit to confirm the diagnosis, classify the diabetes, evaluate for complications and comorbidities, review previous treatments and risk factors, and develop a treatment plan.
5. A complete medical evaluation should include past medical and family history, diabetes history, lifestyle factors, medications, vaccinations, technology use, behavioral and diabetes self-management skills, a physical examination, and a laboratory evaluation.
6. Special attention should be given to evaluating medication adherence and self-management behaviors, psychosocial conditions, and social determinants of health (SDOH) because they significantly affect glycemic control and often go undetected.
7. Diabetic ketoacidosis (DKA) is a state of acute metabolic decompensation manifested by significant hyperglycemia, ketonemia, anion-gap metabolic acidosis, and hypovolemia. DKA most commonly occurs in people with T1D but may also occur sometimes in those with T2D and other types of diabetes.
8. Hyperglycemic hyperosmolar syndrome (HHS) most often occurs in elderly people with T2D and is characterized by severe hyperglycemia and hyperosmolality, profound hypovolemia, and absent/minimal ketonemia without metabolic acidosis.
9. Effective DKA management consists of careful attention to each of the following: intravenous (IV) fluid administration, insulin therapy in sufficient amounts, potassium replacement at the appropriate times, bicarbonate therapy when acidosis is severe, and identification and treatment of the precipitating cause.
10. Delayed resolution or recurrence of DKA or HHS may result from premature IV insulin discontinuation, failure to start subcutaneous (SQ) insulin prior to stopping IV insulin, and failure to identify and treat the precipitating cause. Neurologic complications can result from excessively rapid correction of hyperglycemia, resulting in cerebral edema.
11. Diabetic nephropathy is a progressive disease marked by the transition from glomerular hyperfiltration to albuminuria to progressive chronic kidney disease (CKD) and, finally, end-stage kidney disease.
12. In diabetic nephropathy, overactive renin-angiotensin-aldosterone system (RAAS) activity and direct vasoactive activity mediated by tubuloglomerular feedback (TGF) lead to disproportional afferent arteriolar vasodilation and efferent arteriolar vasoconstriction, thereby altering glomerular hemodynamics, resulting in hyperfiltration.
13. RAAS inhibitors (angiotensin-converting enzyme [ACE] inhibitors or angiotensin receptor blockers [ARBs]) and sodium–glucose cotransporter 2 (SGLT-2) inhibitors are renoprotective agents through the preservation of glomerular hemodynamics.
14. Diabetic retinopathy is the leading cause of blindness in working-age adults worldwide.
15. The most important risk factors for developing diabetic retinopathy are a long duration of diabetes, inadequate glucose control, and elevated blood pressure.
16. Treatment of diabetic retinopathy can be divided into observation, intravitreal injections, laser therapies, and surgery. Most affected patients may be observed, but treatment is warranted for diabetic macular edema (DME) and proliferative retinopathy.
17. Diabetic neuropathy is classified into different syndromes, including distal symmetric polyneuropathy; diabetic autonomic neuropathy; radiculoplexus neuropathy; and focal neuropathies, including cranial neuropathies.
18. Diabetic neuropathy is present in up to 50% to 66% of people with diabetes, with distal symmetric polyneuropathy being the most common pattern of disease.
19. Symptomatic treatment of diabetic neuropathy focuses on the management of neuropathic pain, in addition to other supportive measures to prevent further health consequences.
20. Macrovascular complications, most commonly manifested as atherosclerotic cardiovascular disease (ASCVD) and heart failure (HF), are very common in people with diabetes and are the leading cause of morbidity and mortality.

21. Hyperglycemia is an independent risk factor for macrovascular complications. People with diabetes, particularly those with T2D, often have comorbidities such as hypertension, dyslipidemia, and central adiposity that also contribute to increasing the risk of macrovascular complications.

22. Addressing modifiable ASCVD risk factors in people with diabetes through lifestyle modifications (dietary habits, physical activity, smoking cessation), weight loss, and appropriate medication use has been shown to significantly reduce the risk of cardiovascular complications.

23. Aggressively treating elevated blood pressure to recommended goals using ACE inhibitors or ARBs (but not both), dihydropyridine calcium channel blockers, and thiazide diuretics, alone or in combination, can significantly reduce the risk of macrovascular complications. Similarly, the routine use of lipid-lowering therapy, especially moderate- to high-potency statins, has been shown to reduce the development and progression of ASCVD and prevent cardiovascular (CV) events.

24. Nonalcoholic fatty liver disease (NAFLD) has emerged as the most common cause of chronic liver disease, including advanced fibrosis, and is prominent in people with T2D.

25. Currently, lifestyle modifications to promote weight loss are the cornerstone in NAFLD management, with bariatric procedures in appropriate individuals and certain medications also having benefit.

26. Dietary changes designed to achieve and maintain at least 5% weight loss are recommended for overweight or obese people with diabetes. Weight-loss interventions should focus on calorie restriction to achieve a 500- to 750-kcal/day energy deficit.

27. There is no ideal calorie distribution among carbohydrates, proteins, and fats; however, carbohydrate counting is recommended for people with T2D to reduce postmeal glucose excursions. Common goals are ≤45 to 60 g of carbohydrates per meal (or no more than 1/4 of the plate as starch or grain) and no more than 15 g per snack. In T1D, carbohydrate counting is used to determine mealtime insulin doses.

28. Physical activity and exercise are integral to the prevention and management of T2D. Adults with prediabetes or diabetes should engage in 150 minutes/week of moderate to vigorous physical activity with no more than 2 consecutive days without physical activity.

29. A combination of aerobic and resistance exercise is optimal for maximizing the benefits of exercise therapy in diabetes and can help minimize glucose variability and attenuate hypoglycemia risk.

30. There are physical, pathophysiological, socioeconomic, and complication-related barriers to physical activity in people with diabetes. Identification of these barriers and individualization of exercise regimens based on comorbidities and diabetes complications are key to maximizing the benefits and reducing the risks of exercise in patients with diabetes.

31. The impact of each insulin product on the blood glucose (BG) profile is determined by its pharmacokinetic/pharmacodynamic profile. Basal insulins have long durations of action and minimal peak effects, providing consistent insulin levels to help manage BG during periods of fasting. Bolus insulins have rapid onsets and short durations of action and are typically used to cover meals or correct high BG levels.

32. The approach to insulin therapy differs between T1D and T2D. Treatment of T1D typically requires intensive insulin therapy with either multiple daily injections of insulin or an insulin pump. In contrast, in T2D, insulin is typically added in a stepwise fashion when glycemic goals are not met with noninsulin medications.

33. Common adverse effects of insulin include hypoglycemia, weight gain, injection-site reactions, and lipohypertrophy. Appropriate counseling on the prevention, detection, and treatment of hypoglycemia; lifestyle measures to minimize weight gain; and appropriate insulin injection technique can help mitigate these adverse effects.

34. Numerous factors must be considered when selecting an appropriate insulin product, including diabetes type (T1D vs. T2D), pharmacokinetic/pharmacodynamic properties, total insulin requirements and degree of insulin resistance, number of required injections, and affordability.

35. Noninsulin options for the treatment of T2D include metformin, sulfonylureas, meglitinides, bromocriptine, alpha-glucosidase inhibitors, thiazolidinediones, glucagon-like peptide-1 (GLP-1) receptor agonists, dipeptidyl peptidase-4 (DPP-4) inhibitors, and SGLT-2 inhibitors. Decisions about which to add should depend on whether the person has ASCVD, HF, or CKD, in addition to other individual and drug considerations, such as glycemic efficacy, risk of hypoglycemia, effect on weight, ease of use, mechanism of delivery, cost, and side effects.

36. The most common side effect of metformin is diarrhea. This side effect is usually transient and can be minimized by starting at a low dose (500 mg once daily) and titrating the dose slowly over time to a target dose of 2000 mg daily (usually 1000 mg twice daily), taking the medication with food, and using the extended-release formulation.

37. Certain SGLT-2 inhibitors and GLP-1 receptor agonists have beneficial effects in people with T2D and ASCVD or ASCVD risk. Empagliflozin, canagliflozin, liraglutide, dulaglutide, and semaglutide have demonstrated significant reductions in major adverse ASCVD events (MACE; a composite of CV death, nonfatal myocardial infarction, and nonfatal stroke) in CV outcome trials.

38. Certain SGLT-2 inhibitors and GLP-1 receptor agonists have beneficial effects in people with T2D and CKD. Both classes can delay the onset and progression of CKD.

39. Some SGLT-2 inhibitors have beneficial effects in people with T2D and HF; SGLT-2 inhibitor use in these individuals may decrease hospitalizations for HF and CV death.

40. Precise mealtime insulin dosing requires accurate carbohydrate counting and an appropriate carbohydrate-to-insulin ratio (C:I ratio) that produces premeal to 2-hour postmeal BG excursions of 30 to 50 mg/dL.

41. The C:I ratio is an estimate of the grams of carbohydrate that each 1 unit of rapid-acting insulin will cover; a C:I ratio of X:1 means that 1 unit of insulin should be given for every X grams of carbohydrate to be consumed. The initial C:I ratio for each person is often calculated as follows: 500/Total daily dose (TDD) of insulin.

42. A correction factor (CF) is the amount of rapid-acting insulin that should be added to the mealtime dose when the premeal BG is above the target range or that is taken alone between meals to correct high-BG values. The CF is an estimate of the expected BG drop for each 1 unit of insulin given when the BG is elevated above the goal; a CF of N:1 means that a person should take 1 unit of insulin for every N mg/dL the current BG level is above the individualized target. We calculate an initial CF for each person as 1650/TDD.

43. The American Diabetes Association (ADA) recommends a general A1c goal of <7.0% for many nonpregnant adults with diabetes, whereas the American Association of Clinical Endocrinologists (AACE)/American College of Endocrinology (ACE) recommends an optimal goal of ≤6.5% if it can be achieved safely and affordably.

44. General glycemic goals are recommended for people with T2D, but targets should always be individualized based on patient-specific considerations that may affect the risks and/or benefits of intensive treatment. Factors that may warrant less stringent glycemic goals include a high risk for hypoglycemia or other drug side effects, a long duration of diabetes, limited life expectancy (long-term benefits of a more intensive goal will likely not be realized), a high comorbidity/complications burden, and patient preferences.

45. The ADA recommends comprehensive lifestyle management and metformin as first-line therapy in people with T2D. Metformin should be continued as long as it is tolerated.

46. Initial combination therapy can be considered to extend the time to treatment failure or when more than one glucose-lowering agent is needed to achieve glycemic targets.

47. Early initiation of insulin therapy is recommended in people presenting with a BG of ≥300 mg/dL or an A1c of >10%, and/or if the individual is experiencing symptoms of overt hyperglycemia (polydipsia, polyuria) or catabolism.

48. GLP-1 receptor agonists and SGLT-2 inhibitors with proven CV and renal benefit are recommended for use in people with comorbid ASCVD, HF, and/or CKD. SGLT-2 inhibitors are preferred in the setting of HF and/or CKD. The addition of these agents to mitigate CV and kidney risk is recommended regardless of the current A1c or A1c goal.

49. Thiazolidinediones and one DPP-4 inhibitor, saxagliptin, should be avoided in people with HF; these medications have been reported to increase the risk of hospitalization for HF.

50. When intensifying therapy to improve glycemic control, major considerations for medication selection include (1) avoidance of hypoglycemia, (2) minimization of weight gain or promotion of weight loss, and (3) cost considerations.

51. GLP-1 receptor agonists and DPP-4 inhibitors should not be used in combination because they exert their actions through the same incretin pathway.

52. The ADA recommends consideration of a GLP-1 receptor agonist as the first injectable agent in people with T2D because of drug efficacy, low hypoglycemia risk, and beneficial weight effects. For those requiring insulin therapy to meet individualized goals, the stepwise addition of basal insulin and, if needed, mealtime bolus insulin is recommended.

53. Prediabetes is an easily identifiable metabolic disorder that predicts a significant future risk for T2D development. Diagnosing prediabetes is critical so that measures can be instituted to proactively prevent T2D and its attendant emotional, socioeconomic, and medication burdens and the chronic complications that T2D promotes.

54. For people with prediabetes, intense lifestyle interventions that result in sustained weight loss of ≥7% and include ≥150 minutes/week of moderate-intensity physical activity are effective and essential for preventing progression to T2D.

55. Metformin can be considered for the treatment of prediabetes, especially if body mass index (BMI) is ≥35 kg/m², age is <60 years old, or there is a history of gestational diabetes mellitus (GDM). Shared decision making is crucial for these vulnerable people.

56. Women with T1D or T2D who are considering pregnancy can reduce the risk for congenital abnormalities to the baseline population risk if A1c is ≤6.5% prior to conception (or before 5–8 weeks of gestation).

57. Insulin requirements decrease in the first pregnancy trimester but increase (two- to fourfold) in the second and third trimesters as a result of pregnancy-induced insulin resistance. Adding metformin to decrease insulin requirements is not the standard of care and may be associated with an increased risk of small-for-gestational-age (SGA) infants.

58. Insulin requirements drastically drop upon placental delivery; women with diabetes are at high risk of hypo-glycemia postpartum, requiring less insulin than they did prepregnancy.

59. Pregnancy is a ketogenic state; women with diabetes can develop DKA at lower BG levels (<200 mg/dL) in pregnancy ("euglycemic diabetic ketoacidosis").

60. GDM management with oral agents is controversial because of the ability of glyburide and metformin to cross the placenta, leading to unknown long-term effects on the fetus.

61. Women with GDM are at increased risk of developing T2D in later life. They should be screened for T2D at 6 weeks postpartum and then every 1 to 3 years thereafter.

62. Diabetes is associated with an increased risk of cancer and cancer mortality.

63. Uncontrolled hyperglycemia in patients with cancer is associated with increased infection risk, higher symptom burden, malnutrition, and worse cancer outcomes.

64. Numerous cancer therapies may cause hyperglycemia, including immune checkpoint inhibitors, tyrosine kinase inhibitors, mechanistic target of rapamycin (mTOR) inhibitors, phosphoinositide 3-kinase (PI3K) pathway inhibitors, and glucocorticoids.

65. Checkpoint inhibitor-associated diabetes mellitus (CIADM) is distinct from T1D, with a rapid C-peptide decline and a low association with diabetes-associated autoantibodies.

66. Glycemic targets should be individualized in older adults to minimize the risk of hypoglycemia while still preventing microvascular diabetic complications.

67. Age-related changes can complicate the management of diabetes in older adults and should be considered when selecting appropriate medication regimens.

68. Deprescribing diabetes medications in appropriate people can simplify treatment regimens and reduce the risk of hypoglycemia.

69. Blood pressure targets for most older adults are similar to those recommended in younger people, although antihypertensives should be titrated cautiously to avoid hypotension.

70. Statins and aspirin are recommended for secondary ASCVD prevention in older adults. The benefits of statins for primary ASCVD prevention in older adults with diabetes are less clear, and aspirin should not routinely be used for primary prevention in older adults.

71. Aerobic exercise lowers BG levels during and after exercise in most people with diabetes. Resistance exercise causes less initial BG decline but smoother and more prolonged reductions of postexercise BG. Intermittent high-intensity exercise reduces BG less than moderate, consistent exercise. BG levels increase with resistance and high-intensity exercise in some people and often rise significantly during competition.

72. The primary drivers of hypoglycemia during exercise are non–insulin-mediated glucose uptake by muscle, inability to lower circulating insulin levels during exercise, more rapid insulin absorption from SQ sites, inadequate carbohydrate intake during exercise, and variable insulin sensitivity during and after exercise.

73. The key elements of diabetes management during exercise are frequent BG testing, adequate nutritional intake, appropriate insulin adjustments, anticipation of exercise effects, and adequate hydration.

74. Use of a continuous glucose monitor (CGM) plus an algorithm that makes carbohydrate intake recommendations based on current glucose levels and trend arrows has been reported to significantly improve exercise glucose control in adolescents with T1D.

75. Insulin pump therapy limits postexercise hyperglycemia without increasing the risk for hypoglycemia compared with multiple daily insulin injections. Basal rate reductions starting 60 to 90 minutes before exercise and continuing for 60 to 90 minutes after exercise usually work well for moderate exercise of $\geq$60 minutes or strenuous exercise of $\geq$30 minutes.

76. Target BG levels during hospitalization are 140 to 180 mg/dL for critically ill and noncritically ill patients; the goals can be lowered to 110 to 140 mg/dL in select individuals as long as hypoglycemia is carefully avoided. Glycemic goals in pregnant women are lower: fasting $<$ 95 mg/dL, 1 hour postmeal $<$ 140 mg/dL, 2 hours postmeal $<$ 120 mg/dL.

77. Several important principles of hyperglycemia management in hospitalized patients should be followed. Insulin is the most appropriate agent for treating hyperglycemia in the hospital. IV insulin infusions are best for critically ill patients. Basal/bolus (prandial and correction) insulin regimens are best for noncritically ill patients. BG patterns should be evaluated daily and insulin adjusted as needed.

78. Elements that should be part of all inpatient insulin infusion protocols include setting appropriate glucose targets; nurse-driven, easy-to-use insulin titration protocols; frequent point-of-care glucose measurements; insulin titration based on current glucose levels and the direction and velocity of glucose changes; and acute hypoglycemia management guidelines that include insulin dosing adjustments to prevent further hypoglycemia.

79. A CGM has three components: (1) a sensor that is inserted under the skin and measures interstitial glucose levels almost continuously (every 1–5 minutes), (2) a transmitter that wirelessly transmits glucose values to a receiver, and (3) a receiver that displays glucose values in real time or intermittently and shows trend arrows to inform the user about the direction and magnitude of glucose changes.

80. Professional CGM devices are owned by providers and loaned to users for 1 to 2 weeks at a time, either recording blinded glucose patterns or displaying real-time glucose values that can be downloaded for analysis by providers and/or certified diabetes education specialists.

81. Personal CGM devices are prescribed by the provider and are owned by the user to be worn every day (preferably) or intermittently. Without the need for fingerstick glucose testing or only twice-a-day testing (for calibration), personal CGM provides people with real-time or intermittent interstitial glucose values; trend arrows showing the direction and magnitude of glucose changes; and alarms that alert for hypoglycemia, predicted hypoglycemia, hyperglycemia, and predicted hyperglycemia.

82. The ambulatory glucose profile (AGP) is generated from the CGM download and consists of the glucose management indicator (GMI), an estimate of the equivalent A1c for the preceding 2-week period; the average glucose value; the percentage of time in range (TIR) at various levels; indices of glucose variability; and active CGM wear time.

83. Multiple studies in people with T1D, treated with multiple daily insulin injections or insulin pumps, have demonstrated that the use of CGM reduces A1c, increases glucose time in target range, reduces time in hypoglycemia, improves hypoglycemia awareness in people who have hypoglycemia unawareness, and improves quality of life.

84. Insulin pumps consist of an insulin reservoir, a pumping mechanism, and an infusion set through which insulin is delivered continuously into a subcutaneous site. Rapid-acting insulin analogs are the most common type of insulin used in pumps.

85. Two basic components of insulin delivery by an insulin pump are basal insulin and bolus insulin. Basal insulin is a continuous background insulin infusion to control hepatic glucose production overnight and between meals. Bolus insulin consists of acute insulin doses given to cover meals and/or to correct high BG levels.

86. Bolus insulin has two discrete components: a nutritional dose and a correction dose. The nutritional dose is given to cover the meal a person is preparing to eat. The correction dose is the extra insulin that is added to the nutritional dose if the premeal BG is high; correction boluses may also be taken alone between meals for high-BG values.

87. Hyperglycemia developing suddenly in someone who usually has good BG control on pump therapy requires careful evaluation for potential causes, such as infection; stress; changes in diet, physical activity, or medications; missed doses; insertion-site problems (scar tissue); infusion-set issues (occlusion, kinking); and bad insulin.

88. A hybrid closed-loop system is in integrated system in which CGM data are transmitted directly to an insulin pump, which uses an embedded algorithm to adjust the basal insulin infusion rate and/or give correction boluses to maintain glucose levels within a prespecified target range. These are called hybrid closed-loop systems because the CGM-responsive algorithms can drive basal rates and correction doses but do not yet have the capability to deliver accurate mealtime boluses.

89. Do-it-yourself (DIY) artificial pancreas systems (APSs) are not approved by the U.S. Food and Drug Administration. Some people use these systems to achieve their desired glycemic control. The systems are built by the user with various external equipment requirements, including older insulin pumps, which can be out of warranty; the design of each system is individualized by the user, but DIY APSs still require user inputs that rely on a fundamental understanding of diabetes.

90. Hypoglycemia is a common occurrence in diabetes management and is often a barrier to achieving more intensive glycemic targets. Hypoglycemia is classified into three levels. Level 3 is the most severe and requires assistance from another person.

91. Consuming fast-acting carbohydrates is the treatment of choice for hypoglycemia if a person is able to eat or drink. When a person cannot eat or drink, glucagon can be administered by another person, or IV dextrose can be given by the healthcare team.

92. Most people with T2D also have comorbid obesity, and various management options exist to simultaneously improve both conditions.

93. Antihyperglycemic agents may result in weight gain, weight loss, or weight stability. Discussions with individuals about the impact of different agents on their weight during the treatment of diabetes are of paramount importance.

94. Several antiobesity medications are FDA approved for long-term use and often produce 5% to 10% weight loss when used as an adjunct to lifestyle modification.

95. Bariatric surgery is the most effective treatment modality for achieving long-term weight loss and T2D remission.

96. There are many potential barriers to achieving glucose control, with the root of the problem stemming from clinical and therapeutic inertia.

97. The healthcare team should engage with people who have diabetes through shared decision making, communicate at an appropriate level for the person's health literacy, and express empathy and compassion for all affected individuals.

98. The impact of social determinants of health (SDOH) and psychosocial factors on glycemic control can be significant, yet these barriers are often underappreciated. Providers should routinely screen people for SDOH and psychosocial barriers using validated screening questions or tools.

99. Eighty percent of people with diabetes live in low- and middle-income countries. The International Diabetes Federation (IDF) Africa region has more than 19.4 million people with diabetes (prevalence of 3.9%), and this number will increase 143% by 2045.

100. The prevalence of acute diabetes complications is high in Africa, attributed to decreased awareness and limited resources. Related to delays in diagnosis, vascular complications tend to occur sooner after the diagnosis of diabetes.

CHAPTER 1

DIABETES MELLITUS: CLASSIFICATION, ETIOLOGY, AND PATHOGENESIS

Michael T. McDermott, MD and Jennifer M. Trujillo, PharmD

1. **What are the diagnostic criteria for diabetes mellitus and prediabetes?**
   Table 1.1 lists the diagnostic criteria for diabetes mellitus. In the absence of unequivocal hyperglycemia, the diagnosis requires two abnormal test results from the same sample or from two separate samples. If the test results are discordant, the abnormal one should be repeated. If the A1c is discordant, consider the presence of a hemoglobinopathy.

2. **How common is diabetes mellitus?**
   Diabetes mellitus affected approximately 30 million people in the United States in 2020; prediabetes affected nearly 84 million. The prevalence was highest among those of Native American and Native Alaskan descent (~15%) and lowest among non-Hispanic Caucasians.

3. **What are the different types of diabetes mellitus?**
   The most common types are type 1 diabetes and type 2 diabetes. Less common types include latent autoimmune diabetes in adults (LADA), pancreatic diabetes (type 3c), ketosis-prone type 2 diabetes, posttransplant diabetes, and maturity-onset diabetes of the young (MODY). Diabetes can also occur secondary to other diseases, such as Cushing's syndrome, acromegaly, glucagonoma, and pheochromocytoma.
   Hyperglycemia or diabetes can also result from the use of medications, especially glucocorticoids, atypical antipsychotic drugs, statins, tyrosine kinase/vascular endothelial growth factor (VEGF) inhibitors, epidermal growth factor receptor (EGFR) inhibitors, anaplastic lymphoma kinase (ALK) inhibitors, *BCR-ABL* inhibitors, phosphoinositide 3-kinase (PI3K) inhibitors, and immune checkpoint inhibitors (especially programmed cell death protein 1 [PD-1] and programmed cell death protein 1 ligand [PD-L1] inhibitors). Most drug-induced hyperglycemia resembles or is type 2 diabetes, whereas immune checkpoint inhibitors more often cause what appears to be autoimmune or type 1 diabetes.

4. **What is type 1 diabetes mellitus? What is the etiology and pathogenesis?**
   Type 1 diabetes mellitus is an autoimmune disease in which the immune system destroys pancreatic beta cells, causing absolute insulin deficiency. The disorder results from a genetic predisposition with a superimposed precipitating cause or event. The concordance for type 1 diabetes among identical twins is 30% to 70%, whereas the risk for a nonidentical twin or nontwin sibling of an affected person is 6% to 7%, and the risk for children of a parent with diabetes is 1% to 9%. Roughly 50% of the heritability can be linked to specific human leukocyte antigen (HLA) haplotypes (DR3 and DR4-DQ8), but over 60 non-HLA genes (mostly immune system genes) have also been associated with the risk for type 1 diabetes. Precipitating events that trigger the development of diabetes in genetically predisposed individuals are largely unknown; leading theories include diet in infancy, viral infections (especially enteroviruses), and alterations of the intestinal microbiome.

5. **Describe the development of type 1 diabetes mellitus.**
   Type 1 diabetes develops in stages, starting with the appearance of islet-cell antibodies, followed by progressive loss of beta-cell mass and function. Type 1 diabetes is often diagnosed clinically when there has been a loss of at least 80% of beta-cell mass. Fig. 1.1 depicts the events occurring during the development of type 1 diabetes mellitus.

6. **What tests are best to establish a diagnosis of type 1 diabetes mellitus?**
   Once diabetes is diagnosed according to the criteria outlined previously, identifying type 1 diabetes as the cause is best done by measuring serum C-peptide and two or more islet-cell autoantibodies. C-peptide is a breakdown product of proinsulin that is cosecreted with insulin and that serves as a marker of endogenous insulin secretion; C-peptide levels are low (for the ambient glucose level) or undetectable in people with type 1 diabetes. The islet-cell autoantibodies that are most commonly positive include antibodies to glutamine acid decarboxylase (GAD), insulin, islet antigen-2 (IA-2), and zinc transporter 8 (ZnT8). The presence of these antibodies can also predict the eventual development of type 1 diabetes in family members of an affected person. Those with only a single positive antibody often do not develop type 1 diabetes, but the presence of two or more positive antibodies in children confers an 84% risk of developing type 1 diabetes by adulthood.

Table 1.1 Diagnostic Criteria for Diabetes Mellitus

DIABETES MELLITUS	
Fasting plasma glucose	≥126 mg/dL (7.0 mmol/L)
2-hour plasma glucose[a]	≥200 mg/dL (11.1 mmol/L)
Hemoglobin A1c[b]	≥6.5% (48 mmol/mol)
Random plasma glucose	≥200 mg/dL (11.1 mmol/L) in a patient with symptoms of hyperglycemia or hyperglycemic crisis

[a]Two-hour oral glucose tolerance test: 75 g anhydrous glucose in water.
[b]Hemoglobin A1c: use a method certified by National Glycohemoglobin Standardization Program (NGSP) and standardized to the Diabetes Control and Complications Trial (DCCT).

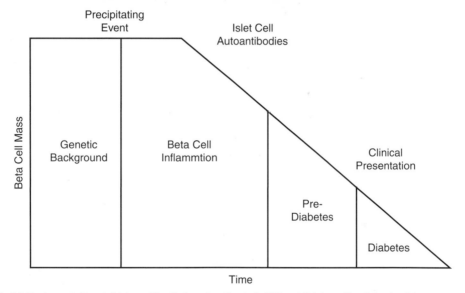

Fig. 1.1 Development of type 1 diabetes mellitus. (Redrawn from Eisenbarth GS. Type 1 diabetes mellitus. A chronic autoimmune disease. *N Engl J Med.* 1986;314:1360-1368.)

7. **What is type 2 diabetes mellitus? What are the etiology and pathogenesis?**

   Type 2 diabetes mellitus has an even stronger genetic predisposition (~90% concordance rate for identical twins) but is clearly polygenic, and the highest-risk genes are still poorly defined. On this genetic background, superimposed acquired factors such as obesity, stress, pregnancy, and glucocorticoid use can precipitate the development of type 2 diabetes. The pathogenesis of type 2 diabetes is multifactorial and complex. The classical triad includes insulin resistance in the liver (excess hepatic glucose production), insulin resistance in muscle (impaired glucose uptake), and progressive beta-cell failure (relative insulin deficiency). The "ominous octet," described by Dr. Ralph DeFronzo in the 2009 Banting Lecture, added five additional abnormalities: fat cells (increased lipolysis), gastro-intestinal tract (incretin hormone deficiency), pancreatic alpha cells (hyperglucagonemia), kidneys (increased glucose reabsorption), and brain (insulin resistance). Many of these defects are present, to a greater or lesser degree, in people with prediabetes and in nondiabetic people with a strong family history of type 2 diabetes.

8. **Explain a recent classification suggesting that there are five main types of diabetes mellitus.**

   Using six variables (GAD antibodies, age, body mass index [BMI], A1c, homeostatic model assessment [HOMA] insulin sensitivity, HOMA beta-cell function), a recent data-driven cluster analysis identified five diabetes clusters, which are shown in Table 1.2. Whereas the traditional classification of diabetes into type 1 and type 2 has a

Table 1.2 Proposed Classification of Diabetes Into Five Distinct Clusters
Cluster 1 (severe autoimmune diabetes [SAID]): early onset, low BMI, poor control, insulin deficiency, GAD antibodies positive. **Cluster 2** (severe insulin-deficient diabetes [SIDD]): similar to cluster 1, but GAD antibodies negative. **Cluster 3** (severe insulin-resistant diabetes [SIRD]): high BMI and insulin resistance. **Cluster 4** (mild obesity-related diabetes [MOD]): high BMI but no insulin resistance. **Cluster 5** (mild age-related diabetes [MARD]): similar to cluster 4, but higher age and more modest metabolic derangements.

BMI, body mass index; *GAD*, glutamine acid decarboxylase.

Table 1.3 Diagnostic Criteria for Prediabetes	
	PREDIABETES
Fasting plasma glucose	100–125 mg/dL (5.6–6.9 mmol/L)
2-hour plasma glucose[a]	140–199 mg/dL (7.8–11.0 mmol/L)
Hemoglobin A1c[b]	5.7%–6.4% (39–47 mmol/mol)

[a]Two-hour oral glucose tolerance test: 75 g anhydrous glucose in water.
[b]Hemoglobin A1c: use a method certified by National Glycohemoglobin Standardization Program (NGSP) and standardized to the Diabetes Control and Complications Trial (DCCT).

distribution of approximately 94% type 2 and 6% type 1 diabetes, this proposed classification suggests a distribution of 7.6% in cluster 1, 14.6% in cluster 2, 15.2% in cluster 3, 21% in cluster 4, and 41.7% in cluster 5.

9. **What is prediabetes?**
   Prediabetes is the precursor to overt diabetes. The diagnostic criteria for prediabetes are shown in Table 1.3. Approximately 11% of people with prediabetes develop overt diabetes each year. People with polycystic ovary syndrome (PCOS), a history of gestational diabetes mellitus (GDM), and a history of steroid-induced hyperglycemia are also at high risk of eventually developing type 2 diabetes mellitus. A structured education program about diabetes and lifestyle modification (diet, exercise, weight loss) has been consistently and unequivocally effective in preventing the progression of prediabetes to diabetes. This approach is strongly endorsed in the Standards of Medical Care in Diabetes of the American Diabetes Association.

10. **What is latent autoimmune diabetes of adults (LADA)?**
    LADA is autoimmune beta-cell destruction that occurs later in life, causing diabetes but often with some minimal residual beta-cell function. The diagnostic criteria are vague but include age >30 years, positive islet-cell antibodies, and significant beta-cell destruction but with some persistent insulin secretion that may allow patients to avoid insulin treatment for more than 6 months. Some experts consider this to be just one end of the spectrum of type 1 diabetes and not really a distinct entity. These authors agree with that view.

11. **What is ketosis-prone type 2 diabetes mellitus?**
    Ketosis-prone type 2 diabetes mellitus often presents with diabetic ketoacidosis (DKA) as a result of a severe but reversible beta-cell (insulin) deficiency and partially reversible insulin resistance. Insulin therapy is required to treat DKA and to control hyperglycemia immediately after DKA but can eventually be stopped and replaced by more typical type 2 diabetes medications in most patients. Nonetheless, DKA can be recurrent. Islet-cell antibodies are absent, and the insulin secretory defect is transient. Insulin resistance is also reversible and may be partially attributable to initial glucose toxicity. This is likely just part of the spectrum of type 2 diabetes. Other names for this condition include *atypical type 2 diabetes, type 1.5 diabetes*, and *Flatbush diabetes*.

12. **What is posttransplant diabetes mellitus?**
    Posttransplant diabetes mellitus occurs in 10% to 50% of people after organ transplantation and appears to result from an underlying disorder of glucose metabolism with superimposed systemic inflammation plus the effects of immunosuppressive medications. Insulin therapy is usually required. The condition worsens the prognosis for the transplanted tissue and overall patient survival. A previous name for this disorder was *new-onset diabetes after transplant* (NODAT), but the preferred term now is *posttransplant diabetes mellitus*.

13. **What are the characteristics of diabetes caused by pancreatic insufficiency?**
    Chronic pancreatitis and surgical pancreatic resection, depending on the extent, can lead to both exocrine and endocrine pancreatic insufficiency. The development of diabetes in this setting has been referred to as *pancreatic, pancreatogenic, pancreatogenous*, and *type 3c diabetes mellitus.* Affected people tend to be very insulin sensitive and prone to hypoglycemia, related partly to their concomitant glucagon deficiency. Other risk factors for hypoglycemia may include coexisting liver disease, malabsorption, poor dietary intake, and alcohol abuse. Because of these individuals' higher hypoglycemia risk, target A1c values tend to be set higher in these individuals than in those with other types of diabetes.

14. **Describe diabetes related to cystic fibrosis (CF).**
    Diabetes mellitus occurs in approximately 50% of people with CF after age 35. People with CF-related diabetes tend to produce adequate amounts of basal insulin but have reduced or delayed insulin secretion in response to meals, causing them to have significant postprandial hyperglycemia. Therefore an oral glucose tolerance test is usually employed to diagnose this condition. Because of their tendency to have pulmonary infections and require glucocorticoid treatment, many individuals have concomitant insulin resistance.

15. **Explain MODY.**
    MODY is characterized by diabetes that is usually diagnosed at a young age (<25 years), with autosomal dominant transmission and lack of autoantibodies; it is the most common type of monogenic diabetes and accounts for 2% to 5% of all diabetes cases. Several different genetic abnormalities have been identified. The affected genes control pancreatic beta-cell development, function, and regulation; the mutations cause impaired glucose sensing and insulin secretion with minimal or no defect in insulin action. Table 1.4 lists the MODY subtypes with their frequencies and optimal treatment strategies.

16. **What is checkpoint inhibitor-associated autoimmune diabetes mellitus (CIADM)?**
    CIADM Is an Insulin-deficient form of diabetes that can develop during or after treatment with immune checkpoint inhibitors; the most commonly implicated agents are PD-1 and PD-L1 inhibitors, such as nivolumab and pembrolizumab. It may develop within 3 months of initial PD-1/PD-L1 inhibitor exposure. This type of diabetes is much like typical type 1 diabetes, although preexposure antibody status has not yet been well studied. Although some affected people have positive islet-cell antibodies, others are antibody negative and lack the higher-risk HLA haplotypes. Antibody-positive individuals tend to have a more abrupt onset and a higher risk of DKA than those who are antibody negative. However, both antibody-positive and antibody-negative individuals exhibit beta-cell failure with severe insulin deficiency and require intensive insulin therapy. See Chapter 17, "Diabetes Management in Cancer Patients."

17. **What is GDM?**
    GDM is defined by the American College of Obstetrics and Gynecology (ACOG) as a "condition in which carbohydrate intolerance develops during pregnancy." Women with GDM have an increased risk of later developing type 2 diabetes mellitus and cardiovascular disease. Adverse perinatal outcomes are also associated with GDM. It is currently recommended that all pregnant women be tested for GDM between weeks 24 and 28 of pregnancy. GDM is discussed in more depth in Chapter 16.

KEY POINTS

1. Diabetes mellitus is diagnosed by any of the following criteria: fasting plasma glucose ≥126 mg/dL (7.0 mmol/L), 2-hour plasma glucose ≥200 mg/dL (11.1 mmol/L), hemoglobin A1c ≥6.5% (48 mmol per mol), or random plasma glucose ≥200 mg/dL (11.1 mmol/L) in a patient with symptoms of hyperglycemia or hyperglycemic crisis.

Table 1.4 Subtypes of Maturity-Onset Diabetes of the Young (MODY)

MODY TYPE	MUTATION	TREATMENT
Type 1 (<10%)	Hepatocyte nuclear factor 4 alpha	Sulfonylurea
Type 2 (15%–30%)	Glucokinase gene	Diet, lifestyle
Type 3 (50%–65%)	Hepatocyte nuclear factor 1 alpha	Sulfonylurea
Type 4 (rare)	Insulin promoter factor 1	
Type 5 (rare)	Hepatocyte nuclear factor 1 beta	Insulin
Type 6 (rare)	Neurogenic differentiation factor 1	Insulin

2. Prediabetes is diagnosed by any of the following criteria: fasting plasma glucose of 100 to 125 mg/dL (5.6–6.9 mmol/L), 2-hour plasma glucose of 140 to 199 mg/dL (7.8–11.1 mmol/L), and hemoglobin A1c of 5.7% to 6.4% (39–47 mmol per mol).
3. Type 1 diabetes mellitus is an autoimmune disease characterized by pancreatic beta-cell destruction, resulting in absolute insulin deficiency. It is best diagnosed by finding a low or undetectable C-peptide and one or more positive islet-cell antibodies: GAD antibodies, insulin antibodies, IA-2 antibodies, or ZnT8 antibodies.
4. Type 2 diabetes mellitus is a heterogeneous metabolic disorder characterized by the pathophysiologic triad of excessive hepatic glucose production, peripheral insulin resistance, and progressive beta-cell failure; other contributing features include increased lipolysis, excessive glucagon secretion, deficient incretin hormone secretion, increased renal glucose reabsorption, and insulin resistance in the brain.
5. Less common types of diabetes include posttransplant diabetes, diabetes resulting from pancreatic insufficiency or pancreatectomy, CF-related diabetes, MODY, and various types of medication-induced diabetes.

BIBLIOGRAPHY

Ahlqvist E, Storm P, Karajamaki A, et al. Novel subgroups of adult-onset diabetes and their association with outcomes: a data-driven cluster analysis of six variables. *Lancet Diabetes Endocrinol*. 2018 May;6(5):361–369.

Aksit MA, Pace RG, Vecchio-Pagan B, et al. Genetic modifiers of cystic fibrosis-related diabetes have extensive overlap with type 2 diabetes and related traits. *J Clin Endocrinol Metab*. 2020;105:1401–1415.

Akturk HK, Kahramangil D, Sarwal A, et al. Immune checkpoint inhibitor-induced type 1 diabetes: a systematic review and meta-analysis. *Diabet Med*. 2019;36;1075–1081.

American Diabetes Association. 2 Classification and diagnosis of diabetes: Standards of Medical Care in Diabetes – 2020. *Diabetes Care*. 2020 Jan;43(Suppl 1):S14–S31.

Atkinson MA, Eisenbarth GS, Michels AW. Type 1 diabetes. *Lancet*. 2014;383(9911):69–82.

Balasubramanyam A, Nalini R, Hampe CS, Maldonado M. Syndromes of ketosis-prone diabetes mellitus. *Endocr Rev*. 2008 May;29(3):292–302.

Bridges N, Rowe R. Holt RIG. Unique challenges of cystic fibrosis-related diabetes. *Diabet Med*. 2018;35(9):1181–1188.

Brooks-Worrell BM, Iyer D, Coraza I, et al. Islet-specific T-cell responses and proinflammatory monocytes define subtypes of autoantibody-negative ketosis-prone diabetes. *Diabetes Care*. 2013 Dec;36(12):4098–4103.

Buzzetti R, Tuomi T, Mauricio D, et al. Management of latent autoimmune diabetes in adults: a consensus statement from and international expert panel. *Diabetes*. 2020 published online Aug 26, 2020. https://doi.org/10.2337/dbi20-0017.

Castelblanco E, Hernández M, Castelblanco A, et al. Low-grade inflammatory marker profile may help to differentiate patients with LADA, classic adult-onset type 1 diabetes, and type 2 diabetes. *Diabetes Care*. 2018 Apr;41(4):862–868.

Christensen AS, Haedersdal S, Stoy J, et al. Efficacy and safety of glimepiride with or without linagliptin treatment in patients with HNF1A (Maturity Onset Diabetes of the Young Type 3): a randomized, double-blinded, placebo-controlled, crossover trial (GLIMLINA). *Diabetes Care*. 2020;43:2025–2033.

Defronzo RA. Banting Lecture. From the triumvirate to the ominous octet: a new paradigm for the treatment of type 2 diabetes mellitus. *Diabetes*. 2009 Apr;58(4):773–795.

DiMeglio LA, Evans-Molina C, Oram RA. Type 1 diabetes. *Lancet*. 2018;391:2249–2262.

Domecq JP, Prutsky G, Elraiyah T, et al. Medications affecting the biochemical conversion to type 2 diabetes: a systematic review and meta-analysis. *J Clin Endocrinol Metab*. 2019;104:3986–3995.

Ewald N, Hardt PD. Diagnosis and treatment of diabetes mellitus in chronic pancreatitis. *World J Gastroenterol*. 2013 Nov 14;19(42):7276–7281.

Firdous P, Nissar K, Ali S, et al. Genetic testing of maturity-onset diabetes of the young current status and future perspectives. *Front Endocrinol (Lausanne)*. 2018 May 17;9:253 eCollection 2018.

Hart PA, Bellin MD, Andersen DK, et al. Type 3c (pancreatogenic) diabetes mellitus secondary to chronic pancreatitis and pancreatic cancer. *Lancet Gastroenterol Hepatol*. 2016 Nov;1(3):226–237.

Hattersley AT. Molecular genetics goes to the diabetes clinic. *Clin Med (Lond)*. 2005 Sep-Oct;5(5):476–481.

Holt RIG. Cystic fibrosis-related diabetes: the missing evidence. *Diabet Med*. 2019 Nov;36(11):1327–1328.

Langenberg C, Lotta LA. Genomic insights into the causes of type 2 diabetes. *Lancet*. 2018 Jun 16;391(10138):2463–2474.

Luo S, Lin J, Xie Z, et al. HLA genetic discrepancy between latent autoimmune diabetes in adults and type 1 diabetes: LADA China Study No. 6. *J Clin Endocrinol Metab*. 2016;101:1693–1700.

Naylor R, Philipson LH. Who should have genetic testing for maturity-onset diabetes of the young? *Clin Endocrinol (Oxf)*. 2011;75:422.

Ode KL, Chan CL, Granados A, Moheet A, Moran A, Brennan AL. Cystic fibrosis related diabetes: medical management. *J Cyst Fibros*. 2019 Oct;18 Suppl 2:S10–S18.

Pearson ER, Flechtner I, Njølstad PR, et al. Switching from insulin to oral sulfonylureas in patients with diabetes due to Kir6.2 mutations. *N Engl J Med*. 2006 Aug 3;355(5):467–477.

Pozzilli P, Pieralice S. Latent autoimmune diabetes in adults: current status and new horizons. *Endocrinol Metab (Seoul)*. 2018 Jun;33(2):147–159.

Sanyoura M, Philipson LH, Naylor R. Monogenic diabetes in children and adolescents: recognition and treatment options. *Curr Diab Rep*. 2018 Jun 22;18(8):58.

Sharif A, Cohney S. Post-transplantation diabetes – state of the art. *Lancet Diabetes Endocrinol*. 2016;4:337–349.

Shivaswamy V, Boerner B, Larsen J. Post-transplant diabetes mellitus: causes, treatment, and impact on outcomes. *Endocr Rev*. 2016 Feb;37(1):37–61.

Thanabalasingham G, Owen KR. Diagnosis and management of maturity onset diabetes of the young (MODY). *BMJ*. 2011;343:d6044.

Thomas NJ, Jones SE, Weeden NJ, et al. Frequency and phenotype of type 1 diabetes in the first six decades of life: a cross-sectional, genetically stratified survival analysis from UK biobank. *Lancet Diabetes Endocrinol*. 2018;6:122–129.

Triolo TM, Fouts A, Pyle L, et al. Identical and nonidentical twins: risk factors involved in development of islet autoimmunity and type 1 diabetes. *Diabetes Care*. 2019;42:192–199.

Tsang VHM, McGrath RT, Clifton-Bligh RJ, et al. Checkpoint inhibitor-associated autoimmune diabetes is distinct from type 1 diabetes. *J Clin Endocrinol Metab*. 2019;104:5499–5506.

Vellanki P, Umpierrez GE. Diabetic ketoacidosis: a common debut of diabetes among African Americans with type 2 diabetes. *Endocr Pract.* 2017 Aug;23(8):971–978.

Venessa H, Tsang M, McGrath RT, et al. Checkpoint inhibitor-associated autoimmune diabetes is distinct from type 1 diabetes. *J Clin Endocrinol Metab.* 2019;104(11):5499–5506.

Vijan S. In the Clinic: Type 2 diabetes. *Ann Intern Med.* 2019 Nov 5;171(9):ITC65–ITC80.

Zaharia OP, Strassburger K, Strom A, et al. Risk of diabetes-associated diseases in subgroups of patients with recent-onset diabetes: a 5-year follow-up study. *Lancet Diabetes Endocrinol.* 2019;7:684–694.

CHAPTER 2

COMPREHENSIVE MEDICAL EVALUATION OF PERSONS WITH DIABETES

Jennifer M. Trujillo, PharmD, BCPS, FCCP, CDCES, BC-ADM, Elizabeth Ko, PharmD and Shasta Tall Bull, PharmD

1. **What are some important components of successful patient-centered collaborative care?**
   Patient-centered collaborative care depends on your ability to communicate effectively and your patient's ability to take an active role in their own healthcare. For your patient to make the most of the tools available to them, they must be ready to receive care and able to understand the information they are given. In some cases, it may be valuable to assess your patient's health literacy and numeracy, which can be done with a quick, 3-minute assessment called "The Newest Vital Sign" (available at https://www.pfizer.com/health/literacy/public-policy-researchers/nvs-toolkit). This tool has been validated and translated into multiple languages.

   A multidisciplinary team with a variety of health professionals can provide thorough treatment and a comprehensive perspective on long-term goals of care. All team members should use patient-centered language such as "person with diabetes" (PWD) instead of "diabetic." Use active listening and motivational interviewing to help your patient identify barriers to change. Each patient will have unique preferences, values, and belief systems that may affect the way the healthcare team provides recommendations for treatment. Work with your patient and any caregivers to promote shared decision making to optimize health outcomes and quality of life.

2. **What are the key components of a diabetes assessment and treatment plan?**
   After confirming and classifying the patient's diabetes, at the initial visit, you should assess the risk of diabetes complications, determine patient-specific goals, and initiate appropriate therapeutic treatments as part of an assessment and treatment plan. It is important to take a comprehensive approach when reviewing your patient's medical history for comorbidities because certain pharmacologic agents for diabetes also have proven benefits in other disease states. The presence of certain comorbid conditions may affect your initial therapeutic decisions in diabetes management. Determine the presence of established atherosclerotic cardiovascular disease (ASCVD) and heart failure (HF). If the patient does not have established ASCVD, use the 10-year ASCVD risk estimation to identify whether the patient has a high ASCVD risk (see question 3). The presence and stage of chronic kidney disease (CKD) should also be considered. Aside from the comorbidities, the patient's risk of hypoglycemia and their weight-management plan should be reviewed. When establishing your treatment plan, work with your patient to build a collaborative relationship to ensure patient buy-in and improve outcomes.

3. **How do you calculate and interpret the ASCVD risk score?**
   An ASCVD risk estimation tool is available online and as a smartphone application (Risk Estimator Plus by American College of Cardiology: http://tools.acc.org/ASCVD-Risk-Estimator-Plus/#!/calculate/estimate/). This estimator takes into account age, gender, race, blood pressure, cholesterol levels, history of diabetes, smoking history, and treatment for these conditions. The tool provides a 10-year risk for ASCVD for patients ages 40 to 79, categorized as low risk (<5%), borderline risk (5%–7.4%), intermediate risk (7.5%–19.9%), and high risk (≥20%).

4. **What are the key components of the comprehensive diabetes medical evaluation?**
   A comprehensive diabetes medical evaluation should start with a thorough past medical and family history (diabetes history, family history, personal history of complications and common comorbidities). At follow-up visits, changes in medical and family history since the last visit should be obtained. Other components to be gathered include lifestyle factors, medications and vaccinations, technology use, and behavioral and diabetes self-management skills. A thorough physical examination should be completed, and appropriate laboratory tests should be evaluated. Each of these will be discussed in more detail in the following sections. Considering the depth and breadth of a comprehensive medical evaluation of diabetes, it is important to prioritize the most crucial aspects of the evaluation at follow-up visits, based on the needs and characteristics of the patient.

5. **What information should be gathered regarding past medical and family history?**
   At a patient's first comprehensive diabetes medical evaluation, complete a thorough collection of your patient's past medical and family history. The patient's diabetes history includes characteristics at onset (age and symptoms), previous treatment regimens and response, and any past hospitalizations. When collecting your patient's family history, look for diabetes in any first-degree relatives and any autoimmune disorders. You should also identify if your patient has a personal history of any macrovascular or microvascular complications, common

comorbidities, hypertension, hyperlipidemia, or presence of anemia or coagulation disorders. Finally, you should determine your patient's date of last dental visit and eye exam, along with any specialist visits. During follow-up appointments, you should collect information regarding changes to medical or family history that may have occurred since your last meeting. At the patient's annual visit, you'll want to repeat a thorough evaluation of complications and common comorbidities as outlined previously.

6. **What information should be gathered regarding lifestyle and social history?**
During a comprehensive diabetes evaluation, a variety of components must be assessed. Although it may be tempting to focus on clinical characteristics and comorbidities, it is important to recognize that lifestyle, cultural, and socioeconomic factors play an important role in your patient's successful management of their disease. The decisions your patient makes throughout their day will affect their glycemic control. These lifestyle factors should be assessed at every visit, including eating patterns, weight history, physical activity, and sleep behavior. Social history should also be assessed, including tobacco, alcohol, and substance use.

These are sensitive topics that may require a referral in patients who appear to be suffering from eating disorders, substance use disorders, sleep disorders, or unsafe living conditions. Although the appointment time with patients is often limited, you can frame your evaluation questions in a conversational context to build a trusting relationship with your patient. Intersperse plenty of open-ended questions to give the patient space to provide the information they feel is most pertinent to their care. Empathize with your patient's individual struggles, and encourage their positive progress so that their healthcare visits can become a place they trust to learn more about collaborating with their team and improving their health.

7. **What information should be gathered regarding medications and vaccinations?**
During the initial visit and at every follow-up, a complete review of your patient's current medications, medication adherence, medication tolerance, and side effects should be performed. A thorough medication reconciliation should be completed each visit because it can reduce potential hospitalization and emergency department visits in PWD. When collecting medication-use information, always ask open-ended questions that are free from judgment and use patient-empowering language. For example, instead of asking, "Are you taking your long-acting insulin every day?" ask, "In the last week, how many times did you miss a dose of your long-acting insulin?" Be sure to document a thorough list of your patient's complete medication regimen, which includes the full medication name, dose, frequency, and route. Make sure to ask about tolerability and experiences with side effects, especially after a new medication is initiated. Remember that many side effects can be transient. If a medication has clear therapeutic benefits, explain to your patient how they can manage side effects and how continuing the medication with good adherence will improve their disease state. Depending on your practice setting, other healthcare professionals, such as pharmacists, can work collaboratively to complete medication reconciliation, guide the patient's medication use, and gather important medication-related information to assist in patient care. Finally, to make an appropriate recommendation for vaccines, an assessment of the patient's risk for preventable diseases and need for a vaccine should be completed at the initial visit and annually thereafter.

8. **What immunizations should be recommended?**
The goal for routine immunizations is to reduce the incidence of preventable diseases in PWD. Table 2.1 summarizes the recommended vaccinations according to age group. The Centers for Disease Control and Prevention (CDC) currently recommends against using a live attenuated influenza vaccine (LAIV, the nasal spray flu vaccine) for patients with diabetes because of the risk of developing flu-related complications.

9. **What should be included in the assessment of treatment-associated hypoglycemia?**
When evaluating treatment-associated hypoglycemia, you should assess the following risk factors:
- Use of insulin or insulin secretagogues (e.g., sulfonylureas, meglitinides)
- Kidney or liver dysfunction
- Longer duration of diabetes
- Older age
- Cognitive impairment
- Hypoglycemia unawareness
- Physical or intellectual disability that may impair behavioral response to hypoglycemia
- Alcohol use

One episode of hypoglycemia puts your patient at greater risk of future events; repeated episodes can affect cognitive function. When collecting the patient's personal history of hypoglycemia, be sure to ask about frequency, causes, and timing of episodes, as well as symptom response or awareness. For example, ask, "How many times in the last week has your blood sugar been below 70 mg/dL?" as opposed to "Do you experience hypoglycemia?" Your choice of questions will be patient specific, depending on medications, age, and lifestyle; the goal is to use open-ended questions that will encourage dialogue. Some patients may fear hypoglycemia to the point that their activities of daily living and medical outcomes are affected. If you suspect your patient is engaging in compensatory behaviors out of fear of hypoglycemia, you can use a screening questionnaire such as the Hypoglycemia

Table 2.1 Recommended Immunizations for Persons With Diabetes

DISEASE	VACCINE	AGE	TIMING/ FREQUENCY	ADDITIONAL INFORMATION
Influenza	Injectable Influenza	≥6 months	Annually	Available influenza vaccine types: 18–64 years • Inactivated influenza vaccine (IIV) • Recombinant influenza vaccine (RIV) • Afluria Quadrivalent—via jet injector or needle • Flublok Quadrivalent—free of egg particle ≥65 yrs: • Fluzone high-Dose • Adjuvanted flu vaccine (Fluad)
Pneumonia	Prevnar (PCV13)	2–5 years	2 doses if unvac- cinated/received an incomplete series with <3 doses 1 dose if received 3 doses after 12 months of age	To complete the vaccine series: Give 1 dose of PPSV23 at ≥8 weeks after the PCV13
		6–18 years	If no prior PCV13: 1 dose (before PPSV23)	Requires 2 doses of PPSV23: 1st dose at ≥8 weeks after any prior PCV13 dose 2nd dose at ≥5 years after 1st PPSV23 dose
	Pneumovax (PPSV23)	19–64 years	1 dose	Regardless of vaccine history, *all* persons with diabetes need PPSV23 dose at age ≥65
Hepatitis B	Hepatitis B	18–59 years	2- or 3-dose series	Consider 3-dose series if ≥60 years of age

Fear Survey–II Worry (HFS-II W) Scale (Table 2.2). A single-item screening question could also be used: "Have you changed any of your life activities because you are worried about getting low blood sugar?" These are quick and widely used tools for framing your conversation about hypoglycemia.

10. **What information should be gathered regarding the use of diabetes-related technology?**
The importance and prevalence of technology are constantly expanding in our patient's lives over time. If your clinic offers telehealth, be sure to ask the patient if they have a computer and privacy at home to access this service. During a comprehensive diabetes evaluation, it is appropriate to assess which forms of technology your patient uses regularly so that you can give them the best available resources within their level of technical understanding. Many of smartphone applications exist for logging food, exercise, and blood sugar trends.
   Advanced technologies associated with insulin delivery, self-monitoring of blood glucose (SMBG), and continuous glucose monitoring can be safe and effective for lowering A1c when your patient is well educated on these devices and all healthcare team members are in communication about which devices are being used. During this part of the assessment, ask your patient what technology they use (insulin pumps, continuous glucose monitors [CGMs], smart pens, etc.) and which model and features they have. Are their devices integrated with each other and/or with their smartphone? If they use an online portal for glucose data collection, be sure to obtain their login information. Whenever you recommend or prescribe new technology to your patient, make sure you allow time for adequate instruction and a means for follow-up questions.

11. **What information should be gathered regarding psychosocial factors and diabetes self-management skills?**
Diabetes self-management education and support (DSMES) is a critical component of effective diabetes care for all patients with diabetes. The need for DSMES should be evaluated at diagnosis, annually, when complicating

Table 2.2 Psychosocial Screening Tools for Patients With Diabetes

SCREENING TOOL	DESCRIPTION AND LINK
Patient Health Questionnaire (PHQ-9)	9-item screening tool for depression https://www.phqscreeners.com/
Generalized Anxiety Disorder (GAD-7)	7-item screening tool for generalized anxiety disorder https://www.phqscreeners.com/
Diabetes Distress Screening (DDS)	17-item screening tool that evaluates diabetes distress across four categories: emotional burden, physician-related distress, regimen-related distress, and interpersonal distress http://www.diabetesed.net/page/_files/diabetes-distress.pdf
Diabetes Eating Problems Survey (DEPS-R)	16-item screening tool that evaluates diabetes-specific disordered eating https://www.ncbi.nlm.nih.gov/pmc/articles/PMC2827495/
Mini-Mental State Evaluation (MMSE)	11-item, 30-point screening tool conducted by a clinician to test a range of everyday mental skills and cognitive function http://www.oxfordmedicaleducation.com/geriatrics/mini-mental-state-examination-mmse/
Social Determinants of Health (SDOH)	26-item screening tool that assesses health-related social needs covering 13 domains of social security and wellness https://innovation.cms.gov/files/worksheets/ahcm-screeningtool.pdf
Hypoglycemia Fear Survey–II W Worry (HFS-II W) Scale	The HFS-II W Scale is an 18-Item questionnaire to assess specific concerns people with diabetes may have related to their risk of having hypoglycemia; see page 89 for the questionnaire. https://www.diabetes.org.uk/resources-s3/2019-03/0506%20Diabetes%20UK%20Australian%20Handbook_P4_FINAL_1.pdf

factors arise, and at transitions of care. DSMES can be provided individually or in a group setting, with or without the use of technology, and in some cases it may be reimbursed by third-party payers. It will be important to ask your patient if they have had diabetes education before, how much, and how long ago. You'll want to assess what gaps exist in their self-management skills and what barriers they currently face to optimal disease self-management. You may need to refer the patient to a Certified Diabetes Care and Education Specialist (CDCES) who can provide expert guidance for your patient's DSMES.

Psychosocial factors that might affect a patient's outcomes include attitudes about diabetes; expectations for medical management and outcomes; affect or mood; financial, social, and emotional resources; and psychiatric history. Consider assessing your patient or referring them for symptoms of diabetes distress, depression, anxiety, eating disorders, and cognitive functions at the initial visit, periodic intervals, and when there is a significant change in disease course, treatment, or life circumstances. There are evidence-based guidelines for psychosocial evaluation and treatment of patients with diabetes, which include an at-a-glance chart to help you determine the intervention mode that will be most helpful. Social determinants of health (SDOH) will also play a critical role in your patient's ability to manage their disease; the Centers for Medicare and Medicaid Services (CMS) have developed a patient questionnaire that can provide a comprehensive snapshot of a patient's SDOH. Table 2.2 provides a summary of helpful screening tools. Also make sure to screen for homelessness and food insecurity when suspected. Single-question screening questions for homelessness and food insecurity are discussed in Chapter 27.

12. **What components should be prioritized in the physical examination?**
Height, weight, body mass index (BMI), and blood pressure should be routinely recorded at each visit. The skin should be examined for acanthosis nigricans, characterized by areas of dark, velvety discoloration of body folds, which can indicate insulin resistance. Insulin injection sites should be inspected for lipohypertrophy. The thyroid should also be palpated. Finally, a comprehensive foot examination should be completed, including pedal pulses; visual inspection of skin integrity, callous formation, foot deformities, or ulcers; and a 10-g monofilament exam.

13. **What labs should be ordered during a comprehensive diabetes evaluation?**
Routine laboratory monitoring is required for the successful management of diabetes. Table 2.3 summarizes the recommended schedule of laboratory evaluations to support a clinical treatment course for patients with diabetes.

Table 2.3 Recommended Laboratory Test Monitoring Schedule

TYPE	TIMING/FREQUENCY	ADDITIONAL GUIDANCE
A1c	At the initial visit, then every 3–6 months	
Urinary albumin-to-creatinine ratio	At the initial visit, then annually	
Serum K+, SCr, eGFR	At the initial visit, then annually	Consider more frequent monitoring in patients with known CKD or change in pharmacologic agents that affect the serum potassium level (ACEi/ARB, diuretics) and/or kidney function.
Lipid panel	At the initial visit, then annually	Consider when suspecting nonadherent to statin therapy or change in LDL-C reduction therapy is required. Annual screening may not be required for patients with normal lipid panel or who are not on cholesterol-reduction therapy.
LFT	At the initial visit, then annually	Consider more frequent monitoring if there is a start or change in medications that affects the lab value.
TSH	At the initial visit, then annually	Especially in patients with T1D. Consider more frequent monitoring with start or change in thyroid medication.
Vitamin B$_{12}$	At the initial visit, then annually	Only in patients taking chronic metformin, T1D, peripheral neuropathy, or unexplained anemia. Consider more frequent monitoring during vitamin B$_{12}$ treatment or changes in medications that can affect vitamin B$_{12}$ level.

ACEi, Angiotensin-converting enzyme inhibitor; *ARB,* angiotensin receptor blocker; *CKD,* chronic kidney disease; *eGFR,* estimated glomerular filtration rate; *LDL-C,* low-density lipoprotein cholesterol; *LFT,* liver function test; *T1D,* type 1 diabetes; *TSH,* thyroid-stimulating hormone; *SCr,* serum creatinine

14. **What other common comorbidities should clinicians be aware of that could complicate diabetes management?**
    Besides assessing diabetes-related comorbidities, there are other common comorbidities that affect PWD and may complicate management. People with type 1 diabetes are at an increased risk of autoimmune diseases, including thyroid disease, celiac disease, and vitamin B$_{12}$ deficiency. Screening for these diseases should be considered, especially if symptoms are present. Diabetes is associated with an increased risk of some cancers of the liver, pancreas, endometrium, colon/rectum, breast, and bladder. Diabetes is also associated with the development of nonalcoholic fatty liver disease and nonalcoholic steatohepatitis. People with diabetes are at an increased risk of pancreatitis, and conversely, people with a history of pancreatitis have a higher risk of developing diabetes.

15. **What referrals should be considered as part of the initial care management of PWD?**
    Referring patients with diabetes to a registered dietitian for medical nutrition therapy may benefit patients through additional support and education for diabetes self-management. Additionally, PWD require routine annual dilated eye exams and biannual dental/periodontal checks. Where relevant, recommend referrals to mental health professionals should be made. Finally, because glucose control is necessary prior to and during pregnancy, women who are considering becoming pregnant should be referred to a family planning counselor.

KEY POINTS

1. A complete medical evaluation should be performed at the initial visit to confirm the diagnosis, classify the diabetes, evaluate for complications and comorbidities, review previous treatments and risk factors, and develop a treatment plan.
2. A complete medical evaluation should include past medical and family history, diabetes history, lifestyle factors, medications and vaccinations, technology use, behavioral and diabetes self-management skills, a physical examination, and laboratory evaluation.
3. A follow-up visit should include most components of a complete medical evaluation but should be prioritized and tailored to meet the needs of the individual patient.
4. Special attention should be given to evaluating medication-taking and self-management behaviors, psychosocial conditions, and SDOH because they significantly affect glycemic control and often go undetected.

BIBLIOGRAPHY

American Diabetes Association. 4 Comprehensive medical evaluation and assessment of comorbidities: Standards of medical care in diabetes—2021. *Diabetes Care*. 2021;44(Suppl. 1):S40–S52.

Beck J, Greenwood DA, Blanton L, et al. 2017 National standards for diabetes self-management education and support. *Diabetes Educator*. 2017;43(5):449–464.

Center for Disease Control and Prevention. (2020). Immunization Schedule. https://www.cdc.gov/vaccines/schedules/. Accessed September 5, 2020.

Young-Hyman D, de Groot M, Hill-Briggs F, et al. Psychosocial care for people with diabetes: a position statement of the American Diabetes Association. *Diabetes Care*. 2016;39:2126–2140.

CHAPTER 3

DIABETIC KETOACIDOSIS AND HYPERGLYCEMIC HYPEROSMOLAR SYNDROME

Michael T. McDermott, MD

1. **What are diabetic ketoacidosis (DKA) and hyperglycemic hyperosmolar syndrome (HHS)?**
   DKA is a state of acute metabolic decompensation manifested by significant hyperglycemia, ketonemia, anion-gap metabolic acidosis, and hypovolemia. DKA typically occurs in people with type 1 diabetes (70%–90%) but may sometimes occur in those with type 2 diabetes (10%–30%) and other types of diabetes. HHS usually occurs in people with type 2 diabetes (especially the elderly) and is characterized by severe hyperglycemia, hyperosmolality, and profound hypovolemia but without significant ketonemia or metabolic acidosis. Table 3.1 lists the diagnostic criteria for DKA and HHS.

2. **What is euglycemic DKA?**
   Euglycemic DKA is the term for a condition in which people have blood glucose (BG) levels <250 mg/dL but have other features of DKA (ketonemia, metabolic acidosis). Although clearly not "euglycemic," BG levels are distinctly lower than those in typical DKA. Euglycemic DKA occurs most often in people taking sodium–glucose cotransporter 2 (SGLT-2) inhibitors, in pregnant women, in starvation, and in those who abuse alcohol.

3. **How common is DKA?**
   Approximately 140,000 hospital admissions occur in the United States each year as a result of DKA. It is the initial presentation for 25% of people with type 1 diabetes. The DKA hospitalization rate in the United States increased by 6.3% per year from 2009 to 2014 and increased dramatically in 2020 during the COVID-19 pandemic. Adults in the 18- to 25-year-old age range have the highest overall incidence of DKA.

4. **Do DKA and HHS ever occur simultaneously?**
   Because the degree of ketosis is related to the severity of insulin deficiency, some people may have insulin deficiency, hyperglycemia, and hyperosmolality severe enough to meet the diagnostic criteria for both DKA and HHS. Furthermore, other types of acidosis may be superimposed; these include lactic acidosis, D-lactic acidosis, alcoholic ketoacidosis, and uremia. People presenting with combined DKA and HHS have a higher mortality rate than those with either condition alone.

5. **What are the most common situations or precipitants for DKA and HHS?**
   The most common situations that precipitate DKA and HHS are listed in Table 3.2.

6. **Explain the pathophysiology of DKA**
   DKA results from absolute or severe insulin deficiency coupled with elevated counterregulatory hormones (glucagon, epinephrine, cortisol, growth hormone). This hormonal milieu impairs tissue glucose utilization, increases hepatic gluconeogenesis and glycogenolysis, enhances adipose tissue lipolysis, and promotes tissue proteolysis. High circulating free fatty acids and insulin deficiency promote hepatic ketogenesis, causing elevated serum ketone levels and ketoacidosis. Hyperglycemia also causes an osmotic diuresis, leading to volume depletion. The overall result is hyperglycemia, ketonemia, metabolic acidosis, and hypovolemia (Fig. 3.1).

7. **Describe the pathophysiology of HHS and how it differs from DKA**
   HHS typically occurs in elderly people with type 2 diabetes, often with concomitant renal disease and/or an impaired thirst mechanism. Because these individuals can still produce insulin, they secrete sufficient amounts of insulin to prevent lipolysis and ketogenesis, thus avoiding ketosis and acidosis. The predominant features, therefore, are more severe hyperglycemia, hyperosmolality, and profound hypovolemia. See Fig. 3.1.

Table 3.1 Diagnostic Criteria for Diabetic Ketoacidosis (DKA) and Hyperglycemic Hyperosmolar Syndrome (HHS)

	DKA			HHS
	MILD	MODERATE	SEVERE	
Glucose	≥ 250 mg/dL	≥250 mg/dL	≥250 mg/dL	≥600 mg/dL
pH	7.25–7.30	7.00–7.24	<7.00	>7.30
HCO₃	15–18 mEq/L	10–14 mEq/L	<10 mEq/L	>18 mEq/L
Ketones	Positive	Positive	Positive	Negative/Small
Sensorium	Alert	Alert/Drowsy	Stupor/Coma	Stupor/Coma

Note: Ketonemia is best detected with a serum beta hydroxybutyrate test. The urine nitroprusside measurement of ketones can underestimate the degree of ketosis because it measures mainly acetoacetate and not beta-hydroxybutyrate, which is the predominant ketone in DKA.

Table 3.2 Common Situations and Precipitating Factors for Diabetic Ketoacidosis (DKA) and Hyperglycemic Hyperosmolar Syndrome (HHS)

New-onset type 1 diabetes mellitus
Omission of insulin therapy in type 1 diabetes mellitus
Infection/sepsis
Adrenal crisis
Acute abdomen
Ischemic extremity
Pulmonary embolism
Myocardial infarction
Cerebrovascular event
Ketosis-prone type 2 diabetes mellitus

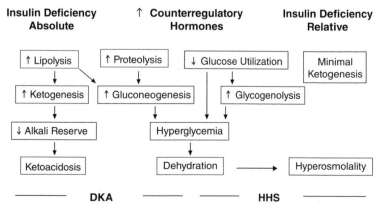

Fig. 3.1 Pathophysiology of diabetic ketoacidosis (DKA) and hyperglycemic hyperosmolar syndrome (HHS).

8. **What water and electrolyte deficits are typically present in DKA and HHS?**

	DKA	HHS
Total water (L)	6	9
Water (mL/kg)	100	100–200
Sodium (mEq/kg)	7–10	5–13
Chloride (mEq/kg)	3–5	5–15
Potassium (mEq/kg)	3–5	4–6
Phosphate (mEq/kg)	5–7	3–7

9. **What equations are useful for diagnosing and monitoring treatment of DKA and HHS?**

$$\text{Anion gap} = Na^+ - (Cl^- + HCO_3^-) \text{ [Normal range: 7–13 mmol/L]}$$
$$\text{Serum osmolality} = 2 \times (Na^+) + (\text{Glucose}/18) + (\text{Blood urea nitrogen [BUN]}/2.8) \text{ [Normal range: 285–295 mOsm/kg]}$$

Note: The diagnosis of anion-gap metabolic acidosis should be made by measurement of serum electrolytes and arterial blood gases simultaneously. Venous blood gas assessment is sufficient for monitoring the course of acidosis during the treatment of these conditions.

10. **What are the key principles of treating DKA and HHS?**
Intravenous (IV) fluid administration
Insulin therapy (IV or subcutaneous [SQ]) in adequate amounts
Potassium replacement at the appropriate time
Bicarbonate therapy when acidosis is severe
Identification and treatment of the precipitating cause

11. **Give recommendations for IV fluid administration in DKA and HHS**
First hour: Normal saline (NS), 15 to 20 mL/kg/hour (1.0–1.5 L)
Maintenance: 1/2 NS, 250 to 500 mL/hour if serum Na is high or normal
NS, 250 to 500 mL/hour if serum Na is low
When BG is <200 mg/dL (DKA) or <300 mg/dL (HHS), change to 5% dextrose-containing fluids.

12. **How important is volume repletion in HHS?**
HHS is associated with more severe hypovolemia than DKA and with some residual insulin secretory capacity. Volume resuscitation is therefore more critical in HHS. Volume repletion and insulin administration are both necessary to treat HHS, but volume repletion is the top priority. Because of the high fluid volumes required and the older age of most individuals with HHS, careful monitoring of volume status is critically important.

13. **How should insulin therapy be given during DKA and HHS?**
Start with an IV bolus of regular insulin, 0.1 unit/kg, followed by an IV infusion of 0.1 unit/kg/hour.
If BG does not decrease 10% in 1 hour, give an additional IV bolus of 0.14 unit/kg and continue the infusion.
When BG is <200 mg/dL (DKA) or <300 mg/dL (HHS), decrease the infusion rate to 0.02 to 0.05 unit/kg/hour.
Our practice is to also administer a long-acting basal insulin 0.25 unit/kg SQ within 10 hours of the start of the IV regular insulin infusion. This low dose of basal insulin reduces the risk of future rebound hyperglycemia without increasing the risk of hypoglycemia.
Note: SQ rapid-acting insulin analogs may be used instead of IV regular insulin in people with mild to moderate DKA in the emergency department or on general medicine wards.

14. **When and how is potassium administered in DKA and HHS?**
Serum potassium (K^+) levels should be checked every 2 hours during the treatment of DKA and HHS because K^+ levels decrease quickly as a result of renal losses and K^+ movement from the extracellular to the intracellular compartment in response to insulin therapy. Serum K^+ can drop to dangerous levels during IV insulin therapy. The following are guidelines for K^+ replacement:
Serum $K^+ \geq 5.2$ mmol/L: Potassium should not be given.
Serum K^+ 3.3 to 5.1 mmol/L: Give potassium chloride (KCl) 20 to 30 mEq/L in the existing IV fluids along with insulin.

Serum K+ <3.3 mmol/L: Insulin should not be given initially. Give KCl 20 to 30 mEq/L in the IV fluids until serum K+ is >3.3 mmol/L. Once serum K+ is >3.3 mmol/L, insulin should be started.

15. **When should bicarbonate be given in the management of DKA and HHS?**
Bicarbonate therapy is not recommended when the serum pH is >6.9. If the pH is ≤6.9, sodium bicarbonate should be given as 2 amps (100 mmol) in 400 mL of water with KCl 20 mEq at 200 mL/hour for 2 hours or until venous pH is >7.0.

16. **When is phosphate replacement indicated in the treatment of DKA and HHS?**
Despite the fall in serum phosphate levels during DKA treatment, phosphate therapy is not indicated in most instances. However, if potential hypophosphatemic complications occur (severe muscle weakness, respiratory failure), 20 to 30 mEq/L can be added to the IV fluids. When IV phosphate is given, it is critical to also monitor serum calcium levels, which can drop quickly with IV phosphate therapy.

17. **Are DKA and HHS considered hypercoagulable states?**
DKA and HHS are considered hypercoagulable states. Prophylactic heparin may be beneficial and should be considered in people with DKA. Full anticoagulation is suggested for those with HHS unless there are contraindications.

18. **What criteria are used to determine when DKA has resolved?**
DKA resolution criteria:
Glucose <200 mg/dL
HCO$_3$ ≥18 mEq/L
pH >7.30
Anion gap ≤13
Ketones negative
        IV insulin can be discontinued when these criteria are met: the individual is clinically improved and able to tolerate oral intake, and the precipitating cause(s) have been addressed. Factors that predict a successful transition from IV to SQ insulin include a stable insulin infusion rate of <2.0 to 2.5 units/hour and BG levels consistently <130 mg/dL. If not already being given, a long-acting basal insulin should be started at least 4 hours before IV insulin is discontinued to prevent rebound hyperglycemia during the insulin gap.

19. **Why can ketones appear to worsen during the treatment of DKA?**
Beta-hydroxybutyrate is the predominant ketone early in DKA but is later converted to acetoacetate during DKA treatment. The nitroprusside test that is commonly used to monitor ketones mainly measures acetoacetate and acetone. Thus, as beta-hydroxybutyrate is converted to acetoacetate during DKA treatment, ketonemia may appear to worsen transiently before it improves.

20. **What pitfalls may occur during the treatment of DKA and HHS?**
IV insulin is discontinued too soon.
SQ insulin is not administered prior to stopping IV insulin.
The precipitating cause of DKA or HHS is not identified or treated.
Cerebral edema may occur if BG is corrected too rapidly (>100 mg/dL/hour).

21. **What is the mortality rate of DKA and HHS?**
Despite appropriate therapy as described previously, the mortality rate is approximately 4% for DKA and nearly 15% for HHS. Adverse prognostic factors for mortality include the presence of coma, hypotension, and extremes of age.

KEY POINTS

1. DKA is a state of acute metabolic decompensation manifested by significant hyperglycemia, ketonemia, anion-gap metabolic acidosis, and hypovolemia. DKA most commonly occurs in people with type 1 diabetes but sometimes occurs in those with type 2 diabetes and other types of diabetes.
2. HHS most often occurs in elderly people with type 2 diabetes and is characterized by severe hyperglycemia and hyperosmolality, profound hypovolemia, and absent or minimal ketonemia and metabolic acidosis.
3. DKA results from absolute or severe insulin deficiency coupled with elevated counterregulatory hormones (glucagon, epinephrine, cortisol, growth hormone), resulting in impaired tissue glucose utilization, increased hepatic gluconeogenesis and glycogenolysis, increased adipose tissue lipolysis and tissue proteolysis, ketogenesis, and hypovolemia resulting from osmotic diuresis.
4. Effective DKA management consists of careful attention to all of the following: IV fluid administration, insulin therapy in adequate amounts, potassium replacement at the appropriate time, bicarbonate therapy when acidosis is severe, and identification and treatment of the precipitating cause.

5. Delayed resolution, recurrence, and complications of DKA or HHS may result from premature discontinuation of IV insulin, failure to administer SQ insulin prior to stopping the IV insulin, failure to identify and treat the precipitating cause, and excessively rapid correction of hyperglycemia that results in cerebral edema.
6. The mortality rate is approximately 4% for DKA and nearly 15% for HHS; factors that predict mortality include the presence of coma, hypotension, and extremes of age.

BIBLIOGRAPHY

Baldrighi M, Sainaghi PP, Bellan M, Bartoli E, Castello LM. Hyperglycemic hyperosmolar state: a pragmatic approach to properly manage sodium derangements. *Curr Diabetes Rev.* 2018;14(6):534–541.

Benoit SR, Zhang Y, Geiss LS, Gregg EW, Albright A. Trends in diabetic ketoacidosis hospitalizations and in-hospital mortality - United States, 2000-2014. *MMWR Morbid Mortal Weekly Rep.* 2018;67(12):362–365.

Desai D, Mehta D, Mathias P, Menon G, Schubart UK. Health care utilization and burden of diabetic ketoacidosis in the US over the past decade: a nationwide analysis. *Diabetes Care.* 2018 Aug;41(8):1631–1638.

Fayfman M, Pasquel FJ, Umpierrez GE. Management of hyperglycemic crises: diabetic ketoacidosis and hyperglycemic hyperosmolar state. *Med Clin North Am.* 2017;101(3):587–606.

Firestone RL, Parker PL, Pandya KA, Wilson MD, Duby JJ. Moderate-intensity insulin therapy is associated with reduced length of stay in critically ill patients with diabetic ketoacidosis and hyperosmolar hyperglycemic state. *Crit Care Med.* 2019 May;47(5):700–705.

Fisher JN, Shahshahani MN, Kitabchi AE. Diabetic ketoacidosis: low-dose insulin therapy by various routes. *N Engl J Med.* 1977 Aug 4;297(5):238–241.

Elangovan A, Cattamanchi S, Farook AR, Trichur RV. Validation of predicting hyperglycemic crisis death score: a risk stratification tool for appropriate disposition of hyperglycemic crisis patients from the emergency department. *J Emerg Trauma Shock.* 2018 Apr-Jun;11(2):104–110.

Haas NL, Gianchandani RY, Gunnerson KJ, et al. The two-bag method for treatment of diabetic ketoacidosis in adults. *J Emerg Med.* 2018 May;54(5):593–599.

Hsia E, Seggelke S, Gibbs J, et al. Subcutaneous administration of glargine to diabetic patients receiving insulin infusion prevents rebound hyperglycemia. *J Clin Endocrinol Metab.* 2012 Sep;97(9):3132–3137.

Kitabchi AE, Umpierrez GE, Fisher JN, Murphy MB, Stentz FB. Thirty years of personal experience in hyperglycemic crises: diabetic keto-acidosis and hyperglycemic hyperosmolar state. *J Clin Endocrinol Metab.* 2008 May;93(5):1541–1552.

Kitabchi AE, Umpierrez GE, Miles JM, Fisher JN. Hyperglycemic crises in adult patients with diabetes. *Diabetes Care.* 2009 Jul;32(7):1335–1343.

Kitabchi AE, Umpierrez GE, Murphy MB, et al. Management of hyperglycemic crises in patients with diabetes. *Diabetes Care.* 2001 Jan;24(1):131–153.

Kreisberg RA. Diabetic ketoacidosis: new concepts and trends in pathogenesis and treatment. *Ann Intern Med.* 1978 May;88(5):681–695.

McCoy RG, Herrin J, Lipska KJ, Shah ND. Recurrent hospitalizations for severe hypoglycemia and hyperglycemia among U.S. adults with diabetes. *J Diabetes Complications.* 2018 Jul;32(7):693–701.

Nyenwe EA, Kitabchi AE. Evidence-based management of hyperglycemic emergencies in diabetes mellitus. *Diabetes Res Clin Pract.* 2011 Dec;94(3):340–351.

Pasquel FJ, Tsegka K, Wang H, et al. Clinical outcomes in patients with isolated or combined diabetic ketoacidosis and hyperosmolar hyperglycemic state: a retrospective, hospital-based cohort study. *Diabetes Care.* 2020 Feb;43(2):349–357.

Stoner GD. Hyperosmolar hyperglycemic state. *Am Fam Physician.* 2017 Dec 1;96(11):729–736.

Ullal J, Aloi JA, Reyes-Umpierrez D, et al. Comparison of computer-guided versus standard insulin infusion regimens in patients with diabetic ketoacidosis. *J Diabetes Sci Technol.* 2018 Jan;12(1):39–46.

Umpierrez GE, Jones S, Smiley D, et al. Insulin analogs versus human insulin in the treatment of patients with diabetic ketoacidosis: a randomized controlled trial. *Diabetes Care.* 2009;32:1164–1169.

Umpierrez G, Korytkowski M. Diabetic emergencies - ketoacidosis, hyperglycaemic hyperosmolar state and hypoglycaemia. *Nat Rev Endocrinol.* 2016 Apr;12(4):222–232.

Vellanki P, Umpierrez GE. Increasing hospitalizations for DKA: a need for prevention programs. *Diabetes Care.* 2018 Sep;41(9):1839–1841.

Wilson JF. In the Clinic: diabetic ketoacidosis. *Ann Intern Med.* 2010 Jan 5;152(1):ITC1–ITC15.

DIABETIC KIDNEY DISEASE

Sophia Ambruso, DO and Isaac Teitelbaum, MD

CHAPTER 4

1. **What is diabetic nephropathy (DN)?**

   The early definition of DN included (1) the presence of albuminuria and (2) concurrent retinopathy in people with type 1 diabetes mellitus (DM1). Over time, with the increased incidence and prevalence of type 2 diabetes mellitus (DM2), it became clear that DN was not limited to those with DM1. The updated definition of DN is used to describe people with pathologic manifestations of classic diabetic glomerulopathy, which include glomerular basement membrane (GBM) thickening, endothelial damage, mesangial expansion, and nodules with podocyte loss (Fig. 4.1).

2. **What is the difference between albuminuria and proteinuria? How are they measured and interpreted?**

   Albuminuria refers to the presence of albumin in the urine, whereas *proteinuria* refers to the presence of all proteins in the urine, including albumin, beta-2 microglobulin, immunoglobulin light chains, retinol-binding protein, and polypeptides. Naturally, proteinuria measurements will be higher than albuminuria measurements for this reason. Albuminuria can be estimated using a spot urine albumin-to-creatinine ratio (ACR) or directly measured via a 24-hour urine albumin collection. Similarly, proteinuria can be estimated using a spot urine protein-to-creatinine ratio (PCR) or directly measured via a 24-hour urine protein collection. Either measurement can be used to evaluate proteinuria, as long as definitions for each are known. A discrepancy between urinary albumin and protein measurements may reflect an underlying pathologic process such as paraproteinemia, in which immunoglobulin light chains are overabundant in the serum and, consequently, in the urine as well.

3. **What do *macroalbuminuria* and *microalbuminuria* refer to in DN?**

   The terms *macroalbuminuria* and *microalbuminuria* were initially adopted to communicate the spectrum of albuminuria in diabetic kidney disease (DKD), representing overt DN and incipient DN, respectively. Because albuminuria was considered an early sign of classical DN, the term *microalbuminuria* was adopted in reference to persistently elevated levels of albuminuria that are often undetectable on dipstick. Although the term continues to be widely used among primary care practitioners, *microalbuminuria* is rarely used by nephrologists. Rather, the more universal description *moderately increased albuminuria* has been adopted to replace the term *microalbuminuria*. Moderately increased albuminuria is defined as 30 to 300 mg/day on 24-hour urine collection or 30 to 300 mg/g for ACR. Likewise, *macroalbuminuria* is now referred to as *severely increased albuminuria*, as defined by >300 mg/day on 24-hour urine or >300 mg/g for ACR (Table 4.1).

4. **What is diabetic kidney disease (DKD)?**

   DKD is an all-encompassing term that includes albuminuric DKD (A-DKD) and nonalbuminuric DKD (NA-DKD). The classical clinical course of DKD is characterized by a progressive increase in albuminuria followed by a decline in the glomerular filtration rate (GFR). However, there is an emerging nonalbuminuric pattern of DKD injury that consists predominantly of tubulointerstitial injury and scarring with nonclassical glomerular lesions.

5. **Describe the features of NA-DKD**

   NA-DKD can occur in both DM1 and DM2; however, it is far more common in DM2. In addition, NA-DKD has a slower trajectory of GFR decline. The emergence of NA-DKD may be a reflection of improved management of diabetes and increased use of the renin-angiotensin-aldosterone system (RAAS) blockade, thus reducing microvascular injury, hyperfiltration, and hyperglycemic-induced injury.

6. **What are the incidence and prevalence of chronic kidney disease (CKD) and end-stage kidney disease (ESKD) in diabetic nephropathy?**

   Diabetes mellitus (DM) affects 10% of the U.S. population, 25% to 30% of whom have DKD. DM is the leading cause of CKD worldwide and accounts for 50% of all patients with ESKD. However, the incidence of ESKD among all individuals with DM is relatively low because of the high rate of cardiovascular mortality in these patients prior to reaching the need for kidney-replacement therapy (KRT).

7. **What are the cardiovascular and mortality outcomes in DN-associated CKD and ESKD?**

   Kidney disease is strongly associated with an increased risk of all-cause and cardiovascular mortality. Known as the *disease multiplier*, CKD has been shown to worsen cardiovascular and noncardiovascular outcomes in people with DM1 and DM2. Notably, most people with DN die of cardiovascular complications prior to reaching the need

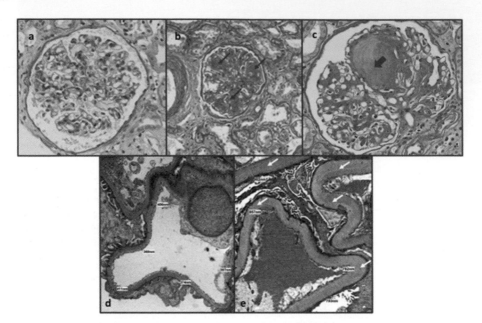

Fig. 4.1 Histologic changes of diabetic nephropathy (DN). (A–C) Light microscopy. (D and E) Electron microscopy. (A) Normal glomerulus. (B) Nodular glomerular sclerosis with mesangial expansion in DN *(thin black arrows)*. (C) Nodular glomerulosclerosis with Kimmelstiel–Wilson nodule in DN *(thick black arrow)*. (D) Normal glomerular basement membrane (GBM) thickness and appearance. (E) Thickened GBM in DN *(white arrows)*.

Table 4.1 Summary of Albuminuria Recommendations

	NORMAL TO MILDLY INCREASED	MODERATELY INCREASED	SEVERELY INCREASED
24-hour urine albumin (mg/day)	<30	30–300	>300
24-hour urine protein (mg/day)	<150	150–500	>500
Albumin-to-creatinine ratio (mg/g)	<30	30–300	>300
Protein-to-creatinine ratio (mg/g)	<150	150–500	>500
Protein dipstick	Negative to trace	Trace to 1+	>1+

Modified from Kidney Disease Improving Global Outcomes. KDIGO clinical practice guideline for lipid management in chronic kidney disease. *Kidney Int. Suppl.* 2013;3(3).

for KRT. The combination of DM and CKD has an additive effect on cardiovascular risk and mortality. Rising albuminuria ($\geq$30 mg/g) and falling GFR independently increase the risk for cardiovascular events and death. For every halving of GFR, the incidence of cardiovascular events is two-fold higher. For every 10-fold increase in baseline urine albumin, the incidence of cardiovascular events is 2.5-fold higher.

8. **What are the nonmodifiable risk factors contributing to DKD and its progression?**
   Genetic predisposition, age, race, and gender all have implications in disease progression. Although a true genetic locus has not been identified, a genetic predisposition to disease progression has been identified for both DM1 and DM2. If a first-degree relative with DM1 has DN, there is an 83% chance that offspring with DM1 will develop DN. A similar predisposition occurs in DM2, but the rates are unknown. Additionally, the offspring of women who are hyperglycemic during pregnancy have a higher risk of DN. Age is directly related to the prevalence of DKD and GFR loss; however, a large component of this is confounded by age-related GFR loss. African American, Latino, and American Indian persons have higher rates of albuminuria, GFR loss, and ESKD, which is only partially explained by socioeconomic disparity. Lastly, although women have a higher risk of DKD, men incur a higher risk of late-stage DKD progression to ESKD.

9. **What are the modifiable risk factors contributing to DKD and its progression?**
Socioeconomic status, education level, obesity, smoking, uncontrolled hyperglycemia, uncontrolled hypertension, and prior episodes of acute kidney injury (AKI) are the identified modifiable risk factors in DKD. Albuminuria and GFR < 60 mL/min/1.73 m^2 are more common among those with lower levels of education, despite controlling for socioeconomic factors. After controlling for race, ESKD was 4.5-fold more common among the 25% living below the poverty line. Obesity and smoking can independently cause direct kidney injury, contributing to DKD progression. Similar to DN, obesity causes increased glomerular hyperfiltration, progressive albuminuria, and podocyte injury, with resultant secondary focal segmental glomerular sclerosis (FSGS). Smoking often leads to nodular sclerosis, which is histologically indistinguishable from diabetic glomerulosclerosis. Poor glycemic control is associated with incident and progressive DKD. Systolic blood pressure > 140 mm Hg increases the risk for the development of severely increased albuminuria and stage III CKD. Finally, AKI increases the risk for DKD as a result of maladaptive repair processes. Interestingly, DKD also increases the risk for AKI.

10. **What are the pathophysiologic changes of DN?**
In DM, the overactive RAAS system, specifically angiotensin II and downstream mediators, results in an increased GFR, also known as hyperfiltration. Prolonged hyperfiltration and extended exposure to angiotensin II, hyperglycemia, and resultant advanced glycation end products (AGEs) lead to unregulated oxidative stress and inflammation, thereby inducing mesangial, endothelial, and tubulointerstitial injury. With sustained oxidative stress and exposure to inflammatory cells and mediators, the long-term sequelae of fibrosis (glomerulosclerosis), tubular atrophy, and subsequent reduced GFR ensue.

11. **What is the natural progression of DN?**
The earliest identifiable alteration in DN is glomerular hyperfiltration, which is manifested by a 25% increase in GFR. Concurrent glomerular hypertrophy, mesangial expansion, and tubular hypertrophy result in enlarged kidneys, a hallmark of early disease. Hyperfiltration is often followed by albuminuria, typically beginning with moderate albuminuria (30–300 mg/g) and progressing to overt albuminuria (>300 mg/g), progressive CKD, and finally ESKD (Fig. 4.2). The albuminuric alterations can occur within 5 years of diagnosis of DM1 but are more frequently identified within 10 to 15 years of diagnosis. In DM2, the duration between diabetes diagnosis and identification of DN is less predictable. This unpredictability relates to delays in DM2 diagnosis, confounding comorbidities, and age-related kidney senescence.

12. **What mechanisms contribute to glomerular hyperfiltration in DN?**
Disproportional afferent arteriolar vasodilation and efferent arteriolar vasoconstriction lend the greatest contributions to glomerular hyperfiltration. This phenomenon is mediated by tubuloglomerular feedback (TGF) and upregulated RAAS activity, leading to circulating mediators that preferentially cause afferent vasodilation (atrial natriuretic peptide, nitric oxide, and prostaglandins) and efferent vasoconstriction (angiotensin II, thromboxane, and endothelin 1; Fig. 4.3). This imbalance increases intraglomerular pressures, with subsequent hyperfiltration. Further dysregulation of the RAAS cascade and TGF is mediated by the necessary upregulation of glucose reabsorption in the proximal convoluted tubule (PCT) via sodium–glucose cotransporter 2 (SGLT-2). Here, sodium cotransport ensues, reducing sodium delivery to the distal convoluted tubule (DCT) and macula densa, further contributing to TGF-mediated afferent arteriolar vasodilation and upregulated RAAS activity.

13. **How does DKD impair the autoregulatory capability of the kidney?**
Endothelial injury causes long-term remodeling, featuring arteriolar intimal hyaline accumulation termed *arteriolar hyalinosis*. This thickens the vessel wall, narrowing the lumen and creating rigid arterioles, thus impairing the arteriolar response to autoregulatory mechanisms in response to shifts in hemodynamic states such as hypovolemia (Fig. 4.4).

14. **Can hyperfiltration and albuminuria regress?**
Yes! Improved glycemic control, blood pressure control (goal $< 140/90$), and modification of glomerular hemodynamics with RAAS inhibitors (e.g., angiotensin-converting enzyme inhibitors [ACEis] and angiotensin receptor blockers [ARBs]) and SGLT-2 inhibitors will lead to a reversal of hyperfiltration, regression of albuminuria, slowed progression of albuminuria, and slowed decline of GFR. As a result of age-related kidney senescence and the

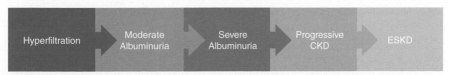

Fig. 4.2 Natural progression of diabetic nephropathy.

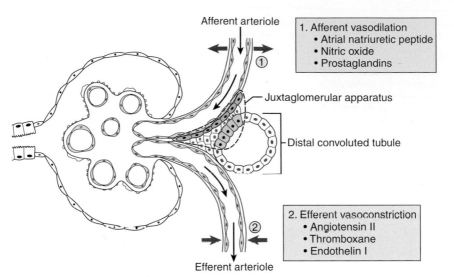

Fig. 4.3 Disproportional afferent arteriolar vasodilation and efferent arteriolar vasoconstriction in hyperfiltration of diabetic nephropathy.

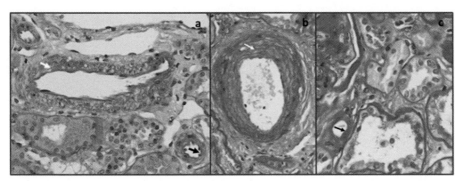

Fig. 4.4 Light microscopy representing a normal artery and arteriole (*thick white and black arrow*, respectively) and thickened artery and arteriole with remodeling and intimal hyalinosis *(pink)* in a kidney with diabetic disease (*thin white and black arrow*, respectively).

presence of confounding comorbidities, regression in DM2 is less common and less predictable than in DM1. Although regression of moderate albuminuria is more common, regression of severe albuminuria has been observed.

15. **What is the prevalence of diabetic retinopathy (DR) among individuals diagnosed with DN?**
    Diabetic retinopathy is present in nearly 100% of people with DM1 and DN. The same is not true in DM2, where only 50% to 60% of individuals exhibit retinopathy. The presence of diabetic retinopathy is part of the criteria for the clinical diagnosis of DN in people with DM1. In fact, in a person with DM1 and presumed DN, the absence of retinopathy should prompt consideration of a kidney biopsy, looking for alternative pathology. This is not the case in DM2.

16. **What are the required criteria to make a clinical diagnosis of DN?**
    See Table 4.2.

17. **What are the indications for biopsy in a patient with diabetes and renal dysfunction?**
    See Table 4.3.

18. **Discuss how worsening GFR affects the phenomenon of "burned-out diabetes" in DM2. What are the underlying mechanisms?**
    In long-standing insulin-requiring DM2, there is a common misperception that a person has "burned-out diabetes" because of the development of increased frequency of hypoglycemic episodes or a decline in insulin

Table 4.2 Criteria for Clinical Diagnosis of Diabetic Nephropathy
1. Duration of disease: DM1 > 10 years or DM2 for any duration
2. Presence of diabetic retinopathy if patient has DM1
3. Previous moderate albuminuria (ACR 30 mg/g–300 mg/g)
4. No macroscopic hematuria, RBC casts, or dysmorphic RBCs (Note: Microscopic hematuria occurs in 10%–15% of patients with diabetic nephropathy. Dysmorphic RBCs also occur but are rare and may suggest an alternate diagnosis.)
5. Enlarged kidneys on ultrasound

ACR, Albumin-to-creatinine ratio; *DM1*, diabetes mellitus type 1; *DM2*, diabetes mellitus type 2; *RBC*, red blood cell.

Table 4.3 Indications for Biopsy in a Patient With Diabetes Mellitus and Kidney Dysfunction
1. Duration of disease: DM1 < 10 years unless diabetic retinopathy is present
2. No retinopathy in DM1 (pattern less predictable in DM2)
3. Nephrotic-range proteinuria without progression through moderate albuminuria
4. Macroscopic hematuria
5. RBC casts or dysmorphic RBCs (Note: Microscopic hematuria occurs in 10%–15% of patients with diabetic nephropathy. Dysmorphic RBCs also occur but are rare and may suggest an alternate diagnosis.)

DM1, Diabetes mellitus type 1; *DM2*, diabetes mellitus type 2; *RBC*, red blood cell.

Table 4.4 Goals of Diabetic Kidney Disease Management
1. Normalization of glomerular hemodynamics and regression of hyperfiltration
2. Regression or slowed progression of albuminuria
3. Halted or slowed progression of diabetic kidney disease

requirements, which in fact may herald worsening kidney function as a result of progressive DN. The mechanisms contributing to this phenomenon are multifaceted but relate to the following: decreased insulin clearance and degradation by the failing kidney, decreased kidney gluconeogenesis, decreased dietary intake (uremia), loss of muscle mass, protein-energy wasting (malnutrition-inflammation complex), and recommended dietary restrictions associated with advancing CKD.

19. **What are the main goals in the management of DKD?**
See Table 4.4.
We recommend addressing the modifiable risk factors for DKD progression by emphasizing glycemic control (A1c goal < 7%), improving blood pressure control (goal < 130/80), and encouraging and facilitating smoking cessation and weight loss. In addition, medicines that preserve glomerular hemodynamics and reduce intraglomerular pressures and glomerular hyperfiltration should be maximized as tolerated; these include ACEis, ARBs, and SGLT-2 inhibitors. There is also some evidence to support the antiproteinuric effect of spironolactone and nondihydropyridine calcium channel blockers, but these are not first-line options.

20. **How is RAAS inhibition effective in DN?**
Disproportional afferent arteriolar vasodilation and efferent arteriolar vasoconstriction lend the greatest contribution to glomerular hyperfiltration in DN and, in part, contribute to the development of albuminuria and subsequent DKD progression. RAAS inhibition with ACEis and/or ARBs provides significant renoprotective properties in both DM1 and DM2 by reducing afferent arteriolar vasodilation and efferent vasoconstriction, thereby decreasing intraglomerular pressures and hyperfiltration. RAAS inhibition has been shown to reduce albuminuria, the progression of albuminuria, the progression of DKD, and the development of ESKD in those with DKD.

Table 4.5 Summary Table of Novel Gastrointestinal Potassium Binders

POTASSIUM BINDER	SODIUM ZIRCONIUM CYCLOSILICATE (LOKELMA)	PATIROMER (VELTASSA)
Mechanism of action	K^+ exchange for Na^+ and H^+	K^+ in exchange for Ca^{2+}
Onset of activity	1 hour	7 hours
Location of drug activity	Entire GI tract	Colon
Side effects	Edema, GI effects, drug interference	GI effects, hypomagnesemia, drug interference
Cost (subject to change)	$675–$730	$850–$925

GI, Gastrointestinal.

21. **In people with advanced CKD initiated on RAAS inhibition, how are the associated declining GFR and hyperkalemia managed?**

    In people with albuminuria, nephrologists try to continue aggressive RAAS inhibition as long as the GFR remains ≥ 20 mL/min. We tend to tolerate the ensuing rise in serum creatinine, provided it does not exceed a 30% to 35% increase and stabilizes within the first 2 to 4 months of drug initiation. If hyperkalemia develops, it is advisable to continue RAAS inhibition while modifying dietary potassium intake. If hyperkalemia persists despite dietary modification, the introduction of one of the novel gastrointestinal (GI) potassium binders—sodium zirconium cyclosilicate (Lokelma) or patiromer (Veltassa)—is recommended while continuing the maximum tolerated dose of RAAS inhibition. See Table 4.5 for the mechanism of action, onset, and location of drug activity; adverse effects; and general cost of the novel GI potassium binders.

22. **What is the mechanism of action of SGLT-2 inhibitors? How are they renoprotective?**

    SGLT-2 inhibitors block SGLT-2 in the PCT. Thus, sodium and glucose remain in the nephron lumen, leading to a robust natriuresis, thereby reducing intravascular volume and blood pressure. Additionally, increased sodium delivery to the DCT and macula densa ensues, downregulating TGF and RAAS activity, thus decreasing afferent arteriole vasodilation, with a resultant reduction of intraglomerular pressures and preservation of glomerular hemodynamics.

23. **What are the mortality, cardiovascular, and kidney outcomes with SGLT-2 inhibitors?**

    SGLT-2 inhibitors reduce the degree of albuminuria and risk of DKD progression, independent of glycemic effects. They lower the risk of ESKD development or kidney disease–associated death, independent of baseline albumin secretion or RAAS inhibition. Finally, SGLT-2 inhibitors reduce the rate of major cardiovascular events in individuals with atherosclerotic disease, regardless of DKD.

24. **What are the adverse drug effects of SGLT-2 inhibitors?**

    Because of increased glycosuria, urogenital infections, typically vulvovaginal candidiasis, are reported to be increased by two- to four-fold. Fournier's gangrene is also known to rarely be associated with SGLT-2 inhibitors. Euglycemic diabetic ketoacidosis has been reported with the use of SGLT-2 inhibitors, requiring appropriate dietary counseling prior to initiating. Finally, there initially appeared to be an increased risk of lower-limb amputations associated with the use of the SGLT-2 inhibitor canagliflozin; however, this was not observed in subsequent trials. In the DAPA-CKD trial, there were no statistically significant differences in severe adverse events between those on dapagliflozin and placebo. In particular, no signal for increased risk of amputations or diabetic ketoacidosis was identified. However, volume depletion was reported in 6% of those taking dapagliflozin compared with 4.2% of those on placebo.

25. **Who are candidates for SGLT-2 inhibitors?**

    Initiation of a SGLT-2 inhibitor is strongly recommended if the criteria in Table 4.6 are satisfied.

26. **How do we interpret the ensuing drop in GFR after initiating SGLT-2 inhibitors?**

    An initial GFR drop, similar to that seen with the initiation of RAAS inhibitors but to a lesser degree, is an anticipated physiologic consequence of SGLT-2 inhibition through alterations in glomerular hemodynamics without causing AKI. Within the first 2 weeks, an approximate 10% decline is expected, followed by stabilization of GFR. However, compared with placebo, long-term GFR decline is reduced with SGLT-2 inhibition.

Table 4.6 SGLT-2 Inhibitor Candidates

INCLUSION CRITERIA	EXCLUSION CRITERIA
1. wi type 2 diabetes mellitus	1. History of recurrent urinary tract infections, chronic indwelling urinary catheter, requirement for self-catheterization, or history of increased postvoid residual measurements
2. GFR 25 to < 60mL/min/1.73m^2 AND/OR albuminuria AND/OR	2. Inability to maintain good genitourinary hygiene
3. Established cardiovascular disease (e.g., CAD, HF, CVA)	3. Significant peripheral vascular disease on exam

CAD, coronary artery disease; *CVA,* cerebrovascular accident; *HF,* heart failure; *SGLT-2,* sodium–glucose cotransporter 2.

27. **Is there a role for GLP-1 receptor agonists in DKD?**

    GLP-1 receptor agonists bind glucagon-like peptide-1 (GLP-1) receptors, slowing gastric emptying and increasing insulin secretion by pancreatic beta cells. In DM2 with moderate to severe CKD, dulaglutide demonstrated a reduced decline in GFR, likely related to associated glycemic control and weight loss. Regardless of mechanism, in patients with persistently elevated albuminuria and worsening DKD, GLP-1 receptor agonists may be considered after first- and second-line agents are exhausted.

28. **Are there therapeutic interventions on the horizon that will benefit those with DKD?**

    Yes! Finerenone is a nonsteroidal, selective mineralocorticoid receptor antagonist with minimal effects on blood pressure and serum potassium compared with the aldosterone receptor blocker counterparts, spironolactone and eplerenone. The FIDELIO DKD trial, recently published in the *New England Journal of Medicine*, compared finerenone to placebo and demonstrated a significant risk reduction in kidney and cardiovascular events in people with DKD.

KEY POINTS

1. DN is a progressive disease, marked by a transition from glomerular hyperfiltration to albuminuria to progressive chronic kidney disease and, finally, ESKD.
2. Overactive RAAS activity and direct vasoactive activity mediated by TGF lead to disproportional afferent arteriolar vasodilation and efferent arteriolar vasoconstriction, thereby altering glomerular hemodynamics, resulting in hyperfiltration.
3. RAAS inhibitors (ACEis/ARBs) and SGLT-2 inhibitors are considered renoprotective agents through the preservation of glomerular hemodynamics.
4. In patients with albuminuric DKD, attempts to maximize and continue ACEi or ARB therapy should be made.
5. In select patient populations, SGLT-2 inhibitors should be initiated and maximized.

BIBLIOGRAPHY

Bakris GL, Agarwal R, Anker SF, et al. Effect if finerenone on chronic kidney disease outcomes in type 2 diabetes. *N Engl J Med.* 2020, Oct 23 (E-pub ahead of print); https://doi.org/10.1056/NEJMoa2025845.

Brenner BM, Cooper ME, de Zeeuw D, et al. Effects of losartan on renal and cardiovascular outcomes in patients with type 2 diabetes and nephropathy. *N Engl J Med.* 2001;345(12):861–869. https://doi.org/10.1056/NEJMoa011161.

de Boer IH, Afkarian M, Rue TC, et al. Renal outcomes in patients with type 1 diabetes and macroalbuminuria. *J Am Soc Nephrol.* 2014;25(10):2342–2350. https://doi.org/10.1681/ASN.2013091004.

Heerspink JHL, Stefansson BV, Correa-Rotter R, et al. Dapagliflozin in patients with chronic kidney disease. *N Engl J Med.* 2020;383(15):1436–1446. https://doi.org/10.1056/NEJMoa2024816.

Hemmelgarn BR, Manns BJ, Lloyd A, et al. Relation between kidney function, proteinuria, and adverse outcomes. *JAMA.* 2010;303(5):423–429. https://doi.org/10.1001/jama.2010.39.

Lewis EJ, Hunsicker LG, Clarke WR, et al. Renoprotective effect of the angiotensin-receptor antagonist irbesartan in patients with nephropathy due to type 2 diabetes. *N Engl J Med.* 2001;345(12):851–860. https://doi.org/10.1056/NEJMoa011303.

Neal B, Perkovic V, Mahaffey KW, et al. Canagliflozin and Cardiovascular and Renal Events in Type 2 Diabetes. *N Engl J Med.* 2017;377(7):644–657. https://doi.org/10.1056/NEJMoa1611925.

Ninomiya T, Perkovic V, de Galan BE, et al. Albuminuria and kidney function independently predict cardiovascular and renal outcomes in diabetes. *J Am Soc Nephrol.* 2009;20(8):1813–1821. https://doi.org/10.1681/ASN.2008121270. (ADVANCE).

Parving HH, Lehnert H, Bröchner-Mortensen J, et al. The effect of irbesartan on the development of diabetic nephropathy in patients with type 2 diabetes. *N Engl J Med.* 2001;345(12):870–878. https://doi.org/10.1056/NEJMoa011489.

Perkovic V, Jardine MJ, Neal B, et al. Canagliflozin and Renal Outcomes in Type 2 Diabetes and Nephropathy. *N Engl J Med.* 2019;380(24):2295–2306. https://doi.org/10.1056/NEJMoa1811744.

Viberti G, Wheeldon NM. MicroAlbuminuria Reduction With VALsartan (MARVAL) Study Investigators. Microalbuminuria reduction with valsartan in patients with type 2 diabetes mellitus: a blood pressure-independent effect. *Circulation.* 2002;106(6):672–678. https://doi.org/10.1161/01.cir.0000024416.33113.0a.

Zoppini G, Targher G, Chonchol M, et al. Predictors of estimated GFR decline in patients with type 2 diabetes and preserved kidney function. *Clin J Am Soc Nephrol.* 2012;7(3):401–408. https://doi.org/10.2215/CJN.07650711.

CHAPTER 5

DIABETIC RETINOPATHY

Jesse M. Smith, MD and Naresh Mandava, MD

1. **What is diabetic retinopathy (DR)?**
   DR is the most common complication of diabetes mellitus and the most common cause of vision loss among working-age adults worldwide. DR is a chronic microangiopathy that primarily involves the retinal circulation. Over time, damage to capillary endothelium leads to vascular occlusion and tissue nonperfusion, retinal ischemia, and vessel leakage (Fig. 5.1).

2. **How common is DR?**
   During the first 20 years of disease, around 60% of people with type 2 diabetes and nearly 100% of those with type 1 diabetes develop DR. Of those affected, one-third have vision-threatening disease.

3. **Name the subtypes of DR**
   DR is split into nonproliferative and proliferative disease. Nonproliferative DR is characterized by microaneurysms, retinal hemorrhages, lipid exudates, and microvascular anomalies that lead to vessel leakage and vessel occlusion. Nonproliferative DR is further separated into mild, moderate, and severe disease (Table 5.1). The hallmark of proliferative DR is the growth and proliferation of abnormal new vessels in response to chronic ischemia. Nonproliferative DR is much more common than proliferative DR. Although both types of DR can cause vision loss, the risk is significantly higher with proliferative DR.

4. **How common is blindness from DR?**
   Legal blindness, as defined by the World Health Organization, is visual acuity of 20/200 or worse in a patient's better-seeing eye. DR is the leading worldwide cause of blindness in working-age adults. In the United States, the 25-year cumulative incidence of blindness in people with type 1 diabetes is around 3%. In people with type 2 diabetes, the incidence is below 1%.

5. **Describe diabetic macular edema (DME)**
   DME is a thickening of the macula caused by the accumulation of fluid in the retinal layers. The fluid comes from damaged and leaky capillaries. The presence of edema in the central portion of the macula disrupts visual function and is the most common cause of vision impairment in DR.

6. **What is neovascularization (NV)?**
   NV is the growth and proliferation of abnormal blood vessels inside the eye. Diabetic damage to the retinal capillary circulation leads to retinal ischemia, which stimulates the release of numerous cytokines, including vascular endothelial growth factor (VEGF). The release of VEGF drives the growth of new vessels in the eye, most commonly on the optic disc, on the retinal surface, into the vitreous gel, and in the anterior chamber angle and the iris. NV is a serious complication of DR and results in vitreous hemorrhage, tractional retinal detachment, and neovascular glaucoma.

7. **What are anterior-segment complications of diabetes?**
   Cataracts form at a younger age and at higher frequency in diabetic eyes. Neovascularization of the iris and the anterior chamber angle cause occlusion of the pathway for aqueous outflow, leading to neovascular glaucoma and resultant blindness.

8. **How does DR cause retinal detachment?**
   Chronic neovascularization on the surface of the retina and optic disc leads to blood vessel growth into the vitreous cavity, using the vitreous cortex as a scaffold. This growth leads to the formation of fibrovascular complexes with strong adherence to both the retinal surface and the vitreous gel. In time, these complexes contract and cause the retina to detach and separate from the retinal pigment epithelium, a monolayer of cells underneath the retina. This type of retinal detachment is called *traction retinal detachment* because it is caused by a mechanical pull from fibrovascular complexes. Traction retinal detachment is a serious complication of DR and commonly causes severe vision loss, even after successful surgical intervention.

9. **What are the major risk factors for developing DR?**
   The most important risk factor is the duration of diabetes. Hyperglycemia and hypertension are important and modifiable risk factors. Tight glucose and blood pressure control have been shown to be effective in preventing vision loss from DR.

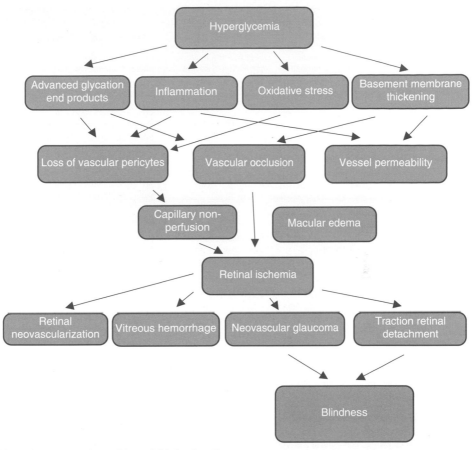

Fig. 5.1 Pathogenesis and natural history of diabetic retinopathy.

Table 5.1 Findings in Subtypes of Diabetic Retinopathy (DR)

DR TYPE	FINDINGS
Mild nonproliferative	Microaneurysms only
Moderate nonproliferative	Microaneurysms, retinal hemorrhages, hard exudates
Severe nonproliferative	Any one of the following: retinal hemorrhages in 4 quadrants, 2 quadrants of venous beading, 1 quadrant of intraretinal microvascular anomaly
Proliferative	Neovascularization (disc, iris, angle, elsewhere), fibrovascular proliferation, traction retinal detachment, neovascular glaucoma

10. **How is DR diagnosed?**
    A diagnosis of DR is made on the basis of a dilated fundus examination by an ophthalmologist or optometrist. Additional imaging modalities, such as fluorescein angiography and optical coherence tomography, can assist in identifying complications of DR, such as neovascularization and diabetic macular edema.

11. **How often should patients with diabetes see an eye doctor for an exam?**
    People with type 1 diabetes should have a dilated fundus exam within 3 to 5 years of first diagnosis, and those with type 2 diabetes should be examined around the time of first diagnosis. Subsequent exam timing is driven by the presence or absence of disease. A patient without any retinopathy or with mild disease may generally follow

Table 5.2 Treatments, Indications, Benefits, and Risks or Downsides in DR			
TREATMENT	**INDICATIONS**	**BENEFITS**	**DOWNSIDES AND RISKS**
Intravitreal anti-VEGF injection	Diabetic macular edema, proliferative diabetic retinopathy	Improvement in VA, prevention of severe vision loss, rapid onset of action	Need for retreatment, infectious endophthalmitis risk, disease progression if lost to follow-up, possible teratogenicity in pregnant patients
Intravitreal steroid injection	Diabetic macular edema	Improvement in VA	Cataract progression, increased intraocular pressure, infectious endophthalmitis risk
Focal laser	Diabetic macular edema	Improvement in VA, durable effect of treatment	Risk of central vision loss, less VA improvement compared with injections, risk of choroidal neovascular membrane development
Panretinal photocoagulation	Proliferative diabetic retinopathy	Prevention of severe vision loss, durable effect of treatment	Postprocedure reduction in visual field and in vision in low-light conditions
Vitrectomy	Traction retinal detachment, vitreous hemorrhage	Prevention of severe vision loss, durable effect of treatment	Infectious endophthalmitis risk, cataract progression, Postprocedure reduction in visual field and in vision in low-light conditions

VEGF, vascular endothelial growth factor; *VA*, visual acuity.

up annually. Patients with more severe disease should establish care with an ophthalmologist and follow up at intervals dictated by disease severity.

12. **How is DR treated?**

Nonproliferative DR without DME can be observed closely without intervention. DME is most commonly treated with serial intravitreal injections of anti-VEGF drugs or corticosteroids at intervals between 1 and 3 months, but long-term treatment success depends on solid patient compliance and follow-up. Proliferative DR is generally treated with panretinal photocoagulation, in which laser pulses are directed to ablate portions of the nonperfused, ischemic peripheral retina while sparing the macula. Panretinal photocoagulation has been shown to decrease the risk of severe vision loss by 50%. Lastly, severe complications of DR, such as vitreous hemorrhage and traction retinal detachment, require vitrectomy by a vitreoretinal surgeon. In this procedure, microsurgical instruments are used to remove the vitreous gel and any fibrovascular complexes, and laser ablative treatment is applied to areas of nonperfused peripheral retina. Table 5.2 reviews treatments, indications, risks, and benefits.

13. **Discuss the risks of treatment**

Intravitreal injection of anti-VEGF agents carries a low risk of infectious endophthalmitis. Intravitreal injection of corticosteroids has a risk of endophthalmitis, cataract formation, and elevated intraocular pressure. Panretinal photocoagulation ablates much of the peripheral retina and therefore causes constriction of the visual field and diminution of night vision. Vitrectomy causes acceleration of cataract formation and also carries a small risk of endophthalmitis.

14. **Does DR correlate to a patient's overall health?**

Yes. Many studies have shown correlations between the severity of DR and systemic complications of DR. For example, one study demonstrated a nearly 50% 10-year all-cause mortality rate in patients with diabetic traction retinal detachment compared with a 2% rate in patients with diabetes without retinopathy.

15. **Can DR be cured?**

No. DR can become inactive in many patients with strict glucose and blood pressure control, but it can also reactivate later. Treatment with anti-VEGF injections can temporarily induce quiescence of DR, but relapse is common when the drug effect fades after several months. Panretinal photocoagulation and vitrectomy are often able to induce long-term or even permanent quiescence of DR, but these procedures are only employed in advanced cases of DR because of risks and side effects.

KEY POINTS

1. DR is the leading cause of blindness in working-age adults worldwide.
2. The most important risk factors for developing DR are a long duration of diabetes, inadequate glucose control, and elevated blood pressure.
3. DR is split into nonproliferative DR and proliferative DR. The highest risk for blindness comes from complications of proliferative DR.
4. Treatment of DR can be divided into observation, intravitreal injections, laser therapies, and surgery. The vast majority of patients may be observed, but treatment is warranted for DME and proliferative DR and its complications.

BIBLIOGRAPHY

Early Treatment Diabetic Retinopathy Study Research Group. Early photocoagulation for diabetic retinopathy. ETDRS report number 9. *Ophthalmology.* 1991;98(5 Suppl):766–785.

Klein R, Klein BE, Moss SE, Cruickshanks KJ. The Wisconsin Epidemiologic Study of diabetic retinopathy. XIV. Ten-year incidence and progression of diabetic retinopathy. *Arch Ophthalmol.* 1994;112(9):1217–1228.

Klein R, Klein BE, Moss SE, Davis MD, DeMets DL. The Wisconsin epidemiologic study of diabetic retinopathy. III. Prevalence and risk of diabetic retinopathy when age at diagnosis is 30 or more years. *Arch Ophthalmol.* 1984;102(4):527–532.

Klein R, Klein BE, Moss SE, Davis MD, DeMets DL. The Wisconsin epidemiologic study of diabetic retinopathy. II. Prevalence and risk of diabetic retinopathy when age at diagnosis is less than 30 years. *Arch Ophthalmol.* 1984;102(4):520–526.

Lee R, Wong TY, Sabanayagam C. Epidemiology of diabetic retinopathy, diabetic macular edema and related vision loss. *Eye Vis (Lond).* 2015;2:17.

Shukla SY, Hariprasad AS, Hariprasad SM. Long-term mortality in diabetic patients with tractional retinal detachments. *Ophthalmol Retina.* 2017;1(1):8–11.

UK Prospective Diabetes Study Group. Tight blood pressure control and risk of macrovascular and microvascular complications in type 2 diabetes: UKPDS 38. *BMJ.* 1998;317(7160):703–713.

UK Prospective Diabetes Study (UKPDS) Group. Effect of intensive blood-glucose control with metformin on complications in overweight patients with type 2 diabetes (UKPDS 34). *Lancet.* 1998;352(9131):854–865.

Wang W, Lo ACY. Diabetic Retinopathy: Pathophysiology and Treatments. *Int J Mol Sci.* 2018;19(6).

CHAPTER 6

DIABETIC NEUROPATHIES

David Stevens, MD, and Dianna Quan, MD

1. **What is neuropathy?**

   Neuropathy or *peripheral neuropathy* is a general term for dysfunction of the peripheral sensory, motor, or autonomic nerves. Afferent inputs from our environment are relayed through sensory nerves to the dorsal root ganglia, through spinal nerve roots, and eventually up to the brain. Efferent motor signals originate in the brain or spinal cord and are carried through spinal nerve roots and along motor nerves to muscles. Neuropathy can also involve the autonomic nervous system, which encompasses the sympathetic, parasympathetic, and enteric nervous systems and regulates involuntary physiologic functions such as heart rate, digestion, and the fight-or-flight response. The clinical manifestations of neuropathy depend on the type of peripheral nerves affected. Nerve disease within the spinal cord and brain is not classified as neuropathy, although symptoms may occasionally be similar.

2. **What are the symptoms associated with neuropathy?**

   Symptoms can be classified broadly as "positive" or "negative." Positive symptoms are sensations normally absent in healthy individuals. Examples include paresthesia, or tingling; allodynia, or discomfort with normally innocuous tactile stimuli; and dysesthesia, or unpleasant distortion of stimulus perception. Pain is the most troublesome positive symptom. In contrast, negative symptoms refer to the loss of normal functions, such as loss of sensation (numbness), loss of strength (weakness), or loss of balance with walking. Patients with neuropathy frequently have both positive and negative symptoms simultaneously.

3. **How common is diabetic neuropathy?**

   Diabetes is the most common cause of peripheral neuropathy in the American population. Prevalence figures vary depending on patient population and definition of neuropathy (based on physical exam findings vs. electrophysiology vs. symptoms). Studies suggest that 50% to 66% of people with diabetes show some objective evidence of neuropathy, and about 20% have symptomatic disease. At the time of diabetes diagnosis, around 10% of people have neuropathy, with this number increasing over disease duration.

4. **How does neuropathy present in diabetes?**

   Diabetic nerve disease can be loosely divided into four basic anatomic patterns or syndromes: distal symmetric polyneuropathy, autonomic neuropathy, plexus or spinal nerve root disease, and focal neuropathies. Patients may have more than one of these patterns simultaneously or at different points during the course of their diabetes.

5. **What is distal symmetric polyneuropathy (DSP)?**

   DSP is a length-dependent sensorimotor peripheral neuropathy that begins distally in the longest nerves going to the toes and feet. It is symmetric and involves multiple different nerves (polyneuropathy). Distal symmetric polyneuropathy is the most common diabetic neuropathy syndrome, with a prevalence of 45% to 54%. Symptoms progress slowly, moving proximally over months and years. Patients initially experience numbness, pain, dysesthesia, or paresthesia. Examination findings include decreased sensation in a classic "stocking-glove" distribution, hyporeflexia, and distal weakness in later stages. Gait imbalance and falls resulting from impaired proprioception may be seen. More severe complications from DSP include repetitive trauma or infections of numb extremities, leading to osteomyelitis and amputations.

6. **What are the features of diabetic autonomic neuropathy (DAN)?**

   This syndrome is caused by damage to the autonomic nerve fibers, leading to gastrointestinal, cardiovascular, or genitourinary dysfunction. Diabetes is the most common cause of autonomic neuropathy, with the prevalence among patients with diabetes estimated at 5% to 7%. Symptomatic dysautonomia is not typically seen in isolation but rather more commonly in combination with DSP. As the disease progresses, patients may have reduced ability or inability to perceive developing hypoglycemia. Limited high-quality data exist in support of most pharmacologic agents, with few drugs having U.S. Food and Drug Administration (FDA) indications for DAN manifestations (Table 6.1).

7. **What is diabetic neuropathic cachexia?**

   Diabetic neuropathic cachexia occurs in patients with uncontrolled diabetes and is characterized by the development of severe generalized peripheral neuropathic pain, autonomic dysfunction, superimposed thoracic and

Table 6.1 Manifestations of Diabetic Autonomic Neuropathy and Commonly Used Treatments

ORGAN SYSTEM	COMMON SYMPTOMS	TREATMENT OPTIONS
Gastrointestinal	Gastroparesis Constipation Nausea Fecal incontinence	Dietary intervention and hydration Promotility agents (e.g., metoclopramide, domperidone, macrolide antibiotics) Dietary intervention, hydration, and bulking agents Antiemetics (e.g., antihistamine, 5HT3 antagonists) Dietary intervention and bulking agents Antidiarrheal agents (e.g., loperamide, bismuth, atropine)
Cardiovascular	Exercise intolerance Orthostasis	Graded exercise program Reduction or elimination of blood pressure–lowering medications, adequate hydration, compression stockings or abdominal binder Mineralocorticoid (e.g., fludrocortisone) Sympathomimetic agents (e.g., midodrine, droxidopa)
Genitourinary	Urinary dysfunction Incontinence Urinary retention Sexual dysfunction	Pelvic muscle strengthening and lifestyle modification Serotonin–norepinephrine reuptake inhibitor (e.g., duloxetine) Alpha-1 blocker (e.g., tamsulosin) Phosphodiesterase 5 inhibitors (e.g., sildenafil, tadalafil, vardenafil, avanafil)
Skin	Abnormal sweating	Lifestyle modification Topical treatments

lumbosacral radiculopathies, and profound weight loss over the course of a few months. With proper glycemic control, these patients often recover to baseline weight with resolution of pain within 1 year, although more prolonged recoveries have been noted. It is considered very rare, and much of the literature describing this syndrome is in the form of case reports. Some clinical features overlap with diabetic radiculoplexus neuropathy (DRPN), although whether there are shared mechanisms of disease is not well understood.

8. **What is DRPN?**

   Plexopathy (damage to the brachial or lumbosacral plexus) and radiculopathy (damage to a spinal root) are uncommon, occurring in an estimated 1% of people with diabetes. Individual peripheral nerves also may be affected in isolation or in association with plexus and spinal root injury. Pain in the distribution of a spinal nerve root, plexus, or individual nerve begins abruptly, most commonly in the proximal leg or hip and often with no obvious antecedent trigger. Pain is often excruciating, affecting daily activities, sleep, appetite, and mood. Symptoms usually begin asymmetrically but sometimes become bilateral. As pain begins to subside slowly, weakness and atrophy become noticeable over days to weeks. Additional examination findings in the affected area include sensory loss and hyporeflexia. The pathophysiology and triggers are unclear, but there appears to be an inflammatory component with nonsystemic microvasculitis in many cases. Blood glucose levels are not clearly correlated with onset, and even patients with well-controlled glucose may be affected. Numerous names have been given to this disorder, including *diabetic amyotrophy, proximal diabetic neuropathy*, and *Bruns–Garland syndrome*.

9. **What focal neuropathies are common in diabetes?**

   People with diabetes are at higher risk of developing focal neuropathies related to entrapment or compression of individual peripheral nerves. The most common nerves affected are the median, ulnar, and fibular nerves (Table 6.2).

10. **What cranial neuropathies (CNs) occur more commonly in diabetes?**

    Diabetic CNs have an acute onset. They are caused by damage to the microvascular blood supply of the nerves and occur in about 1% to 2% of diabetic individuals. The most commonly affected cranial nerves are III, IV, VI, and VII. Deficits related to diabetic CN gradually recover over weeks to months with supportive treatment, including glycemic control, eye patching for diplopia, and protection of the eye with lubrication where lid function is impaired (Table 6.3).

Table 6.2 Compression Neuropathies in Diabetes

NERVE/SITE OF COMPRESSION	SYMPTOMS	EXAMINATION FINDINGS
Median nerve/ wrist (carpal tunnel syndrome)	Numbness in fingers and hand Pain and paresthesia in the hand, often worse with gripping or hyperflexion at the wrist Hand weakness	Decreased sensation of thumb, digits 2 and 3, and lateral aspect of digit 4 Pain or paresthesia with tapping over the nerve at the wrist (Tinel's sign) Pain, numbness, or paresthesia with hyperflexion at wrists (Phalen's sign) Decreased thenar muscle bulk or atrophy and weakness of thumb abduction, opposition, flexion
Ulnar nerve/elbow (cubital tunnel syndrome)	Numbness in fingers and hand Pain and paresthesia in the hand often worse with elbow flexion or pressure on medial aspect of elbow Hand weakness	Decreased sensation of digit 5 and medial aspect of digit 4 Pain or paresthesia with tapping over the nerve at the cubital tunnel (Tinel's sign) Decreased muscle bulk or atrophy on hypothenar hand and intrinsic muscles of hand Weakness finger abduction and flexion digits 4 and 5 Claw-hand appearance
Fibular nerve/ fibular head	Numbness foreleg and foot Pain, paresthesia at lateral knee or foreleg, especially with bending knee or crossing legs when sitting Catching of toe with walking, tripping, falls	Decreased sensation lateral foreleg and dorsolateral foot Pain or paresthesia with tapping over the nerve at the fibular head (Tinel's sign) Weakness of toe and ankle dorsiflexion (foot drop)

Table 6.3 Cranial Neuropathies and Their Associated Findings

CRANIAL NERVE	EXAMINATION FINDINGS
III (oculomotor nerve)	Binocular horizontal or diagonal diplopia Impaired eye adduction, elevation, and depression Classic "down and out" deviation of eye Ptosis Normal pupillary response to light (pupillary sparing)
IV (trochlear nerve)	Binocular vertical diplopia Impaired depression and internal rotation of eye Eye is deviated up Compensatory contralateral head tilt
VI (abducens nerve)	Binocular horizontal diplopia Impaired abduction of eye Eye is deviated inward
VII (facial nerve)	Unilateral weakness of upper and lower face Weakness of eye closure Flattening of nasolabial fold with asymmetrical smile Decreased taste Hyperacusis

11. **What bloodwork is appropriate to evaluate diabetic neuropathy?**
    For DSP, other reversible causes of symmetric, length-dependent peripheral neuropathy should be sought. Routine chemistries, liver function panel, vitamin B_{12} level, and serum protein electrophoresis with immunofixation electrophoresis are adequate for most patients. Additional bloodwork such as rheumatological screening, testing for infections, or other studies can be added as indicated by history. In focal neuropathy syndromes involving the

cranial nerves or lumbosacral or brachial plexus, primary or secondary vasculitides or infectious processes should be considered. Testing should be tailored to the individual based on history and physical findings.

12. **What other diagnostic tools should be utilized when working up diabetic neuropathy syndromes?**
Electromyography (EMG) and nerve conduction studies (NCSs) are often helpful for confirming a diagnosis of peripheral neuropathy, mapping the areas of involvement, and providing quantitative information about severity. Magnetic resonance imaging (MRI) can help exclude other causes of focal neuropathy, plexopathy, or radiculopathy, such as structural disease with nerve or nerve root impingement, tumor, or infection. The use of contrast improves imaging sensitivity when tumor or infection are a concern. A brain MRI should almost always be part of the workup for cranial nerve deficits, especially in the acute presentation. Strokes, tumors, demyelinating lesions, inflammation, infection, causes of increased intracranial pressure, and various other central nervous system disorders should not be overlooked. A patient presenting with multiple cranial neuropathies should always raise a red flag for alternative causes besides diabetes.

13. **What are symptomatic treatment options for diabetic nerve pain?**
There is no single best agent for diabetic nerve pain, and therapy should be tailored for each patient's preferences and comorbidities. Unfortunately, despite numerous medication trials, many patients have persistent pain that interferes with daily function. There is no effective medication that reverses loss of sensation. In all patients with pain, it is important to set expectations, give each medication an adequate trial (both dose and duration), and consider using agents from different classes if results are inadequate with a single agent (Table 6.4). Medications that are clearly ineffective should be discontinued.

14. **What treatments are available for focal diabetic nerve symptoms?**
Focal limb neuropathies may respond to splinting, occupational or physical therapy, or simple avoidance of exacerbating positions or activities. Decompressive surgery may be appropriate if conservative measures are incompletely effective or electrodiagnostic testing demonstrates significant ongoing nerve injury. Durable medical equipment may help with weakness. For instance, a cane or walker can mitigate fall risk, or in patients with foot drop, an ankle–foot orthotic can improve gait stability. For double vision related to cranial nerve III, IV, or VI palsies, eye patching can improve comfort during healing. For cranial nerve VII palsy, lubricating eyedrops, eye patching, or taping the eye closed to protect against corneal abrasion can help.

15. **How should DRPN be managed?**
The natural history of DRPN is spontaneous improvement over weeks to months, although some deficits may persist. Because of possible underlying immune-mediated nerve injury, immunotherapy with steroids, intravenous immunoglobulin (IVIG), and plasma exchange (PLEX) have been used at some centers. There is currently no high-quality evidence for the efficacy of these treatments. Supportive care with pain control, blood sugar management, and physical therapy are important in all patients with DRPN.

Table 6.4 Common Neuropathic Pain Medications and Basic Clinical Considerations

MEDICATION CLASS	CLINICAL CONSIDERATIONS
Antiepileptics	
Gabapentin	May cause weight gain, peripheral edema, sedation
Pregabalin[a]	Renal dosing adjustment needed for renal insufficiency
Serotonin–norepinephrine reuptake inhibitors	
Duloxetine[a]	May cause nausea, sleep impairment, fatigue
Venlafaxine	Avoid concomitant use with tricyclic antidepressants
	Helpful in patients with coexisting depression
Tricyclic antidepressants	
Nortriptyline	Frequent anticholinergic side effects
Amitriptyline	May cause QT prolongation especially in elderly
	Sedative effect may be a benefit when pain prevents sleep
Topicals	
Capsaicin[a]	Burning sensation may limit use with capsaicin
Lidocaine	Temporary relief
	May help when oral polypharmacy is a concern

[a]U.S. Food and Drug Administration indication for diabetic nerve pain.

16. **How does diabetes cause neuropathy?**

The pathophysiology of nerve damage in diabetes is not fully understood but can be divided broadly into the following contributors to nerve dysfunction: hyperglycemia, dyslipidemia, impaired insulin signaling, and metabolic syndrome. The common theme throughout these mechanisms is the promotion of inflammation and oxidative stress leading to neuronal, Schwann cell, and endothelial cell damage.

17. **Can prediabetes cause neuropathy?**

In clinical practice, some people develop neuropathy before an official diagnosis of diabetes. One explanation is that elements of metabolic syndrome are often present before the onset of full-blown diabetes and may contribute to the development of neuropathy on their own. Lag time in the diagnosis of type 2 diabetes itself may also contribute. Regardless of the direct effect of prediabetes on peripheral nerves, the higher risk of morbidity and mortality in prediabetes is reason enough to intervene. The effect of prediabetes management on peripheral neuropathy requires further study.

18. **What disease-modifying treatments are available for diabetic neuropathy?**

Strict glucose control is thought to be a primary mechanism for disease modification in diabetic neuropathy, but results differ between people with type 1 and type 2 diabetes. Strict glucose control has been shown to significantly reduce the incidence and severity of DSP in people with type 1 diabetes. Strict glucose control in type 2 diabetes is not as well correlated with a reduced incidence and progression of DSP. A possible explanation is that type 2 diabetes is associated with more contributors to neuropathy (e.g., hyperlipidemia) than is type 1 diabetes, and thus strict glucose control alone is insufficient to prevent the progression of neuropathy. Currently, no FDA-approved medications are indicated to reverse or prevent the development of DSP. Additional simple measures, such as appropriate footwear, meticulous foot care, and mitigation of fall risk, can also reduce more serious consequences of diabetic nerve disease.

19. **What is treatment-induced neuropathy of diabetes (TIND)?**

Also known as *insulin neuritis*, TIND is a reversible syndrome characterized by severe neuropathic pain and autonomic dysfunction after the initiation of glycemic control (particularly if rapid and strict) in patients with chronically uncontrolled blood glucose levels. Symptoms usually occur within 4 to 8 weeks of treatment initiation, and the risk for developing this syndrome has been correlated with the degree and rapidity of hemoglobin A1c reduction. It can occur in both type 1 and type 2 diabetes. Although previously thought to be quite rare, a study in 2015 estimated the incidence at about 10%. As A1c goals become more stringent, the incidence of TIND may increase. The underlying mechanisms are not well understood. Similar reports of worsened retinopathy and nephropathy in patients with diabetes after the initiation of strict glycemic control suggest a common microvascular pathophysiology. Pain and other symptoms during the initial onset are often refractory to treatment, requiring multiple medications, but most patients improve over months, even with sustained glycemic control. Some experts suggest a more gradual initiation of glycemic control with an A1c reduction of <2 percentage points over 3 months.

20. **What are some future directions for the treatment of diabetic neuropathy?**

There are many ongoing studies that seek to understand the underlying mechanisms of diabetic neuropathies in order to develop preventive and neuroprotective treatments. Diabetic neuropathy also serves as an important model for investigating treatments for chronic neuropathic pain. Ultimately, the prevention of diabetes itself is an area of wide-ranging study that will likely have the greatest impact on diabetic neuropathies.

KEY POINTS

1. Diabetic neuropathy is classified into different syndromes, including distal symmetric polyneuropathy, DAN, radiculoplexus neuropathy, and focal neuropathies, including cranial neuropathies.
2. Diabetic neuropathy is present in up to 50% to 66% of patients with diabetes, with distal symmetric polyneuropathy being the most common pattern of disease.
3. Diabetic neuropathy syndromes can be diagnosed clinically, with supportive tests done to exclude other causes or contributors.
4. Symptomatic treatment focuses on the management of neuropathic pain, in addition to other supportive measures to prevent further health consequences.
5. Disease-modifying treatment consists primarily of strict glucose control, but the management of other contributing comorbidities, especially in patients with type 2 diabetes, is important.

BIBLIOGRAPHY

Callaghan BC, Cheng HT, Stables CL, Smith AL, Feldman EL. Diabetic neuropathy: clinical manifestations and current treatments. *Lancet Neurol.* 2012;11(6):521–534. https://doi.org/10.1016/S1474-4422(12)70065-0.

Callaghan BC, Little AA, Feldman EL, Hughes RA. Enhanced glucose control for preventing and treating diabetic neuropathy. *Cochrane Database Syst Rev.* 2012;6(6):CD007543. https://doi.org/10.1002/14651858.CD007543.pub2. Published 2012 Jun 13.

Chan YC, Lo YL, Chan ES. Immunotherapy for diabetic amyotrophy. *Cochrane Database Syst Rev.* 2017;7(7):CD006521. https://doi.org/10.1002/14651858.CD006521.pub4. Published 2017 Jul 26.

Dyck PJ, Kratz KM, Karnes JL, et al. The prevalence by staged severity of various types of diabetic neuropathy, retinopathy, and nephropathy in a population-based cohort: the Rochester Diabetic Neuropathy Study [published correction appears in Neurology 1993 Nov;43(11):2345]. *Neurology.* 1993;43(4):817–824. https://doi.org/10.1212/wnl.43.4.817.

Feldman EL, Callaghan BC, Pop-Busui R, Zochodne DW, Wright DE, Bennett DL, Bril V, Russell JW, Viswanathan V. Diabetic neuropathy. *Nat Rev Dis Primers.* 2019 Jun 13;5(1):41. https://doi.org/10.1038/s41572-019-0092-1. PMID: 31197153.

Gibbons CH, Freeman R. Treatment-induced diabetic neuropathy: a reversible painful autonomic neuropathy. *Ann Neurol.* 2010;67(4): 534–541. https://doi.org/10.1002/ana.21952.

Gibbons CH, Freeman R. Treatment-induced neuropathy of diabetes: an acute, iatrogenic complication of diabetes. *Brain.* 2015;138(Pt 1):43–52. https://doi.org/10.1093/brain/awu307.

Kelkar P, Masood M, Parry GJ. Distinctive pathologic findings in proximal diabetic neuropathy (diabetic amyotrophy). *Neurology.* 2000;55(1):83–88. https://doi.org/10.1212/wnl.55.1.83.

Wahren J, Foyt H, Daniels M, Arezzo JC. Long-acting C-peptide and neuropathy in type 1 diabetes: a 12-month clinical trial. *Diabetes Care.* 2016;39(4):596–602. https://doi.org/10.2337/dc15-2068.

CHAPTER 7

PREVENTION OF MACROVASCULAR COMPLICATIONS

Stuart T. Haines, PharmD, BCPS, BCACP

1. **What are the incidence and prevalence of macrovascular complications in patients with diabetes?**

   People with type 1 and type 2 diabetes are far more likely to develop macrovascular complications than people without diabetes. Macrovascular complications include coronary artery, cerebral artery, and peripheral artery disease as a result of atherosclerosis, as well as heart failure. Nearly 70% of patients with diabetes over the age of 65 die of heart disease, and 16% die of stroke. Epidemiologic studies suggest that patients with type 2 diabetes are at least two but perhaps four times more likely to die of a cardiovascular (CV) cause than those without diabetes. The majority of patients with type 2 diabetes are obese (>85%) and have comorbid hypertension (>70%) and dyslipidemia (>60%). This quartet of CV risk factors substantially increases the risk of CV morbidity and mortality. Although females are at lower risk of CV disease compared with males of the same age, diabetes appears to largely erase this advantage. More than 30% of all patients with diabetes also have established CV disease. The good news is that the risk of macrovascular complications in patients with diabetes has steadily declined over the past 20 years, likely as a result of intensive management of CV risk factors with effective mediations and other interventions.

2. **What are the most common macrovascular complications associated with diabetes?**

   Among people living with diabetes, nearly 30% have atherosclerotic cardiovascular disease (ASCVD), most often manifested as coronary artery disease, myocardial infarction, or angina. Approximately 15% of people with diabetes have concurrent heart failure, and another 8% have experienced a stroke.

3. **How does diabetes contribute to the pathophysiology of macrovascular disease?**

   The relationship between hyperglycemia and CV disease is complex and multifactorial. Dyslipidemia is highly correlated with atherosclerosis, and the majority of patients with diabetes have abnormal lipid patterns characterized by increased triglycerides, decreased high-density lipoprotein cholesterol (HDL-C), and low-density lipoprotein cholesterol (LDL-C) particles that are smaller and denser than normal. Small, dense LDL-C particles can more easily penetrate and form attachments to the arterial wall. In addition, small, dense LDL-C particles are more susceptible to oxidation. Oxidized LDL-C is proatherogenic because it triggers an immune response, with leukocytes attacking the vessel walls. This in turn leads to a proliferation of endothelial and smooth muscle cells. In addition, LDL-C particles can become glycated, which lengthens the half-life and further increases the availability of LDL-C to promote atherogenesis. Although HDL-C is believed to be protective against the formation of atherosclerotic plaque, glycation of HDL-C shortens its half-life, leading to lower-than-normal concentrations. Hyperglycemia also contributes to endothelial dysfunction. A healthy endothelium regulates blood vessel tone, platelet activation, thrombosis, and inflammation. Diabetes promotes dyslipidemia and increases oxidation, glycosylation, and endothelial dysfunction, all of which contribute to the formation of atherosclerotic plaques.

4. **What are the risk factors for the development of macrovascular complications in patients with diabetes?**

   Hyperglycemia, which is the hallmark of diabetes mellitus; dyslipidemia; hypertension; and central adiposity are all strong, independent, but modifiable risk factors that each contribute to the development of macrovascular complications. Age, sex, and family history of premature CV disease are nonmodifiable risk factors. Smoking and other forms of tobacco use are another strong risk factor for the development of ASCVD. Although overall glycemic control correlates with the risk of macrovascular complications, glycemic variability, the degree to which blood glucose concentrations fluctuate during the day, may be an equally important risk factor. Systemic inflammation appears to be a risk factor, and there is mounting evidence that medications that reduce systemic inflammation can reduce the incidence of major adverse cardiovascular events (MACEs). Patients with diabetes often have elevated levels of high-sensitivity C-reactive protein (hs-CRP), interleukine-1 (IL-1), toll-like receptors (TLRs), and mitogen-activated protein (MAP) kinase. Currently, only hs-CRP is routinely used in clinical practice to assess cardiovascular risk. Lastly, hypercoagulability appears to play a role and increases the risk of thrombosis, vessel occlusion, and ischemia. People with diabetes generally have higher circulating concentrations of platelet coagulation products such as platelet factor 4 and thromboxane B_2, which correlate with platelet hyperactivity. In addition, patients with diabetes often have elevated concentrations of clotting factors (II, VII, VII, XI, and XII), plasminogen activator inhibitor-1 (PAI-1), and prothrombin activation fragment 1 + 2. Although none of these procoagulant markers is routinely measured in clinical practice, antiplatelet therapy is generally recommended in patients with diabetes and at least one additional major CV risk factor and in all patients who have established ASCVD.

5. How do I estimate a patient's risk for developing macrovascular complications?
   The most widely used risk estimator to determine a patient's risk of a major CV event over the next 10 years is the ASCVD Risk Estimator Plus, available on the Internet at http://www.cvriskcalculator.com or http://tools.acc.org/ascvd-risk-estimator-plus/. Several pieces of information are needed to get an accurate risk estimate. In addition to age, sex, and race, the risk estimator requires the patient's most recent total cholesterol and HDL-C measurements, systolic and diastolic blood pressure readings, and whether the patient is receiving treatment for high blood pressure. Diabetes and tobacco use are both important factors considered by the risk estimator. The ASCVD Risk Estimator Plus is not intended for use in patients who already have established CV disease with a history of myocardial infarction or stroke because the estimated 10-year ASCVD risk is already high ($\geq$20%). Moreover, the risk estimator has not been validated in younger adults (<40 years old) or the oldest old ($\geq$80 years old).

6. What are the dietary and exercise recommendations for mitigating CV risk in people with diabetes?
   Intensive lifestyle modification with a focus on weight loss, if the patient is obese or overweight, and regular physical activity are the cornerstones of diabetes management. The Look AHEAD study found that modest weight loss of $\geq$7% of body weight, or approximately 5 to 8 kg for most patients, plus moderately intense physical activity performed for $\geq$175 min/week leads to significant improvements in waist circumference, glycemic control, systolic blood pressure, and HDL-C. The benefits of lifestyle modification appear to be most pronounced in those who do not have preexisting CV disease. Although many epidemiologic studies have found a strong correlation between body weight, physical fitness, and CV events, the Look AHEAD trial failed to demonstrate a clear benefit with increased physical activity and weight loss in the intervention group despite a favorable impact on several CV risk factors. Nonetheless, the American Diabetes Association (ADA) recommends physical activity most days of the week, ideally combining both aerobic and resistance exercises, because it improves glycemic control and assists with weight management.

7. Does tobacco cessation mitigate CV risk?
   Roughly 20% to 25% of people with diabetes smoke tobacco, and another 25% report being ex-smokers. Smoking tobacco increases the risk of not only lung disease and cancer but also the risk of macrovascular and microvascular complications. In patients with diabetes, smoking tobacco increases the risk of CV morbidity and mortality by as much as 50% compared with nonsmokers with diabetes. There are some immediate health benefits from smoking cessation (e.g., reduced risk of upper respiratory tract infections), and the excess CV risk can be largely reversed after a person remains tobacco-free for >10 years. Tobacco is highly addictive, and most patients, even those motivated to quit, find it difficult to stop smoking. Remember the three As: ask, advise, and assist. It is important to ask patients about tobacco use at every encounter and, if they are a current user, to advise them to stop. Clear and consistent messaging about the negative impact of tobacco use, delivered in a nonjudgmental manner, substantially increases quit rates. Assist by identifying the patient's motivations and barriers, offering a referral to a formal smoking cessation program, prescribing effective treatments for smoking cessation, and providing follow-up and psychological support. Relapse is common, and many patients must make multiple quit attempts before they are able to remain tobacco-free long term. Smoking cessation is perhaps the single most powerful intervention to improve any patient's health, but it is particularly potent in the patient with diabetes.

8. Does the treatment of hyperglycemia improve CV risk?
   An abundance of epidemiologic evidence demonstrates a strong association between hyperglycemia and CV risk, with an estimated 10% to 15% increase in events for every 1% increase in the A1C or 18-mg/dL (1-mmol/L) increase in fasting glucose >100 mg/dL. Moreover, these relationships appear to be linear. Long-term follow-up of the participants in the Diabetes Control and Complications Trial (DCCT) and the United Kingdom Prospective Diabetes Study (UKPDS) demonstrated significant reductions in CV event rates and all-cause mortality in those who were randomized to intensive glycemic control (target A1C <7%) compared with usual care (mean A1C 8%–8.5%). However, unlike the improvements in microvascular complications observed with intensive glycemic control, reductions in macrovascular events may require 10 years or more to materialize. See Fig. 7.1.

9. What is the impact of antidiabetes medications on CV risk?
   Although hyperglycemia appears to be a modifiable CV risk factor, not all antidiabetes medications lead to improved CV outcomes, and some may have a detrimental impact. See Table 7.1. Insulin and sulfonylureas, medications that have been used to treat diabetes for decades, have not been tested in a rigorous manner, but epidemiologic studies and a few comparative effectiveness studies suggest that the sulfonylureas and insulin neither reduce nor increase CV risk. Similarly, the dipeptidyl peptidase-4 (DPP-4) inhibitors appear to have a neutral effect on CV outcomes. Long-term metformin use may have a beneficial impact on MACE, but the evidence to support this claim is weak. Unlike rosiglitazone, the thiazolidinedione (TZD) pioglitazone reduces the risk of myocardial infarction and stroke. TZDs increase the risk of heart failure, partly as a result of fluid retention. In general, the glucagon-like peptide-1 (GLP-1) receptor agonists have a positive impact on MACE, and some

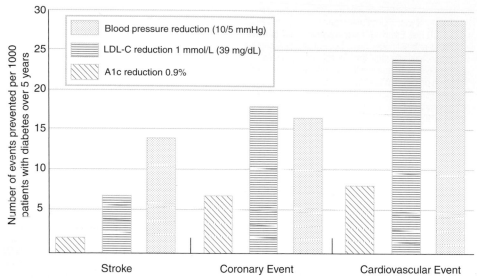

Fig. 7.1 Estimated reductions in major adverse cardiovascular events from treating hyperglycemia, hypertension, and low-density lipoprotein cholesterol.

Table 7.1 Impact of Antidiabetes Medications on Cardiovascular Risk

	MACE	CV DEATH	MYOCARDIAL INFARCTION	STROKE	HEART FAILURE
Insulin	↔	↔	↔	↔	↔
Sulfonylureas	↔	↔	↔	↔	↔
Metformin	↓	↔	↔	↔	↔
Pioglitazone	↓	↔	↓	↓	↑
Rosiglitazone	↔	↔	↔	↔	↑
DPP-4 inhibitors	↔	↔	↔	↔	↔
GLP-1 receptor agonists	↓	↓	↓	↓	↓
SGLT-2 inhibitors	↓	↓	↓	↔	↓

CV, Cardiovascular; *DPP-4*, dipeptidyl peptidase-4; *GLP-1*, glucagon-like peptide-1; *MACE*, major adverse cardiovascular event; *SGLT-2*, sodium-glucose transporter-2.

(e.g., liraglutide) have been shown to reduce CV and/or all-cause mortality. The sodium–glucose transporter 2 (SGLT-2) inhibitors have been shown to have a favorable impact on heart failure outcomes, and some agents in this class (e.g., empagliflozin) have also reduced MACE, CV death, and all-cause mortality.

10. **Which antidiabetes medications are preferred in patients with diabetes who have comorbid CV disease or who are at high risk of CV events?**
    In most patients with established ASCVD or who are at very high risk of CV events (e.g., 10-year risk of major CV event ≥20%), either a GLP-1 receptor agonist or SGLT-2 inhibitor should be considered and preferentially used. Given their favorable impact on MACE and ischemic stroke, the GLP-1 receptor agonists might be a preferential choice in patients who have had an ischemic stroke. Among the GLP-1 receptor agonists, only liraglutide reduced the risk of CV death, and both exenatide extended release and liraglutide significantly reduced all-cause mortality in CV outcome trials. The SGLT-2 inhibitors are particularly useful in patients with comorbid heart failure because they reduce the risk of new-onset heart failure and hospitalizations related to heart failure. Among the SGLT-2 inhibitors, only empagliflozin demonstrated a significant reduction in CV death and all-cause mortality in the CV outcome trials. However, the SGLT-2 inhibitors have not yet demonstrated a favorable impact on the risk of stroke.

Given the differences in the patient populations enrolled in the CV outcome studies, it is not yet known if the CV benefits observed in the clinical trials are a class effect or if significant differences exist. In the absence of comparative effectiveness studies, those agents with proven CV benefits should be preferentially used. Currently, it is unknown whether combination therapy with both an SGLT-2 inhibitor and a GLP-1 receptor agonist would provide additive CV benefit.

11. **What is the evidence that hypertension is a modifiable CV risk factor in patients with diabetes?**

    Hypertension with a sustained blood pressure of ≥140/90 mm Hg contributes to the development of both ASCVD and microvascular complications. Numerous controlled clinical trials have shown that antihypertensive therapy significantly reduces the risk of CV events, particularly the risk of stroke, retinopathy, chronic kidney disease, heart failure, and all-cause mortality. See Fig. 7.1. During pregnancy, elevated blood pressure increases the risk of poor maternal and fetal outcomes. Given the known risks of elevated blood pressure and the clear benefits of antihypertensive treatment, the patient's blood pressure should be measured at every routine clinical visit, and patients who are being treated for hypertension should self-monitor blood pressure at home.

12. **Who should be treated, and what are the goals of treatment, for hypertension in patients with diabetes to reduce CV risk?**

    All patients with diabetes with blood pressure readings of ≥120/80 mm Hg should be encouraged to adopt lifestyle changes if they have not already done so, to limit dietary sodium intake to <2.4 gm per day, increase dietary potassium intake, engage in regular physical activity, and lose 5% to 10% of body weight if overweight or obese. In patients with diabetes who have a confirmed office-based blood pressure reading of ≥140/90 mm Hg, pharmacologic therapy in addition to lifestyle changes should be instituted. If the office-based blood pressure reading is ≥160/100 mm Hg, two antihypertensive drugs or a combination product should be initiated. In all cases, the goal of treatment is to consistently maintain the blood pressure at ≤140/90, but a lower blood pressure target (≤130/80) would be reasonable in those with preexisting CV disease or a 10-year ASCVD risk of ≥15%. During pregnancy, the recommended blood pressure is ≤135/85.

13. **What antihypertensive medications are preferred in patients with diabetes to reduce CV risk?**

    Any of the recommended first-line antihypertensive agents, including angiotensin-converting enzyme (ACE) inhibitors, angiotensin receptor blockers (ARBs), dihydropyridine calcium channel blockers (CCBs), and thiazide diuretics, should be used preferentially, alone or in combination, for the treatment of hypertension in patients with diabetes who are not pregnant or do not plan to become pregnant. All have been shown to significantly reduce the risk of macrovascular and microvascular complications in patients with diabetes. Multiple drugs are often required to achieve the target blood pressure, and certain combinations may offer greater benefit than others. An ACE inhibitor or ARB plus a dihydropyridine CCB has been shown in some studies to be more effective than other combinations. Conversely, a combination of an ACE inhibitor plus an ARB or direct renin inhibitor should be avoided because these combinations do not improve outcomes and increase the risk of hyperkalemia. Given their favorable impact on renal outcomes, ACE inhibitors and ARBs are the recommended choice in patients with proteinuria. After a myocardial infarction and in patients with angina or heart failure, a beta blocker (i.e., carvedilol, metoprolol, or bisoprolol) should be used. In women who are pregnant or plan to become pregnant, ACE inhibitors, ARBs, and spironolactone should be avoided because of their teratogenic effects. Labetalol, methyldopa, and long-acting nifedipine are the drugs of choice during pregnancy. Combination products, when available, should be used to reduce pill burden and cost.

14. **What is the evidence that dyslipidemia is a modifiable CV risk factor in patients with diabetes?**

    Similar to hypertension, dyslipidemia is a strong and independent risk factor for CV morbidity and mortality. For each 1-mmol/L (39-mg/dL) increase in LDL-C, there is a 15% to 30% increase in vascular events, and treatment with lipid-lowering therapy has resulted in significant reductions in CV morbidity and mortality. See Fig. 7.1. Most patients with diabetes have an abnormal lipid profile; poor glycemic control is associated with elevated serum triglycerides and low HDL-C concentrations. Although there is a strong inverse relationship between HDL-C concentrations and CV events, treatment with drug therapies that increase HDL-C has not resulted in reduced event rates.

    A lipid profile should be obtained at the time of diagnosis and, in patients under the age of 40 years who are not being treated with lipid-lowering therapy, remeasured every 3 to 5 years. For patients being treated with lipid-lowering therapy, it is reasonable to obtain a lipid panel 12 weeks after initiating or changing therapy and annually thereafter.

Table 7.2 Recommended Statins and Doses

MODERATE-INTENSITY STATIN THERAPY	HIGH-INTENSITY STATIN THERAPY
Atorvastatin 10–20 mg daily Fluvastatin extended release 80 mg daily Lovastatin 40 mg daily Pitavastatin 1–4 mg daily Pravastatin 40–80 mg daily Rosuvastatin 5–10 mg daily Simvastatin 20–40 mg daily	Atorvastatin 40–80 mg daily Rosuvastatin 20–40 mg daily

15. **Who should be treated, and what are the goals of treatment, for dyslipidemia in patients with diabetes to reduce CV risk?**

   Given that patients with diabetes are at high risk of macrovascular complications, all adults with diabetes aged 40 to 74 years should be treated with a statin unless there is a contraindication (e.g., pregnancy) or the patient is unable to tolerate therapy. It is also reasonable to initiate statin therapy in patients 20 to 39 years of age if they have additional CV risk factors, such as hypertension, a strong family history of premature CV events, or current smoker. If the patient does not have evidence of ASCVD, a moderate-intensity statin plus lifestyle modification will significantly reduce the risk of a CV event. In patients with established ASCVD or age 50 to 70 years who have multiple CV risk factors, a high-intensity statin should be initiated, with the goal of reducing LDL-C by at least 50% from the patient's baseline measurement. If the baseline measurement is unknown, a goal LDL-C of <70 mg/dL is reasonable. Other lipid-lowering therapies can be considered to achieve this goal.

16. **What lipid-lowering medications are preferred in patients with diabetes to reduce CV risk?**

   Statins are the drug of choice for the treatment of dyslipidemia because of their proven efficacy and safety in a wide range of patient populations. See Table 7.2. In a patient without established ASCVD, statin monotherapy is sufficient, and other lipid-lowering therapies are not recommended unless the patient is unable to tolerate a statin. In a patient with established ASCVD who is not able to achieve their LDL-C target, the addition of ezetimibe or a proprotein convertase subtilisin/kexin type 9 (PCSK9) should be considered. Ezetimibe is generally preferred because of its lower cost. In patients with established ASCVD or who have multiple CV risk factors, icosapent ethyl should be added to statin therapy if the patient's triglycerides remain elevated (≥135 mg/dL). Other lipid-lowering therapies, such as niacin and fibrates, have not been shown to improve CV outcomes when used in combination with statins and are, therefore, not recommended. Some patients are unable to tolerate statin therapy because of the development of muscle symptoms. In the absence of muscle breakdown as evidenced by elevated serum creatinine kinase concentrations, an attempt to reinitiate statin therapy after a drug holiday should be strongly considered. Strategies to manage statin intolerance include reducing the statin dose, using alternate-day dosing, switching to a more hydrophilic statin (e.g., rosuvastatin, pravastatin), initiating vitamin D or coenzyme Q-10 supplementation, or a combination of these strategies.

KEY POINTS

1. Macrovascular complications, most commonly manifested as ASCVD, in addition to heart failure, are very common in patients with diabetes and the leading cause of morbidity and mortality.
2. Hyperglycemia is an independent risk factor for macrovascular complications. People with diabetes, particularly those with type 2 diabetes, often have comorbidities such as hypertension, dyslipidemia, and central adiposity that also contribute to ASCVD and increase the risk of macrovascular complications.
3. Addressing modifiable CV risk factors in patients with diabetes through lifestyle modifications (dietary habits, physical activity, and smoking cessation) and appropriate medication use has been shown to significantly reduce the risk of CV complications.
4. Aggressively treating elevated blood pressure to recommended goals using ACE inhibitors or ARBs (but not both), dihydropyridine CCBs, and thiazide diuretics, alone or in combination, can significantly reduce the risk of macrovascular complications. Similarly, the routine use of lipid-lowering therapy, especially moderate- to high-potency statins, has been shown to reduce the development and progression of ASCVD and prevent CV events.
5. In patients with type 2 diabetes and established ASCVD, the use of select SGLT-2 inhibitors and GLP-1 receptor agonists further reduces the risk of macrovascular complications and mortality. The SGLT-2 inhibitors significantly reduce the risk of MACE and the development heart failure and hospitalizations resulting from heart failure exacerbations. The GLP-1 receptor agonists significantly reduce the risk of MACE. However, the benefits and risks may be different among the agents within each of these drug classes.

BIBLIOGRAPHY

2017 ACC/AHA/AAPA/ABC/ACPM/AGS/APhA/ASH/ASPC/NMA/PCNA Guideline for the prevention, detection, evaluation, and management of high blood pressure in adults: executive summary. *Circulation*. 2018;138:426–483.

American Diabetes Association. 10. Cardiovascular disease and risk management: Standards of medical care in diabetes — 2021. *Diabetes Care*. 2021;44(Suppl 1):S125–S150.

Huang X, Phan J, Chen D, et al. Efficacy of lifestyle interventions in patients with type 2 diabetes: a systematic review and meta-analysis. *Eur J Intern Med.* 2016;27:37–47.

Lambrinou E, Hansen TB, Beulens JWJ. Lifestyle factors, self-management and patient empowerment in diabetes care. *Eur J Preventative Cardiology.* 2019;26:55–63.

Lazarte J, Hegele R. Dyslipidemia management in adults with diabetes. *Can J Diabetes.* 2020;44:53–60.

North E, Newman J. Review of cardiovascular outcomes trials of sodium-glucose cotransporter-2 inhibitors and glucagon-like peptide-1 receptor agonists. *Curr Opin Cardiol.* 2019;34:687–692.

Sheen A. Cardiovascular effects of new oral glucose-lowering agents DPP-4 and SGLT-2 inhibitors. *Circulation Research.* 2018;122:1439–1459.

Wang CCL, Hess CN, Hiatt WR, Goldfine AB. Clinical update: cardiovascular disease in diabetes mellitus. Atherosclerotic cardiovascular disease and heart failure in type 2 diabetes—mechanisms, management, and clinical considerations. *Circulation.* 2016;133:2459–2502.

Zhu J, Yu X, Zheng Y, et al. Association of glucose-lowering medications with cardiovascular outcomes: an umbrella review and evidence map. *Lancet Diabetes Endocrinol.* 2020;8:192–205.

CHAPTER 8

DIABETES AND NONALCOHOLIC FATTY LIVER DISEASE

Thomas Jensen, MD, Mark Lindsay, NP, Amanda Wieland, MD, and Emily Folz, MD

1. **What are nonalcoholic fatty liver disease (NAFLD), nonalcoholic steatohepatitis (NASH), and liver fibrosis?**

   NAFLD is defined as the presence of excess liver fat (steatosis) based on biopsy or imaging in the absence of a secondary cause (excess alcohol [meaning >30 g/day for men and >20 g/day for women], certain medications, and disorders such as hepatitis C). Excess steatosis is defined on biopsy as ≥5% of liver cells containing macrovesicular steatosis. The grades of steatosis are determined by the percentage of hepatocytes involved on biopsy: grade 1 (5%–33%), grade 2 (34%–66%), and grade 3 (≥67%). Based on proton magnetic resonance spectroscopy (1H-MRS) from the Dallas Heart Study, the definitions with the 95% confidence intervals (CIs) were the following: normal fat percentage ≤5.56%, grade 1 (11%; 95% CI, 7%–14%), grade 2 (18%; 95% CI, 14%–23%), and grade 3 (25%; 95% CI,10%–28%). Other definitions for modalities such as magnetic resonance imaging (MRI) using proton density fat fraction (PDFF) have also been defined in the literature, with grade 1 (8.9%–9.4%), grade 2 (15.8%–16.3%), and grade 3 (22.1%–25%).

   Nonalcoholic steatohepatitis (NASH) is defined on biopsy according to the NAFLD Activity Score (NAS) with three categories: steatosis (0–3), inflammation (0–3), and ballooning (0–2). NAS scores of <3 are considered negative for NASH, 3 to 4 are a gray zone, and ≥5 are definite NASH. Most authorities recommend that the presence of ballooning should be seen on biopsy to diagnose NASH. Acidophil bodies (compact eosinophilic cells representing apoptotic hepatocytes) and Mallory–Denk bodies (ropey intracytoplasmic inclusions composed of damaged intermediate filaments) are also often seen but are not required for the diagnosis.

   Liver fibrosis results from chronic liver damage and the deposition of extracellular matrix, especially collagen, and by inflammatory cells (hepatic stellate cells in particular) that lead to rigid scar formation. There are four stages of liver fibrosis: stage 1, fibrosis in the perisinusoidal or portal/periportal regions; stage 2, both perisinusoidal and portal/periportal fibrosis; stage 3, bridging fibrosis between perisinusoidal and portal/periportal regions; stage 4, complete distortion of hepatic architecture from scar tissue with nodular regeneration.

   One can have simple steatosis without NASH or fibrosis, NASH with or without fibrosis, and fibrosis with or without NASH.

2. **What is the prevalence of NAFLD in the general population and in those with diabetes?**

   NAFLD is now the leading cause of chronic liver disease around the world, especially in developed countries. Currently, it is estimated to affect 20% to 30% of the adult population, although rates vary, with 24% reported in the United States, 23% in Europe, 27% in Asia, 30% in South America, and 32% in the Middle East; the prevalence is lower in Africa at 14%. This variance likely coincides with the prevalence of obesity and diabetes, as well as genetic factors. In people with diabetes, especially type 2 diabetes (T2D), the rates of NAFLD are much higher than in the general population, with an average prevalence of 55.5% (47.3%–63.7%), again with variation among populations: in the United States, 51.8% (31.3%–71.6%); South America, 56.8% (34.1%–77%); Asia, 52% (45.4%–58.6%); the Middle East, 67.3% (60.4%–73.6%); and Africa, 30.4 (11.6%–67.1%). However, the reported rates depend on which diagnostic modality is used (biopsy vs. radiologic vs. serologic). Rates of NASH are less well established, given the current reliance on biopsy for diagnosis, but derived information in the U.S. data estimates NASH to be present in 21% of patients with NAFLD and in 3% to 4% of the general population. In people with T2D, it is estimated that 37.3% have NASH, and of those with T2D and NAFLD, 17% have advanced fibrosis (stage 3 or 4). The prevalence of the NAFLD spectrum has increased over the years, with an expected rise in NAFLD by 18.3% to 100 million cases in the United States by 2030, an increase in NASH to as many as 43 million cases, and an increase in cirrhosis from 3.5 million cases to 4.5 million. The link between NAFLD and type 1 diabetes (T1D) is less well established, with ranges from 20% to 50%; however, microvascular and macrovascular complications are known to be increased in people with T1D and NAFLD.

3. **What are the risk factors for developing NAFLD?**

   Many risk factors have been linked to NAFLD (Fig. 8.1). The two strongest risk factors are T2D and/or insulin resistance and central obesity. Hypertriglyceridemia accompanied by low high-density lipoprotein cholesterol (HDL-C),

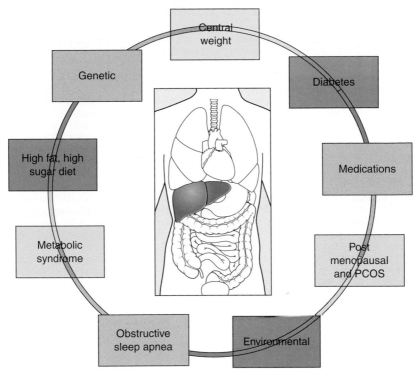

Fig. 8.1 Risk factors.

especially with insulin resistance, is also frequently present. Other risk factors include high blood pressure, age, postmenopausal status in females, polycystic ovarian disease, obstructive sleep apnea, diets rich in saturated fats and simple sugars (especially fructose), and a sedentary lifestyle. In addition, secondary risk factors such as hepatitis C, celiac disease, hypothyroidism, excess alcohol consumption (>21 drinks for males and >14 drinks for females per week), medications (steroids, methotrexate, amiodarone), environmental exposures (heavy metals, petrochemicals, certain weed-killer ingredients), and ethnic background (higher risk in Asian, Hispanic, and Native American people compared with Caucasians and lower rates in African American people) contribute; in part, this is driven by the prevalence of genetic risk factors.

4. **Which genetic risk factors are linked to NAFLD and type 2 diabetes?**
The most common gene variants in NAFLD are Patatin-like phospholipase domain-containing protein 3 *(PNPLA3)* I148M, which regulates hepatic lipid droplet lipolysis; transmembrane 6 superfamily member 2 *(TM6SF2)* E167K variant; and membrane-bound O-acyl transferase protein 7 *(MBOAT7)* rs641738 C > T gene variant. Although these variants have not been found to pose additional risk for T2D beyond traditional risk, other genes have emerged as risk factors for both T2D and NAFLD. The strongest gene association has been the transcription factor 7–like 2 *(TCF7L2)* rs7903146 (C/T) polymorphism, which has been associated with beta-cell dysfunction, impaired incretin responses, increased hepatic glucose production, and an independent risk for NAFLD, although the exact mechanistic pathway has not been fully elucidated. In addition, the sterol regulatory element-binding factor-2 *(SREBF-2)* rs133291 C/T polymorphism, which regulates fatty acid uptake and metabolism, and the sterol regulatory element-binding proteins-2 *(SREBP-2)* rs133291 C/T polymorphism, which regulates cholesterol synthesis, have also been implicated in the development of T2D and NAFLD. Variants in the adiponectin gene *ADIPOQ* that modulates fatty acid oxidation are also linked to T2D and NAFLD. Glucokinase regulatory protein *(GCKR)* rs780094 has also been implicated in the development of NAFLD and T2D, although the association is strongest in Asian populations. On the other hand, the *GCKR* gene P446L variant, which promotes hepatic glucose uptake, leading to increased de novo lipogenesis, appears to offer protection from T2D.

5. **What is the natural progression of NAFLD, and what risk factors are linked to progressive disease?**

Although we do not have a clear picture of the evolution of NAFLD over time because of insufficient longitudinal data and an incomplete understanding of the exact mechanisms leading to progression or regression, data have emerged in the last decade to give us a better understanding of these issues. For instance, evaluating the development of simple steatosis, a 2012 study from the Israeli National Health and Nutrition Examination Survey found at a 7-year follow-up that 19% of participants developed NAFLD (based on ultrasound), with an average weight gain of 5.8 ± 6.1 kg, whereas weight gain was 1.4 ± 5.5 kg in those who did not develop NAFLD. Further, of those with NAFLD, 36.4% saw resolution at 7 years after an average weight loss of 2.7 ± 5.8 kg, or 5% weight loss. It has been shown that simple steatosis, once thought to be a benign process, can progress as well. One study found that 44% of people with simple steatosis developed NASH and 27% developed fibrosis at a median follow-up interval of 6.6 years. People with NASH at baseline appear to be more likely to progress than those with simple steatosis. A meta-analysis of paired biopsies found that patients with NASH advanced one level of fibrosis after 7.1 years on average, whereas those with simple steatosis took 14.3 years on average to progress one level of fibrosis. Another meta-analysis of four studies reported patients with NASH to have a mean annual progression rate of 0.09 fibrosis stages, with roughly 40% progressing at follow-up; 20% of those rapidly progressed from stage 0 to stage 3 or 4 fibrosis over a median of 5.9 years at follow-up. Roughly 25% of patients with NASH will progress to cirrhosis by 9 years and 10% to decompensated cirrhosis at 13 years. The presence of NASH, particularly with advanced fibrosis, increases the risk of hepatocellular carcinoma to an incidence rate of 5.29 per 1000 person-years. Risk factors that predict progression include central obesity and weight gain, insulin resistance, hypertension, obstructive sleep apnea, older age, male gender, hyperuricemia, and the previously mentioned genetic polymorphisms, especially *PNPLA3*. In addition, one of the longest longitudinal studies showed that patients with NAFLD compared with the normal population had increased risks of cardiovascular disease (hazard ratio [HR] = 1.55, CI = 1.11–2.15, $P = 0.01$), cirrhosis (HR = 3.2, CI = $1.05 - 9.81$, $P = 0.041$), and overall mortality (HR = 1.29, CI = $1.04 - 1.59$, $P = 0.020$); however, these findings appear to have been driven mainly by people with stage 3 to 4 fibrosis (HR = 3.3, CI = $2.27 - 4.76$, $P < 0.001$) and were not significant in those with an NAS score of 5 to 8 or stage 0 to 2.

6. **What clues might alert the provider that a person has NAFLD?**

The presence of T2D alone would likely be a strong enough indication to screen for NAFLD. Currently, the European Association for the Study of the Liver, the European Association for the Study of Diabetes, and the European Association for the Study of Obesity (EASL/EASD/EASO) recommend that people with insulin resistance and/or metabolic syndrome be screened for NAFLD. Liver enzyme measurements alone have not been found to adequately identify NAFLD, in part because cutoffs for what is considered normal include some patients with the disease; an alanine aminotransferase (ALT) >17 IU/L in females and >25 IU/L in males has been reported to be sensitive but not specific for NAFLD. The American Diabetes Association (ADA) recently recommended evaluating people with diabetes who have elevated liver enzymes or who are incidentally found to have hepatic steatosis on imaging.

7. **What strategies are currently available to evaluate the presence and severity of NAFLD?**

Presence of NAFLD is often discovered when hepatic steatosis is identified on CT, ultrasound (US), or MRI. On CT, fat within hepatocytes decreases the attenuation of the liver parenchyma proportionate to the quantity of fat. CT is insensitive for detecting <30% fat by histology. However, liver attenuation measuring < 45 Hounsfield Units (HU) on CT performed with or without IV contrast is 100% specific and moderately sensitive for the detection of >30% hepatic steatosis by histology.

On US, hepatic fat increases the echogenicity (brightness) of the liver. US is relatively insensitive for the detection of <20% steatosis; however, it has a reported sensitivity of 84.4% and specificity of 93.6% for the detection of >20% fat by histology. It is often the first-line imaging study to evaluate patients with elevated transaminases because it is widely available, relatively inexpensive, safe, and radiation-free.

Two magnetic resonance imaging (MRI) methods are available to assess presence of hepatic steatosis. Chemical-shift imaging, also called in-phase and out-of-phase imaging, provides a qualitative assessment of hepatic steatosis. Conversely, MRI proton density fat fraction (PDFF) provides a quantitative assessment of liver fat with a PDFF measurement of >6% correlating with >5% fat by histology.

Biomarker panels combining serum biomarkers with clinical parameters have been proposed to noninvasively detect hepatic steatosis but are not widely used in clinical practice. These include the Fatty Liver Index (FLI), the hepatic steatosis index (HSI), the SteatoTest, and the NAFL screening score.

Presence of hepatic fibrosis is the most important predictor of liver-related mortality and can be assessed using:

1. Biomarker panels, such as the FIB-4 and NAFLD fibrosis score (NFS), which combine routinely assessed clinical parameters with standard laboratory tests.
2. Elastography techniques which are based on the premise that collagen deposition associated with fibrosis imparts parenchymal rigidity or stiffness.

The FIB-4 and NFS each have a high negative predictive value for ruling out advanced fibrosis. Elastography, on the other hand, can be used to stratify individuals as those having no or minimal fibrosis versus those having severe fibrosis and cirrhosis. Individuals falling between these two measures require additional testing. Elastography can also be used to monitor disease progression and treatment response.

Transient elastography (TE), also called Fibroscan, is a point of care modality widely available in specialty clinics. It is painless, relatively inexpensive, and has excellent reproducibility. It can reliably exclude severe fibrosis and cirrhosis with a high negative predictive value of approximately 90%. Its applicability had been limited in obese patients, but this has been partly overcome by the development of the XL probe.

Newer ultrasound-based elastography techniques, such as shear wave elastography (SWE) and acoustic radiation force impulse imaging (ARFI), can be implemented on standard US machines and have similar sensitivity and specificity to TE, but they have been insufficiently validated. Like TE, they are poor at discriminating intermediate stages of fibrosis. MR elastography out-performs TE, SWE, and ARFI, with greater accuracy for diagnosing advanced fibrosis; however, its use is limited by cost and accessibility.

8. **When is a biopsy clinically indicated?**
Biopsy is typically indicated for two major reasons:

1. Confirm diagnosis. Biopsy can be helpful if there is a reasonable competing diagnosis that needs to be excluded.
2. Assess for NASH and fibrosis when confirmation will help guide monitoring and clinical care.

Given the high prevalence of NAFLD in the general population (>30% in some estimates), it is not realistic to biopsy all individuals with suspected NAFLD or NASH. Biopsy is the gold standard for diagnosis but is expensive and invasive. If there is a competing diagnosis of the cause of underlying liver abnormalities, the appropriate serologic workup should be done first. If this is unremarkable and no other clear etiology is found, a biopsy may not be needed if it would not change management or recommendations. Noninvasive assessment to evaluate the degree of fibrosis can be helpful to determine the risk for NASH with fibrosis. If NASH and fibrosis are suspected, a biopsy might be important to confirm severity and help guide future treatment options. This should be evaluated on a case-by-case basis.

9. **What is the cornerstone of NAFLD treatment?**
Lifestyle modifications that promote weight loss are the cornerstone of management. Weight loss of <5% body weight results in modest improvements in NASH and fibrosis (10% and 16%, respectively), whereas weight loss of greater than 10% is associated with resolution of NASH in 90% of people, with 45% showing fibrosis regression. Liver fat content can improve even more dramatically, with weight loss of 5% to 10% leading to 50% to 60% resolution of steatosis and >10% weight loss leading to 97% resolution. Less aggressive weight loss, such as 3% to 5%, has also been found to be beneficial in nonobese patients. Data have shown that macronutrient content, notably saturated fats and simple sugars (especially high-fructose corn syrup), contribute to de novo lipogenesis and inflammation. Long-term studies have shown that both low-carbohydrate (10%–30%) and low-fat (20%) diets can improve hepatic triglyceride content. Diets such as the Mediterranean diet and DASH diet with an emphasis on monounsaturated and polyunsaturated fats, reduction of saturated fats and trans fats, and incorporation of complex carbohydrates with fiber can promote improvement in liver fat content. Regardless of the particular diet, a reduction in caloric intake with adherence to meal planning is key for successful weight loss. Exercise also plays a role in the management of NAFLD, assisting with the promotion and maintenance of weight loss in addition to cardiovascular risk reduction and improved insulin sensitivity. Clinicians should encourage moderate-intensity exercise with a goal of 150 minutes per week.

10. **Are there any medications currently approved by the U.S. Food and Drug Administration (FDA) for NAFLD and NASH?**
There are currently no FDA-approved medications for NAFLD/NASH (as of 2020). Multiple medications are currently in phase 3 clinical trials. There is hope that new medications will be approved to target NAFLD/NASH in the next few years. In 2018, the FDA identified two surrogate clinical endpoints that ideally would be met for a therapy to be approved: (1) resolution of steatohepatitis on overall histopathologic reading and no worsening of liver fibrosis; and (2) fibrosis improvement of ≥ 1 fibrosis stage and no worsening of steatohepatitis.

Although there are no FDA-approved pharmacologic treatments for NAFLD/NASH, the American Association for the Study of Liver Diseases (AASLD) guidance from 2018 outlined the use for two agents that have shown improvement in histologic NASH. Risks and benefits should be discussed with patients, given the concern for toxicity and side effects with long-term use. Pioglitazone can be considered in patients with biopsy-proven NASH with and without T2D. Vitamin E can be considered for patients with biopsy-proven non-cirrhotic nondiabetic NASH.

11. **What role does bariatric surgery have in the management of NAFLD and NASH?**
Weight-loss surgery has been found to be an effective intervention to promote regression and reversal of NAFLD in the setting of sustained weight loss. Both Roux-en-Y gastric bypass (RYGB) and sleeve gastrectomy (SG) improve the pathology of NAFLD early on by reducing caloric intake, which improves hepatic insulin resistance. Glucagon-like peptide-1 (GLP-1) levels increase significantly after bariatric surgery; along with weight loss, this improves peripheral insulin resistance, leading to reduced lipolysis and influx of fat to the liver. A recent meta-analysis of 32 cohort studies with biopsy data (mean follow-up of 15 months [3–55 months]) reported resolution of steatosis in 66%, inflammation in 50%, ballooning in 76%, and fibrosis in 40%; mean NAS decreased an average of 2.39 points. RYGB appears to be superior, showing 80% resolution in steatosis, 57% in inflammation, 80% in ballooning, and 50% in fibrosis. However, worsening of disease in some participants, including fibrosis progression in 12%, was also observed. A recent study of 35 patients with advanced fibrosis (stages 3 and 4) reported that despite 23% weight loss after bariatric surgery, 46% had persistent advanced fibrosis after a mean 6 years of follow-up. Reversal of fibrosis was more significant with RYGB than with SG and was not related to the amount of weight loss. Thus, in people with more advanced disease and especially those with significant insulin resistance and the use of insulin, RYGB might be the procedure of choice. Finally, recent endoscopic bariatric procedures have been shown to improve liver enzymes, NAS, liver steatosis, and even fibrosis (limited to imaging). It should be noted that patients with cirrhosis had an in-hospital mortality rate of 1.2% after bariatric surgery. Therefore this likely should be limited to people without decompensated cirrhosis who are classified as Child–Pugh class A.

12. **At what point should referral to a specialist be considered?**
Referral to a gastroenterologist, hepatologist, or someone specializing in the NAFLD field is recommended in the setting of chronically elevated liver enzymes (3 months or more), when another comorbid liver condition is known or suspected, in people with more advanced liver disease (stage 3 or 4 fibrosis), or if a biopsy is being considered.

KEY POINTS
1. NAFLD has emerged as the most common cause of chronic liver disease, including advanced fibrosis, and is prominent in people with T2D.
2. New diagnostic tools have emerged to better assist in the diagnosis and grading of NAFLD disease severity.
3. Currently, lifestyle modifications to promote weight loss are the cornerstone of NAFLD management, with certain medications and bariatric surgery in appropriate populations also having benefit.

BIBLIOGRAPHY

Barr RG, et al. Elastography assessment of liver fibrosis: Society of Radiologists in ultrasound consensus conference statement. *Radiology.* 2015;276(3):845–861.
Bataller R, Brenner DA. Liver fibrosis. *J Clin Invest.* 2005;115(2):209–218.
Buzzetti E, et al. Noninvasive assessment of fibrosis in patients with nonalcoholic fatty liver disease. *Int J Endocrinol.* 2015: 343828.
Chalasani N, et al. The diagnosis and management of nonalcoholic fatty liver disease: practice guidance from the American Association for the Study of Liver Diseases. *Hepatology.* 2018;67(1):328–357.
Cusi K, et al. Long-term pioglitazone treatment for patients with nonalcoholic steatohepatitis and prediabetes or type 2 diabetes mellitus: a randomized trial. *Ann Intern Med.* 2016;165(5):305–315.
Ekstedt M, et al. Fibrosis stage is the strongest predictor for disease-specific mortality in NAFLD after up to 33 years of follow-up. *Hepatology.* 2015;61(5):1547–1554.
Goh GB, et al. Considerations for bariatric surgery in patients with cirrhosis. *World J Gastroenterol.* 2018;24(28):3112–3119.
Hallsworth K, Adams LA. Lifestyle modification in NAFLD/NASH: facts and figures. *JHEP Rep.* 2019;1(6):468–479.
Lee Y, et al. Complete resolution of nonalcoholic fatty liver disease after bariatric surgery: a systematic review and meta-analysis. *Clin Gastroenterol Hepatol.* 2019;17(6):1040–1060. e1011.
Petaja EM, Yki-Jarvinen H. Definitions of normal liver fat and the association of insulin sensitivity with acquired and genetic nafld-a systematic review. *Int J Mol Sci.* 2016;17(5):633.
Salomone F, et al. Endoscopic bariatric and metabolic therapies for non-alcoholic fatty liver disease: evidence and perspectives. *Liver Int.* 2020;40(6):1262–1268.

Sanyal AJ, et al. Pioglitazone, vitamin E, or placebo for nonalcoholic steatohepatitis. *N Engl J Med.* 2010;362(18):1675–1685.

Spengler EK, Loomba R. Recommendations for diagnosis, referral for liver biopsy, and treatment of nonalcoholic fatty liver disease and nonalcoholic steatohepatitis. *Mayo Clin Proc.* 2015;90(9):1233–1246.

Younossi ZM, et al. Global epidemiology of nonalcoholic fatty liver disease: meta-analytic assessment of prevalence, incidence, and outcomes. *Hepatology.* 2016;64(1):73–84.

CHAPTER 9

DIABETES MANAGEMENT: LIFESTYLE MEASURES—NUTRITION

Shannon Lynn Christen, RD, CDCES

1. **What are the goals for medical nutrition therapy (MNT) for those with diabetes?**
The goal for MNT is to design an individualized meal pattern that meets targets for body weight, blood pressure, lipids, and glycosylated hemoglobin (A1c), ultimately to lower the risk of developing disease-related complications. It is best to get a detailed diet history, including the patient's preferences. It is also crucial to get shared buy-in from the primary food preparer and purchaser. Dietary changes need to be a part of the shared decision-making process. The focus should be more on an eating pattern instead of good foods versus bad foods. A variety of eating patterns can achieve dietary goals related to diabetes.

2. **What meal patterns should those with diabetes lean toward?**
Nutrition therapy for those with diabetes is crucial; however, there is not a "one-size-fits-all" eating pattern for diabetes. Many eating patterns have demonstrated achievement of positive outcomes, including weight loss. Those meal patterns include Mediterranean-style, plant-based or vegetarian, carbohydrate-controlled, or even low-/very low-carbohydrate strategies. Importantly, it appears that no single approach has been proven to be consistently superior. When constructing an individualized meal plan, consider the importance of incorporating nutrient-dense foods (e.g., vegetables, whole fruits, legumes, dairy, lean sources of protein, nuts, seeds, and whole grains) and achieving the desired energy deficit for weight loss (see question 4).

   Most importantly, the meal pattern should be one that has been customized to the individual, focusing on personal preferences, needs, and goals and the likelihood of long-term adherence. A meal pattern that is too far from a practical and achievable approach is unlikely to be sustainable. Patients should work closely with a registered dietitian nutritionist (RD/RDN) while creating meal-pattern changes. In addition, close monitoring of blood glucose levels may be needed because medication adjustments may be necessary.

3. **What is the simplest strategy to teach a person how to follow a meal plan?**
There is no single ideal distribution of calories among carbohydrates, fats, and proteins, but carbohydrate counting is routinely recommended in type 2 diabetes (T2D) to prevent glucose excursions after meals. A simple strategy for carbohydrate counting is the plate plan (Fig. 9.1). The diabetes plate includes half of the plate as nonstarchy vegetables (with limited added fat), one-quarter of the plate as a lean protein, and one-quarter of the plate as a starch or grain. One to two more servings of carbohydrate foods (e.g., a fruit and/or dairy serving) can be included as well. This works well for meal patterns that aren't combined foods, such as lasagna or casseroles. It can provide at least a visual approach of how to organize a simple meal.

   More specific carbohydrate counting may be useful in some patients. This training would include reading food labels, using measuring tools, and using carbohydrate-counting resources such as Calorie King (http://www.calorieking.com). Common goals for patients with T2D are to limit carbohydrate intake to no more than 45 to 60 g per meal and no more than 15 g per snack. In type 1 diabetes (T1D), carbohydrate counting is important so that the mealtime insulin dose can be matched to the food consumption and timing of the meal.

4. **What should be the initial weight-loss goal for people with diabetes who are overweight or obese?**
An initial weight loss goal of 5% is recommended for those with diabetes who are overweight or obese for targeted improvement of lipids, blood pressure, and glucose control. Weight loss is achieved through the consumption of fewer calories to create a calorie deficit. The initial approach may be a 500- to 750-calorie-per-day reduction to achieve a 1.0- to 1.5-pound weight loss per week.

5. **What dietary fats should those with diabetes include in their dietary pattern?**
The strongest evidence still points to the consumption of monounsaturated and polyunsaturated fats and less saturated fats. To achieve metabolic and cardiovascular disease goals, the percentage of total calories from saturated fats should be limited. The popularity of the saturated fat coconut oil has become a common theme in those following a meal pattern that may be lower in carbohydrates. Coconut oil is more than 90% saturated in the form of lauric acid. It is unclear if there are any meaningful health benefits of lauric acid. Instead, suggest the use of oils like olive, peanut, avocado, canola, sunflower, and safflower oils. Trans fats should also be avoided. It is also important to point out to patients that regardless of the type of fat, the calorie count of all fats is the same for all fats for the same quantity.

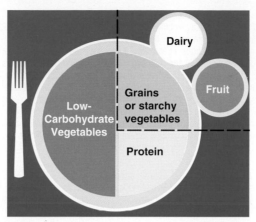

Fig. 9.1 Plate method for meal planning.

6. **Can alcohol be a part of a meal pattern for a person with diabetes?**
   Yes, people with diabetes can follow the same guidelines on alcohol intake as those without diabetes. For women, no more than one drink per day, and for men, no more than two drinks per day is recommended. One serving of alcohol is 1.5 oz of hard alcohol, 12 oz of beer, or 5 oz of wine. Patients should be educated about the risks, which include hypoglycemia, hyperglycemia, and weight gain. Increased alcohol intake can decrease hepatic glucose output and could increase the risk of hypoglycemia in those taking insulin or insulin secretagogues. Maintaining close glucose monitoring, wearing medical identification, and having access to quick-acting treatment for hypoglycemia are all important. Alcohol contains calories; therefore, increased alcohol consumption could lead to weight gain or could make it difficult for patients to successfully lose weight. Also, mixers such as margarita mix may be high in calories, carbohydrates, and/or added sugars and can lead to hyperglycemia.

7. **What is the sodium goal for those with diabetes?**
   The target is <2300 mg per day. This goal can be tricky to reach if the patient's meal pattern includes routine consumption of processed foods, frequent restaurant meals, or adding salt when preparing meals at home. Consider limiting added sodium at the table and in the cooking process, and have the patient use tools like a salt packet instead of a salt shaker to better determine the amount of sodium they add. Encourage whole, fresh foods instead of processed or canned foods whenever possible, and encourage patients to cut back on restaurant or fast-food meals.

8. **Can nonnutritive sweeteners be a part of the meal plan for those with diabetes?**
   Nonnutritive sweeteners are considered safe based on U.S. Food and Drug Administration (FDA) guidance. Low-calorie and nonnutritive beverages are still a better substitution than their calorie-filled counterparts, especially if the goal is to reduce calorie intake or glucose excursions. For example, one 12-oz can of diet soda contains 0 calories, carbohydrates, and sugars, whereas one 12-ounce can of regular soda contains 131 calories, 34 g of carbohydrates, and 32 g of sugar. The concern is that those consuming diet beverages may then adjust their eating pattern to still include more calories because they have chosen to consume a beverage with few calories, thus sabotaging their weight and blood sugar goals. Overall, water is still recommended as the best beverage for consumption over nonnutritive sweetened beverages.

9. **How effective is MNT at lowering A1c?**
   MNT provided by an RD/RDN is associated with an A1c improvement of 1.0% to 1.9% in those with T1D and 0.3% to 2.0% in those with T2D. Many insurance companies allow for annual MNT benefits for patients with diabetes, and patients should be offered an appointment routinely. A referral is typically required, and resources available in or near your community can be found at http://www.eatright.org or http://www.diabeteseducator.org.

10. **How do social determinants of health (SDOH) affect nutrition?**
    SDOH are strong predictors of morbidity and mortality because they contribute to poor nutritional choices, poor access to healthy food, and lack of support for physical activity. Those in more complicated situations may be in an environment that leads to less informed healthcare choices and lower health literacy. Food deserts are common in the United States, and for many patients, the closest food resource could be a local convenience store, which may provide very few fresh or frozen high-quality nutritional foods such as fruits and vegetables.

11. **What role does food insecurity play in nutrition?**
    Food insecurity occurs whenever the availability of nutritionally adequate and safe foods or the ability to acquire acceptable food in socially acceptable ways is limited or uncertain. Food insecurity affects approximately 13% of households in the United States and is a contributor to poor glycemic control in people with diabetes. Food insecurity can lead to glucose variability and both hyper- and hypoglycemia. Programs that may benefit those with food insecurity include the Supplemental Nutrition Assistance Program (SNAP), formerly called the Food Stamp Program; the Special Supplemental Nutrition Program for Women, Infants, and Children (WIC); school meal programs; summer food-service programs; and community-based food and nutrition assistance programs. Some evidence suggests that when comparing food items purchased with SNAP benefits to items available at food banks/shelters, the food at food banks was slightly more nutritious. Providing resources to patients that include a phone number to the Hunger-Free Hotline could make a difference in a patient's ability to provide self-care.

KEY POINTS

1. Dietary changes designed to achieve and maintain at least 5% weight loss are recommended for any overweight or obese person with diabetes. Weight-loss interventions should focus on calorie restriction to achieve a 500- to 750-kcal/day energy deficit.
2. There is no single ideal distribution of calories among carbohydrates, fats, and proteins, but carbohydrate counting is routinely recommended in T2D to prevent glucose excursions after meals. Common goals are no more than 45 to 60 g of carbohydrates per meal (or no more than one-quarter of the plate as the starch or grain) and no more than 15 g per snack. In T1D, carbohydrate counting is used to determine mealtime insulin doses.

BIBLIOGRAPHY

American Diabetes Association. 5. Facilitating behavior change and well-being to improve health outcomes: Standards of Medical Care in Diabetes – 2021. *Diabetes Care*. 2021;44(Suppl. 1):S53–S72.

Evert AB, Dennison M, Gardner CD, et al. Nutrition therapy for adults with diabetes or prediabetes: a consensus report. *Diabetes Care*. 2019;42:731–754.

Fan L, Gundersen C, Baylis K, Saksensa M. The use of charitable food assistance among low-income households in the United States. *J Acad Nutr Diet*. 2021;121(1):27–35.

CHAPTER 10

EXERCISE AND DIABETES

Layla A. Abushamat, MD, MPH, and Jane E.B. Reusch, MD

1. **What is the difference between physical activity and exercise, and which has a greater impact on diabetes?**
   Physical activity refers to all forms of movement that lead to energy expenditure. Exercise is a structured form of physical activity with the goal of improving fitness. Both physical activity and exercise play a role in the prevention and management of diabetes mellitus (DM). In type 2 DM (T2DM), physical activity and exercise play an important role in improving glycemic control and preventing the progression of diabetes complications. However, the role of physical activity in type 1 DM (T1DM) is less well defined.

2. **What are physical activity guidelines for people with DM?**
   The American Diabetes Association (ADA) recommends that most people with DM (T1DM and T2DM) should engage in at least 150 minutes of moderate to vigorous physical activity per week, similar to the general population. This guidance is outlined in detail in the *Physical Activity Guidelines for Americans*, 2nd edition. Despite this recommendation, 40.8% of people with T2DM are considered physically inactive (<10 minutes per week).

3. **How do demographic factors, such as gender, race, and ethnicity, affect the ability of people with dm to meet physical activity guidelines?**
   The National Health and Nutrition Examination Surveys (NHANES) from 2007 to 2016 show that women in the general population have lower physical activity levels than men across all age groups and settings; this difference is also seen in people with DM. Additionally, meeting physical activity guidelines in DM differs by race and ethnicity, with 42.6% of African Americans, 44.2% of whites, and 65.1% of Hispanic individuals meeting the recommended threshold for physical activity.

4. **What is the role of sedentary time in T2DM?**
   Higher sedentary time correlates with increased morbidity and mortality in the general population and in people with DM. Sedentary time increases risk even in the context of meeting the guidelines for moderate to vigorous physical activity. In those with T2DM, higher sedentary time correlates with worse glycemic control; breaking up this time every 30 minutes with light physical activity, or even standing, can improve glycemic control. It may also prevent T2DM in those at risk.

5. **What is the role of exercise in the prevention of T2DM?**
   There is an inverse relationship between physical activity and T2DM: higher levels of physical activity are associated with a lower risk of developing T2DM. Individuals who are obese and have low physical activity levels have a 7.4-fold increased risk of developing T2DM. Exercise as a regular form of physical activity reduces the risk of developing T2DM in the general population by an average of 42%. Exercise can improve cardiorespiratory fitness (CRF), weight management, and other cardiovascular risk factors (hypertension, cholesterol and triglyceride levels), all of which are implicated in an increased risk of T2DM incidence.

6. **Identify the benefits of physical activity/exercise in T2DM**
   Exercise, along with medical nutrition therapy, forms the foundation of all T2DM management. Exercise enhances the efficiency of glucose disposal via stimulation of glucose transporter translocation by muscle contraction. These effects promote improved glucose uptake into muscle and augmented insulin action, both of which aid in acute glycemic control. The effect of a bout of exercise on glucose disposal lasts for up to 2 hours, and the insulin sensitivity effect lasts for up to 48 hours after exercise. Insulin sensitivity is linked to exercise duration and intensity. Shorter (<20 minutes), high-intensity bouts or longer (>60 minutes), low-intensity bouts can increase insulin action for up to 24 hours. Each individual needs to learn how a specific type of exercise (running, walking, weights) and exercise intensity (light, moderate, vigorous) affects their blood glucose. Over time, people with T2DM who engage in any type of regular exercise can decrease their hemoglobin A1c by an average of 0.67%.

7. **What are the optimal duration and frequency of exercise in those with DM?**
   Aerobic exercise should be done for at least 10 minutes per day most days, with moderate- to vigorous-intensity exercise optimally being done 30 minutes on most days. The goal for all people with DM is to increase exercise frequency, duration, and intensity over time in order to meet physical activity guidelines of 150 minutes/week.

Given the 48-hour effect of exercise on insulin sensitivity, there should be no more than 2 days between exercise sessions. Resistance exercise should be done on 2 to 3 nonconsecutive days per week. Flexibility and balance training should also be considered 2 to 3 times per week in older adults with DM.

8. **Review key strategies for increasing physical activity in adults with T2DM**
   The key strategies for improving physical activity include the following:
   1. Identifying barriers
   2. Pinpointing when/where to perform exercise
   3. Using follow-up prompts
   4. Focusing on past success
   5. Reviewing goals and revising goals if the current strategy is not working

9. **What common barriers do people with DM encounter when exercising?**
   Fear of exercise-related hypoglycemia is the number-one barrier to exercise. Further, people with DM report discomfort with physical activity, related to fitness level and weight status. Women with T2DM report a higher rate of perceived exertion (RPE) during submaximal exercise compared with their nondiabetic counterparts. Additionally, those who use insulin pump therapy may report difficulties with skin irritation, pump tubing, and concern with pump visibility. Similarly, diabetes distress, depression, and other psychosocial factors (community and family support, socioeconomic status, etc.) may affect motivation to exercise. The new hybrid closed-loop insulin-delivery systems differ from conventional insulin pumps in the adjustments required to safely manage blood glucose during and after exercise. These issues are best discussed with the provider helping to manage the patient's DM.

10. **How do DM complications contribute to barriers to exercise in DM?**
    The presence of DM complications is associated with a high incidence of depression, which may affect motivation to exercise. Specific complications inflict barriers that further reduce the incentive to exercise. For instance, those with nephropathy are predisposed to anemia, which leads to decreased oxygen-carrying capacity and potential dyspnea with exertion. Other barriers related to specific complications include the following:
    1. Vision impairment (retinopathy)
    2. Poor proprioception and balance and risk for injury (neuropathy)
    3. Pain and discomfort (diabetic foot ulcers)
    4. Dyspnea with exertion (cardiovascular disease and heart failure)
    5. Fear of hypoglycemia (insulin dependence, hypoglycemia unawareness)

11. **Identify the pathophysiological barriers to exercise in DM**
    Exercise intolerance in DM is associated with both physiologic and behavioral factors. People with T2DM have a dissociation between oxygen substrate delivery and extraction, potentially as a result of vascular, endothelial, and mitochondrial dysfunction leading to impaired blood flow. Insulin sensitivity and CRF are directly related. Furthermore, women with uncomplicated T2DM have been shown to have abnormal diastolic parameters while exercising (particularly, increased pulmonary capillary wedge pressure), suggestive of subclinical heart failure. These factors can contribute to perceived exercise difficulty.

12. **Discuss the relationship between exercise and CRF in those with T2DM and the impact this relationship has on morbidity and mortality**
    Exercise is a modifiable risk factor for impaired CRF. Even small increases in physical activity predict improvements in cardiovascular outcomes and mortality. Exercise improves insulin sensitivity; as mentioned previously, insulin sensitivity directly correlates with CRF. Additionally, youth and adults with uncomplicated T1DM and T2DM have lower CRF levels compared with the general population and when matched for body mass index (BMI) and baseline activity level, even in the absence of cardiovascular disease (CVD). Lower CRF levels predict greater short-term mortality risk in people with DM, as with the general population. Furthermore, lower CRF levels in people with DM have been associated with future risk of CVD events. In epidemiologic studies in youth and adults, low CRF levels also predict the development of DM.

13. **How does exercise affect micro- and macrovascular outcomes in people with T2DM?**
    Higher levels of physical activity are associated with a reduced risk of future diabetic nephropathy, retinopathy, neuropathy, and CVD. This inverse relationship has been shown in people with T1DM and in those with T2DM who progress to requiring insulin. Additionally, moderate to vigorous physical activity is associated with lower rates of CVD and overall mortality. Therefore exercise and level of physical activity have value as prognostic factors in people with DM.

14. **Discuss exercise as a therapeutic adjunct to pharmacologic therapy in T2DM**
    Lifestyle intervention through medical nutrition therapy and exercise form the foundation for T2DM treatment. Therefore they must be the initial step for therapy but should also be readdressed each time therapy is intensified.

Notably, the addition of exercise training to metformin monotherapy has been shown to reduce postprandial hyperglycemia by ~20%, an effect comparable to the addition of a sulfonylurea, thiazolidinedione, or dipeptidyl peptidase-4 inhibitor.

15. **How does exercise affect glycemic control in those with DM?**
The effect of different types of exercise on glycemic control is highly variable, particularly in T1DM. Generally, continuous aerobic exercise is associated with decreases in blood glucose levels, particularly if done postprandially in the setting of insulin. Therefore there is a high risk of hypoglycemia with this type of exercise, particularly in people with T1DM. Hypoglycemia can occur during exercise but more commonly is seen 6 to 15 hours after exercise. Because of the prolonged effects of exercise on insulin action (up to 48 hours), exercise has been associated with nocturnal hypoglycemia and impaired counterregulatory responses to hypoglycemia in T1DM. High-intensity aerobic activity in short bursts (as with high-intensity interval training [HIIT]) and resistance training are associated with increases in blood glucose levels. Hyperglycemia can also result from fear of hypoglycemia that leads to insulin underdosing or overconsumption of carbohydrates prior to the exercise session. Therefore care should be taken to inform people with DM about the risks associated with each modality and strategies to prevent increased glucose variability with exercise sessions. The bottom line is that the glycemic impact varies for each individual based on the type, timing, intensity, and duration of the exercise session and the current diabetes medications. The goal is to help people exercise safely, and this commonly requires trial and error.

16. **What exercise modality produces optimal results in individuals with DM?**
This question should be approached as aspirational. The simple answer is whatever the individual prefers and will do regularly. As noted previously, different types and intensities of exercise affect blood glucose differently. Less glucose variability is seen with HIIT and resistance training in some but not all reports. Given the benefits of aerobic exercise, the provider should work with an interested individual to plan for safe exercise. There is evidence that performing resistance exercise prior to aerobic exercise may mitigate increased glucose variability and attenuate the risk of hypoglycemia.

17. **Discuss the advantages of using an insulin pump compared with multiple daily injections for insulin users who exercise**
With either delivery modality, the amount of insulin on board is the primary factor to consider. High levels of insulin on board mean the individual will be at risk for hypoglycemia and should have carbohydrates available. Low levels of insulin on board increase the risk of hyperglycemia (particularly with vigorous activity). The advantage of using an insulin pump is the ability to make small adjustments in the basal rate prior to and during exercise, in addition to the ability to suspend insulin delivery if needed; these actions can help mitigate the risk of hypoglycemia during aerobic activity. At the same time, there may be more rapid absorption of the subcutaneous insulin provided by the pump. An advantage to using multiple daily injection (MDI) therapy is that absorption of long-acting basal insulin is unaffected. It should be noted that with the newer hybrid closed-loop systems, high blood glucose prior to exercise may generate increased basal rates and a large amount of insulin on board.

18. **What specific safety measures regarding hypoglycemia should be advised for those with DM who exercise?**
Given the high variability in glycemic responses to exercise therapy, it is important to focus on each individual's response to exercise. The blood glucose level should always be checked prior to exercise in people with T1DM; an ideal range prior to exercise is 90 to 250 mg/dL. In general, to reduce the risk of hypoglycemia, people with DM may need to ingest carbohydrates prior to exercise and/or decrease insulin dosing prior to and after the session. For low- or moderate-intensity activity done while fasting, an average additional 10 to 15 g of carbohydrates should be ingested; for activities done with rapid-acting insulin on board, 30 to 60 g of carbohydrates may be needed. The amount of carbohydrates needed will also be affected by the blood glucose level prior to exercise. A 25% to 75% reduction in insulin doses prior to or after exercise may also be warranted. Particular attention should be given to common medications used in DM and its comorbidities that may lead to hypoglycemia. These include insulin secretagogues and beta blockers. Glucose tablets and gels should be readily available during exercise sessions for those individuals who are at high risk of hypoglycemia during activity. Continuous glucose monitors (CGMs) can alleviate the fear of hypoglycemia for these individuals.

19. **What other safety measures should be recommended for those with DM who exercise?**
No medical clearance is needed to initiate physical activity in those with DM who are asymptomatic. Exercise stress testing can be considered in individuals at high risk for CVD, but practically speaking, if the individual can climb three flights of stairs, no cardiovascular testing is warranted. In people with DM and coronary artery disease (CAD), a supervised cardiac rehabilitation program can be considered when initiating physical activity. There are increased risks of dehydration and hypotension during exercise with some antihypertensive agents. Careful blood pressure monitoring and adequate hydration during exercise can help mitigate these risks. For those with diabetic neuropathy, special care should be taken to use appropriate footwear and examine the feet before and after

exercise. In those with foot ulcers or other foot deformities (Charcot joint), pressure on the joint or ulcer should be minimized, and non-weight-bearing activity may be optimal. Vigorous exercise should be avoided in those with proliferative retinopathy because they are at increased risk of vitreous hemorrhage and retinal detachment.

20. Are there any contraindications to exercise in DM?

Contraindications to exercise in DM include vitreous hemorrhage, acute chest pain or shortness of breath concerning for myocardial infarction, or any signs of acute cerebrovascular accident.

KEY POINTS

1. Physical activity and exercise are integral to the prevention and management of type 2 diabetes. Adults with diabetes should engage in 150 minutes/week of moderate to vigorous physical activity with no more than 2 consecutive days without physical activity.
2. A combination of aerobic and resistance exercise is optimal for maximizing the benefits of exercise therapy in patients with diabetes and can help with minimizing glucose variability and attenuate hypoglycemia risk.
3. There are physical, pathophysiological, socioeconomic, and complication-related barriers to physical activity in patients with diabetes. Identification of these barriers and individualization of exercise regimens based on comorbidities and diabetes complications are key to maximizing the benefits of exercise and reducing the risks of exercise in patients with diabetes.

BIBLIOGRAPHY

1. Abushamat LA, McClatchey PM, Scalzo RI , Reusch JEB. The role of exercise in diabetes. In: Feingold KR, Anawalt B, Boyce A, et al., eds. *Endotext*. South Dartmouth (MA) 2020.
2. Abushamat LA, McClatchey PM, Scalzo RL, et al. Mechanistic causes of reduced cardiorespiratory fitness in type 2 diabetes. *J Endocr Soc*. 2020;4(7):bvaa063.
3. American Diabetes A 5. Facilitating behavior change and well-being to improve health outcomes: standards of medical care in diabetes-2020. *Diabetes Care*. 2020;43(Suppl 1):S48–S65.
4. Avery L, Flynn D, Dombrowski SU, van Wersch A, Sniehotta FF, Trenell MI. Successful behavioural strategies to increase physical activity and improve glucose control in adults with Type 2 diabetes. *Diabet Med*. 2015;32(8):1058–1062.
5. Colberg SR, Sigal RJ, Yardley JE, et al. Physical activity/exercise and diabetes: a position statement of the American Diabetes Association. *Diabetes Care*. 2016;39(11):2065–2079.
6. Magkos F, Hjorth MF, Astrup A. Diet and exercise in the prevention and treatment of type 2 diabetes mellitus. *Nat Rev Endocrinol*. 2020;16(10):545–555.
7. Piercy KL, Troiano RP, Ballard RM, et al. The physical activity guidelines for Americans. *JAMA*. 2018;320(19):2020–2028.
8. Wake AD. Antidiabetic effects of physical activity: how it helps to control type 2 diabetes. *Diabetes Metab Syndr Obes*. 2020;13:2909–2923.

CHAPTER 11

DIABETES MANAGEMENT: INSULIN THERAPY

Lindsay A. Courtney and Jennifer M. Trujillo

1. **How do the pharmacokinetic (PK) and pharmacodynamic (PD) properties of insulin products compare?**

   Appreciating the PK and PD properties of insulin products is crucial to understanding how insulin will affect the glucose profile. Table 11.1 provides a summary of key properties of insulin products available in the United States, and Fig. 11.1 compares the general PK/PD profiles of different insulin products. Insulin products are categorized by their PK/PD profiles as ultrarapid-acting, rapid-acting, short-acting, intermediate-acting, and long-acting insulins. Short-acting, rapid-acting, and ultrarapid-acting insulins are categorized as bolus insulins because they have fast onsets and short durations of action. Intermediate and long-acting agents are categorized as basal insulins because they typically have long durations of action with less of a peak effect.

2. **What factors can affect the PK/PD properties of insulin?**

   Several factors affect the PK/PD properties of insulin. Over the years, insulin analogs have been developed in different ways to enhance PK/PD features and make insulin products that more closely mimic physiologic insulin secretion. For example, rapid-acting insulin analogs (aspart, lispro, glulisine) have a faster onset of action and shorter duration of action compared with the traditional regular insulin. Since then, ultrarapid-acting insulin analogs (aspart [Fiasp] and lispro-aabc [Lyumjev]) have been formulated to have an even faster onset. Similarly, longer-acting basal insulin products (glargine U-300 and degludec) were developed with flatter profiles and longer durations of action to provide more consistent basal insulin concentrations. Other external factors can affect the PK/PD of insulin. Insulin absorption is affected by the site of injection, the thickness of subcutaneous (SC) tissue, the amount of adipose tissue, subcutaneous blood flow, skin temperature, and the amount of insulin administered.

3. **What is bolus insulin?**

   Bolus insulin options include short-acting regular insulin, rapid-acting analogs (aspart, glulisine, and lispro), and ultrarapid acting analogs (faster-acting insulin aspart, lispro-aabc, and inhaled insulin; see Table 11.1). All bolus insulin agents are effective in lowering postprandial glucose (PPG) levels and glycosylated hemoglobin (A1c). Rapid-acting agents have a faster onset of action and shorter duration of action compared with short-acting insulin. Because of this, current guidelines recommend the use of rapid-acting agents over short-acting agents in patients with type 1 diabetes (T1D) to reduce the risk of hypoglycemia; however, cost may necessitate the use of regular insulin in some patients. Ultrarapid-acting agents may be an option for patients who have rapid rises in glucose after meals and desire a bolus insulin with a faster onset. Faster-acting insulin aspart (Fiasp) is insulin aspart formulated with niacinamide, which aids in speeding the initial absorption of insulin. Insulin lispro-aabc (Lyumjev) uses two excipients to accelerate the absorption of insulin lispro at the injection site: a microdose of treprostinil; a prostacyclin analog, which increases local vasodilation; and citrate, which enhances local vascular permeability.

4. **What is basal insulin?**

   Basal insulin options include long-acting analogs (detemir, glargine U-100, glargine U-300, degludec) and neutral protamine Hagedorn (NPH) insulin (see Table 11.1). All basal insulin agents are effective at lowering fasting plasma glucose (FPG) levels and A1c. The PK/PD profile of NPH insulin makes it a less ideal basal insulin because it has a distinct peak effect and does not last a full 24 hours. It must be administered twice daily in patients with T1D and may also need twice-daily dosing in patients with type 2 diabetes (T2D). Insulin detemir and glargine U-100 have improved PK/PD profiles compared with NPH but may still exhibit a peak effect and may not last a full 24 hours in all patients. Insulin glargine U-300 and insulin degludec are newer basal insulins without peak effects and durations of action that exceed 24 hours. These PK/PD benefits are appealing because they permit once-daily dosing without wearing off, allow for more dosing flexibility, and are less likely to cause hypoglycemia. Studies have shown that these agents result in similar reductions in FPG and A1c but result in less nocturnal hypoglycemia compared with insulin glargine U-100.

5. **What is the difference between basal and bolus insulin coverage?**

   Basal insulin secretion suppresses hepatic glucose production to control blood glucose levels in the fasting state and premeal periods. Normal basal insulin secretion from the pancreas varies slightly throughout the day, responding to changes in activity, blood glucose levels, and regulatory hormones. Basal coverage is usually accomplished with injections of long-acting preparations or with the basal infusion function on the insulin pump.

Table 11.1 The Pharmacodynamics of Insulin Preparations

PREPARATIONS (U-100 UNLESS OTHERWISE NOTED)	ONSET	PEAK[a]	DURATION[a]
Bolus Insulin Products			
Ultrarapid acting			
Insulin aspart (Fiasp)	15–20 min[b]	90–120 min	5–7 hours
Insulin lispro aabc (Lyumjev)	15–17 min[c]	120–174 min	4.6–7.3 hours
Insulin human—inhaled (Afrezza)	3–7 min	12–15 min	2.5–3 hours
Rapid acting	10–20 min	30–90 min	3–5 hours
Insulin aspart (NovoLog)			
Insulin lispro U-100, U-200 (Humalog, Admelog)			
Insulin glulisine (Apidra)			
Short acting			
Regular (Humulin R, Novolin R)	30–60 min	2–4 hours	5–8 hours
Basal Insulin Products			
Intermediate acting			
NPH (Humulin N, Novolin N)	2–4 hours	4–10 hours	10–24 hours
Long Acting			
Insulin detemir (Levemir)	1.5–4 hours	6–14 hours[d]	16–20 hours
Insulin glargine (Lantus, Basaglar)	2–4 hours	No peak	20–24 hours
Insulin glargine U-300 (Toujeo)	6 hours	No peak	36 hours
Insulin degludec U-100, U-200 (Tresiba)	1 hour	No peak	42 hours
Combination Products			
70% NPH, 30% regular (Humulin 70/30, Novolin 70/30)	30–60 min	Dual	10–16 hours
75% NPL, 25% lispro (Humalog 75/25)	5–15 min	Dual	10–16 hours
50% NPL, 50% lispro (Humalog 50/50)	5–15 min	Dual	10–16 hours
70% aspart protamine, 30% aspart (Novolog 70/30)	5–15 min	Dual	15–18 hours
Concentrated Human Regular Insulin			
Regular U-500	30 min	4–8 hours	13–24 hours

[a]The peak and duration of insulin action are variable, depending on injection site, duration of diabetes, renal function, smoking status, and other factors.
[b]Onset of appearance is 2.5 minutes.
[c]Onset of appearance is 1 minute.
[d]Long-acting insulins are considered "peakless," although they have exhibited peak effects during comparative testing.

NPH, Neutral protamine Hagedorn; *NPL*, insulin lispro protamine suspension.

Bolus insulin doses consist of two components: the nutritional dose, which is the amount of insulin required to manage glucose excursions after meals; and the correction dose, which is the amount of insulin required to reduce a high glucose level detected before a meal. Bolus coverage is accomplished with the administration of ultrarapid-acting, rapid-acting, or short-acting insulin preparations or with the use of the bolus function on the insulin pump.

6. **How is insulin used in the treatment of T1D?**
T1D is caused by autoimmune destruction of the pancreatic beta cells, which leads to an absolute deficiency of insulin. Therefore the mainstay of treatment of T1D is intensive insulin therapy (IIT). IIT is the use of multiple daily injections (MDIs) of insulin (both basal and bolus formulations) or an insulin pump in an effort to mimic the normal physiologic secretion of insulin by the pancreas. IIT may also be referred to as *physiologic, multiple-component*, or *basal-bolus insulin therapy*.

IIT includes continuous basal coverage in addition to bursts of insulin to regulate the rise in glucose after food intake (Fig. 11.2). A long-acting insulin is injected either once or twice daily to provide the basal insulin

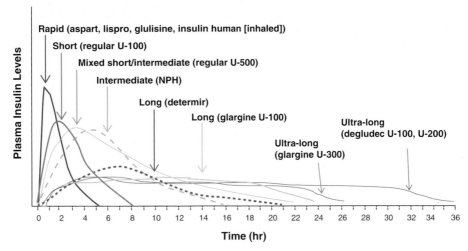

Fig. 11.1 Pharmacokinetic profiles of currently available insulin products.

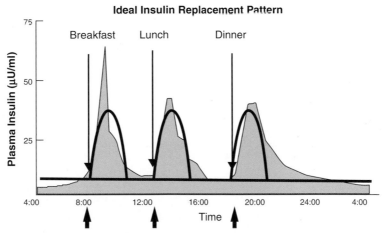

Fig. 11.2 Intensive insulin therapy pattern. Schematic representation of insulin therapy pattern provided by once-daily long-acting basal insulin and rapid-acting bolus insulin before each meal to mimic normal physiologic insulin secretion. (From White RD. Insulin pump therapy (continuous subcutaneous insulin infusion). *Prim. Care.* 2007;34:845–871.)

portion of an MDI regimen, which is approximately 50% of a patient's total daily dose. Ideally, basal insulin should cover background insulin needs only, independent of food intake. A rapid, ultrarapid, or short-acting insulin is injected before meals to provide the bolus insulin portion of an MDI regimen (see Fig. 11.2). Rapid-acting or ultra-rapid-acting insulin is preferred over short-acting insulin because of the more rapid onset and shorter duration of action. A patient can adjust each bolus dose to match the carbohydrate intake and to correct for high glucose levels before the meal, whereas the basal dose remains constant from day to day.

When initiating insulin therapy in someone with T1D, the starting dose is generally calculated based on weight, starting with a total daily insulin dose of 0.4 to 1.0 units/kg. After calculating the total daily dose, approximately half is given as basal insulin, and the other half is given as bolus insulin, distributed across meals. Insulin doses are then titrated based on blood glucose monitoring data, and bolus doses can be further refined based on carbohydrate counting and correctional dosing.

IIT is complex because it requires multiple injections or pump boluses per day in addition to basal insulin doses, routine monitoring, and collaborative decision making. The most successful insulin therapy is adjusted based on changes in nutritional intake, glucose levels, stress levels, and physical activity. Critical components include the use of self-monitoring of blood glucose (SMBG) or continuous glucose monitoring to identify glucose patterns and adjust insulin doses, a carbohydrate-to-insulin (C:I) ratio according to food intake, and the use of correction factors (CFs) for the adjustment of insulin according to glucose levels. Precise insulin dosing for T1D is reviewed in Chapter 13.

7. How is insulin used in the treatment of T2D?

The approach to insulin use in T2D is different than in T1D. People with T2D can often be managed with noninsulin medications and lifestyle modifications for years before insulin is required. However, because of the progressive nature of T2D, many patients will eventually require insulin to achieve glycemic control. Current treatment guidelines suggest a stepwise approach. Once injectable therapy is needed, a GLP-1 receptor agonist should be considered preferentially before insulin because of its comparable glucose-lowering effects, lower risk of hypoglycemia, and preferred effect on weight. If additional glucose lowering is needed after the GLP-1 receptor agonist has been maximized, basal insulin is the next recommended step, followed by a stepwise addition of bolus insulin if needed based on the A1c and glucose profile.

Early initiation of insulin therapy is preferred in patients with extremely elevated glucose levels (e.g., A1c > 10% or glucose > 300 mg/dL), evidence of ongoing catabolism, and symptoms of hyperglycemia. Although those patients may need insulin initially, they can likely transition from insulin to other medications once the acute hyperglycemia and glucotoxicity have resolved.

8. How should insulin be intensified in the treatment of T2D?

When a patient with T2D requires intensification to insulin therapy, basal insulin is typically the first step. Basal insulin is added to the medication regimen at a starting dose of 10 units (or 0.1–0.2 units/kg) per day. The dose is then up-titrated, typically by 2 to 4 units twice weekly, using a validated dose-titration method until FPG levels are within the target range (80–130 mg/dL for patients with an A1c goal of <7%). Many approaches to up-titration have been validated. A common approach is increasing the dose by 3 units every 3 days until FPG levels are within 80 to 130 mg/dL, without hypoglycemia. It is important to determine whether your patient is capable and willing to titrate the dose at home on their own or if they require more guidance, such as weekly phone calls to review glucose data and titrate the dose collaboratively. Either way, a dose-titration plan is crucial to avoid clinical inertia and attain glucose control. Patients should also be educated about glucose goals and the anticipated basal insulin dose. Knowing what to expect in this setting can improve adherence to the titration plan. Dose titration should continue until FPG levels are reached or until the dose reaches approximately 0.5 units/kg/day. At that time, if additional therapy is needed to achieve glycemic goals, prandial insulin can be added. A bolus insulin product can be added to the largest meal or the meal leading to the largest glucose excursions, at a starting dose of 4 units. The dose can then be titrated by 1 to 2 units twice weekly based on postprandial glucose levels. A reasonable recommended target PPG level for most patients is <180 mg/dL. Additional doses of bolus insulin can be added to the other meals if needed to achieve glycemic goals.

9. What are the most common adverse effects of insulin?

Hypoglycemia is the most common and serious adverse effect of insulin therapy and a major limiting factor in the glycemic management of diabetes.

- Level 1 hypoglycemia = glucose <70 mg/dL but ≥54 mg/dL
- Level 2 hypoglycemia = glucose <54 mg/dL
- Level 3 hypoglycemia = a severe event characterized by altered mental status and/or physical status requiring assistance

The newer rapid-acting and long-acting insulin analogs are associated with less hypoglycemia than the older short- and intermediate-acting human insulin products. Common symptoms of hypoglycemia include shakiness, irritability, confusion, tachycardia, and hunger. Hypoglycemia can lead to impaired concentration, cognition, and reaction time. Frequent episodes of hypoglycemia can lead to the loss of clinical warning symptoms, which is known as *hypoglycemia unawareness*. Mild hypoglycemia can be treated with the "rule of 15," which includes the immediate ingestion of 15 g of fast-acting carbohydrates (e.g., 1/2 cup of fruit juice, 1 Tbsp honey, 3 glucose tablets, 5–6 hard candies), followed by a repeat glucose check in 15 minutes. If hypoglycemia persists, additional carbohydrates should be ingested. Severe hypoglycemia that cannot be treated with oral carbohydrates may require the administration of glucagon by a third party. More information about hypoglycemia is provided in Chapter 25.

Weight gain is another adverse effect of insulin. Patients should be informed about the potential for weight gain with insulin, particularly those with T2D who are overweight or obese. Using GLP-1 receptor agonists prior to or in combination with basal insulin can help mitigate the weight gain caused by insulin. Patients should also be encouraged to implement lifestyle modifications to minimize weight gain from insulin.

Insulin can also cause injection-site reactions and lipohypertrophy. Proper injection technique and injection-site rotation are crucial for patients on long-term insulin therapy to avoid lipohypertrophy.

10. What insulin products are currently available in the United States?
    Each insulin product is unique in terms of its formulation and availability. Some insulin products are available in vials, disposable pen devices, or cartridges to insert into reusable pen devices. Some newer products are only available in pen devices and do not come in vials. Products vary in terms of concentration, units per pen, maximum dose per injection, and storage (Table 11.2). Most insulin products are U-100, meaning their concentration is 100 units/mL; however, some insulin products have higher concentrations (U-200: 200 units/mL, U-300: 300 units/mL, U-500: 500 units/mL). Syringes, pen needles, or insulin pump supplies must be prescribed separately. Understanding these differences is crucial to ensure that prescriptions are written and dispensed correctly.

11. What education tips should be included when counseling a patient on the appropriate use of insulin?
    Counseling on the use of insulin must include appropriate storage; proper administration (dose, injection technique, and timing of injection); glycemic targets; SMBG; dose titration; and the prevention, detection, and treatment of hypoglycemia. Insulin should be stored in the refrigerator until ready for use. Prior to injecting, insulin should be removed from the refrigerator and allowed to warm to room temperature to avoid painful injections. After initial use, insulin can be stored at room temperature for the duration specified for each product (see Table 11.2). Before each use, NPH insulin and all suspension-based insulin preparations need to be resuspended by inverting or rolling gently at least 20 times. Improper mixing of the suspension prior to administration can lead to glycemic variability.

    Injection technique varies slightly depending on whether an insulin pen or a syringe is used. When using an insulin pen, patients first need to remove the pen cap, attach a pen needle, and prime the pen to ensure unobstructed flow. The recommended pen needle length is 4 mm to reduce pain and decrease the risk of intramuscular injection. The pen is then dialed to the correct dose, and the needle is inserted perpendicularly into the skin of the abdomen, thigh, or outer arm at a 90-degree angle. Injecting into a lifted skinfold is typically not recommended except in very young children (≤6 years old) and very thin adults. Once the needle is fully inserted, the button of the pen should be depressed completely and held for 10 seconds. When giving higher doses, the pen may need to be held in the skin longer than 10 seconds to prevent medication leakage.

    When using a syringe to inject insulin from a vial, the appropriate syringe and needle size must be prescribed. Each syringe has markings appropriate for a certain concentration of insulin, ranging from U-100 to U-500. The shortest needle available is 6 mm and is recommended for most people. When syringe needles are used in children (≥6 years old), adolescents, or slim to normal-weight adults (body mass index [BMI] of 19–25 kg/m²), injections should be given into a lifted skinfold. To draw up insulin from a vial, air should first be drawn into the syringe at a dose equal to or slightly greater than the dose of insulin to be given. The air should then be pushed into the vial, creating positive pressure and allowing for the insulin to be easily drawn up. Once the correct dose is drawn up, the needle is inserted into the skin of the abdomen, thigh, or outer arm, and the plunger is depressed completely to administer the full dose. With both insulin pens and syringes, patients should be advised to rotate injection sites to prevent lipohypertrophy.

12. When should bolus insulin be taken?
    - Rapid-acting insulin should be taken within 15 minutes before meals and snacks.
    - Rapid-acting insulin can be taken as follows:
      - 15 to 30 minutes before meals if the premeal BG is higher than 130 mg/dL
      - Immediately after eating if gastroparesis or a concurrent illness is present
      - Upon arrival of food if unfamiliar with meal size, content, or timing (i.e., in a restaurant or hospital)
    - Fast-acting insulin aspart (Fiasp) and insulin lispro-aabc (Lyumjev) should be taken at the beginning of the meal or within 20 minutes after starting the meal.
    - Inhaled insulin should be taken at the beginning of the meal.
    - Human regular insulin should be taken approximately 30 minutes before meals.

13. When should basal insulin be taken?
    - Insulin glargine U-100, detemir, glargine U-300, and degludec should be taken once a day at the same time each day.
    - Insulin glargine U-100 or detemir may be taken at bedtime if a dawn phenomenon is present.
    - Basal insulin analogs (glargine, detemir, or degludec) cannot be mixed with other insulins.
    - If nocturnal hypoglycemia results from taking a full dose of glargine or detemir at bedtime, an option would be to split the dose so that 50% is taken in the morning and the other 50% is taken in the evening, approximately 12 hours apart.
    - NPH insulin is given in the morning and at bedtime to avoid nocturnal hypoglycemia.
    - Doses of insulin glargine U-300 and insulin degludec should not be adjusted more frequently than every 3 to 4 days because of their longer half-lives.

Table 11.2 Insulin Product Availability

INSULIN	COMPOUND NAME (U-100 UNLESS OTHERWISE NOTED)	PRODUCT AVAILABILITY	UNITS PER PEN	MAXIMUM DOSE (UNITS) PER INJECTION (PENS ONLY)	PEN STORAGE AT ROOM TEMPERATURE (DAYS)	MEDIAN AWP COST (PREFILLED PEN UNLESS OTHERWISE NOTED)[a]
Ultrarapid acting	Aspart (Fiasp)	Vial, cartridge, prefilled pen	300	80	28	$447
	Lispro aabc U-100, U-200 (Lyumjev)	Vial, cartridge, prefilled pen	300 (U-100) 600 (U-200)	60	28	$424
	Human—inhaled (Afrezza)	Inhalation cartridge	N/A	N/A	N/A	$924
Rapid-acting	Aspart (NovoLog)	Vial, cartridge, prefilled pen	300	80	28	$223
	Lispro (Humalog)	Vial, cartridge, prefilled pen	300	60	28	$212
	Lispro (Admelog)	Vial, prefilled pen	300	80	28	$202
	Lispro U-200 (Humalog)	Prefilled pen	600	60	28	$424
	Glulisine (Apidra)	Vial, prefilled pen	300	80	28	$439
Short-acting	Regular (Humulin R, Novolin R)	Vial	N/A	N/A	N/A	N/A
Intermediate-acting	NPH (Humulin N, Novolin N)	Vial, prefilled pen	300	60	14	$208

Continued

Table 11.2 Insulin Product Availability—cont'd

INSULIN	COMPOUND NAME (U-100 UNLESS OTHERWISE NOTED)	PRODUCT AVAILABILITY	UNITS PER PEN	MAXIMUM DOSE (UNITS) PER INJECTION (PENS ONLY)	PEN STORAGE AT ROOM TEMPERATURE (DAYS)	MEDIAN AWP COST (PREFILLED PEN UNLESS OTHERWISE NOTED)[a]
Long-acting	Detemir (Levemir)	Vial, prefilled pen	300	80	42	$370
	Glargine (Lantus)	Vial, prefilled pen	300	80	28	$340
	Glargine(Basaglar)	Prefilled pen	300	80	28	$190
	Glargine U-300(Toujeo)	Prefilled pen	450 (SoloStar) 900 (Max SoloStar)	80 (SoloStar) 160 (Max SoloStar)	56	$340
	Degludec(Tresiba)	Vial, prefilled pen	300	80	56	$407
	Degludec U-200(Tresiba)	Prefilled pen	600	160	56	$407
Combination	70% NPH, 30% Regular (Humulin 70/30, Novolin 70/30)	Vial, prefilled pen	300	60	28	$208
	75% NPL, 25% lispro (Humalog 75/25)	Vial, prefilled pen	300	60	10	$212
	50% NPL, 50% lispro (Humalog 50/50)	Vial, prefilled pen	300	60	10	$424
	70% aspart protamine, 30% aspart (Novolog 70/30)	Vial, prefilled pen	300	60	14	$224
Concentrated	Regular U-500	Vial, prefilled pen	1,500	300	28	$229

[a]AWP data do not include vials of regular human insulin and NPH available at Walmart for approximately $25 per vial.

AWP, Average wholesale price; *N/A,* not applicable; *NPH,* neutral protamine Hagedorn.

14. **How do you switch from one insulin product to another?**

Switching between insulins requires consideration of the PK/PD profile of each product. Because rapid-acting insulin analogs have similar PK/PD properties, they can be switched on a unit-to-unit basis. Similarly, 1:1 conversion is recommended when converting rapid-acting insulin analogs to ultrarapid-acting insulin based on clinical trials demonstrating similar dosing requirements between these agents. The recommended ratio between rapid-acting insulin and inhaled human insulin (Afrezza) is 1.5 units Afrezza:1 unit rapid-acting insulin. Afrezza is only available in 4-unit increments; therefore, additional adjustments may be needed.

When switching between basal insulins, a 1:1 unit conversion is typically recommended. However, in some cases, data from clinical trials and real-world clinical experience show that a straight 1:1 conversion may not be optimal. When switching from twice-daily NPH to long-acting insulin glargine 100 U/mL (Gla-100) or insulin glargine 300 U/mL (Gla-300), the dose should be reduced to 80% of the total daily dose of NPH to reduce the risk of hypoglycemia. Conversion from once-daily NPH to Gla-100 or Gla-300 can be done on a 1:1 unit basis. A higher total daily dose of Insulin detemir (IDet) may be needed compared with Gla-100, particularly in those needing twice-daily IDet. When switching from Gla-100 to Gla-300, an approximately 10% to 18% higher dose of Gla-300 may be needed to achieve equivalent glycemic control. Conversion from Gla-300 to Gla-100, requires a 20% dose reduction. Initial dosing of insulin degludec (IDeg) should be reduced by approximately 20% when switching from other insulins. As a result of the longer time to achieve steady state with longer-acting insulins such as IDeg or Gla-300, clinicians and patients should be aware of the potential for hyperglycemia during the first few days after switching to these agents. When switching from longer-acting insulin to shorter acting agents, the risk of hypoglycemia may be greater because of the greater time needed to clear long-acting insulins. With any insulin product switch, patients should be monitored closely for significant changes in glycemic control and the incidence of hypoglycemia.

15. **What is U-500 insulin, and when should it be considered?**

U-500 regular insulin is concentrated insulin containing 500 units/mL, which is five times more concentrated than U-100 insulin. The use of U-500 insulin reduces the volume of insulin injected, resulting in fewer injections, less discomfort, and potentially improved insulin absorption. Based on its unique PK/PD properties (see Table 11.1), U-500 insulin provides both basal and prandial coverage, allowing for dosing two to three times per day with meals. All other insulins should be stopped when starting U-500 insulin.

Caution should be taken to ensure appropriate dosing and administration of U-500 insulin to avoid potentially severe overdose errors. The availability of U-500 insulin pens and U-500 syringes has improved the safety of this insulin product, and these dedicated U-500 devices should be used for administration whenever possible. However, if U-100 syringes are used, patients should be instructed on appropriate dosing because they will need to draw up the insulin to one-fifth of their U-500 units. Because of its unique PK properties and potential for significant safety concerns if dosed incorrectly, U-500 insulin is typically reserved for individuals with T2D and severe insulin resistance requiring greater than 200 units of insulin per day.

16. **What is inhaled insulin, and when should it be considered?**

Inhaled insulin is formulated to be inhaled and absorbed through the lungs. The only commercially available inhaled insulin, Afrezza, is a rapid-acting human insulin. It comes as a dry powder adsorbed onto Technosphere microparticles, which facilitate delivery deep into the lungs and rapid dissolution into the bloodstream. Because of its rapid absorption, Afrezza has a more rapid peak and shortened duration of action compared with rapid-acting insulin analogs. Safety concerns regarding pulmonary function have limited the routine use of Afrezza. It is contraindicated in patients with chronic lung disease, such as asthma or chronic obstructive pulmonary disease (COPD), because of the risk of bronchospasm. When Afrezza is used, pulmonary function tests should be monitored at baseline, after the first 6 months, and yearly thereafter regardless of pulmonary symptoms. Consider discontinuation of the product if forced expiratory volume (FEV_1) declines $\geq$20% or in patients who develop persistent respiratory symptoms such as wheezing, cough, or bronchospasm. Based on these considerations, inhaled insulin should generally be reserved for patients with T1D who need a faster-acting agent for meals or correction.

17. **What is mixed insulin, and when should it be considered?**

Certain insulin products can be combined in the same syringe or may come as premixed solutions. NPH and other intermediate-acting insulins (lispro protamine and aspart protamine) can be mixed with regular human insulin or rapid-acting insulin analogs. This combination creates a PK/PD profile that provides both basal and prandial coverage while minimizing the number of injections required. Refer to Table 11.2 for a complete list of available premixed insulins. Although premixed insulin provides the convenience of fewer injections without the need for mixing, these products provide less dosing flexibility because of the fixed ratios of basal and prandial insulin. Current guidelines recommend considering self-mixed or premixed insulin for patients with T2D whose A1c is above target after optimizing basal insulin plus prandial insulin with at least one meal of the day. Premixed NPH/regular insulin may also be considered as a cost-effective alternative to insulin analogs.

18. **What is the cost of insulin?**

Refer to Table 11.2 for a complete list of insulin pricing. The affordability of insulin is currently a significant concern, with the cost of insulin nearly tripling between 2002 and 2013. The high cost of insulin can lead to medication nonadherence because patients with diabetes are often forced to choose between paying for their medications or paying for other necessities. In 2017, the Insulin Access and Affordability Working Group published recommendations for addressing issues with insulin affordability through a multifaceted approach involving providers, pharmacies, insurers, manufacturers, researchers, and regulatory bodies. The American Diabetes Association has endorsed the Insulin Price Reduction Act (H.R. 4906/S.2199), which aims to reduce insulin costs by providing incentives for manufacturers to decrease the list price of all insulin products. Despite efforts to pass legislation at the federal and state levels, insulin cost remains a major unresolved issue. Refer to Chapter 27 for strategies to help patients with overcoming barriers to medication access.

KEY POINTS

1. The impact of each insulin product on the glucose profile is guided by its PK/PD profile. Basal insulins have a long duration of action and minimal peak effect, providing consistent levels of insulin to help manage blood glucose during periods of fasting. Bolus insulins have fast onsets and short durations of action and are typically used to cover meals or correct high blood sugar levels.
2. The approach to insulin therapy differs between T1D and T2D. Treatment of T1D typically requires intensive insulin therapy with either multiple daily injections of insulin or an insulin pump. In contrast, in T2D, insulin is typically added in a stepwise fashion when glycemic goals are not met with noninsulin medications.
3. Common adverse effects of insulin include hypoglycemia, weight gain, injection-site reactions, and lipohypertrophy. Appropriate counseling on the prevention, detection, and treatment of hypoglycemia; lifestyle measures to minimize weight gain; and appropriate insulin injection technique can help mitigate these adverse effects.
4. There are various insulin products on the market. Numerous factors must be considered when selecting an appropriate agent, including diabetes diagnosis (e.g., T1D vs. T2D), PK/PD properties, total insulin requirements and degree of insulin resistance, number of required injections, and affordability.

BIBLIOGRAPHY

American Diabetes Association. Bills addressing drug and insulin affordability endorsed by American Diabetes Association. Press Release. January 15, 2020. Available at: https://www.diabetes.org/newsroom/press-releases/2020/drug-insulin-affordability#:~:text=The%20American%20Diabetes%20Association%20(ADA,Chronic%20Condition%20Copay%20Elimination%20Act. Accessed December 10, 2020.

American Diabetes Association. 6. Glycemic targets: Standards of medical care in diabetes – 2021. *Diabetes Care.* 2021;44(Suppl 1): S73–S84.

American Diabetes Association. 9. Pharmacologic approaches to glycemic treatment: Standards of medical care in diabetes – 2021. *Diabetes Care.* 2021;44(Suppl 1):S111–S124.

Anderson SL, Trujillo JM, Anderson JE, Tanenberg RJ. Switching basal insulins in type 2 diabetes: practical recommendations for health care providers. *Postgrad Med.* 2018;130(2):229–238.

Cefalu WT, Dawes DE, Gavlak G, et al. Insulin access and affordability working group: conclusions and recommendations. *Diabetes Care.* 2018;41(6):1299–1311.

Frid AH, Kreugel G, Grassi G, et al. New insulin delivery recommendations. *Mayo Clin Proc.* 2016;91(9):1231–1255.

Johnson EL, Frias JP, Trujillo JM. Anticipatory guidance in type 2 diabetes to improve disease management: next steps after basal insulin. *Postgraduate Medicine.* 2018;130(4):365–374.

Neumiller J. American Diabetes Association. 2020–2021 Guide to medications for the treatment of diabetes mellitus. White JR, Editor. American Diabetes Association, 2020, pp 27–48.

Patel D, Triplett C, Trujillo J. Appropriate titration of basal insulin in type 2 diabetes and the potential role of the pharmacist. *Adv Ther.* 2019;36:1031–1051.

Pettus J, Santos Cavaiola T, Edelman SV. Recommendations for Initiating Use of Afrezza inhaled insulin in individuals with type 1 diabetes. *Diabetes Technol Ther.* 2018;20(6):448–451.

Reutrakul S, Wroblewski K, Brown RL. Clinical use of U-500 regular insulin: review and meta-analysis. *J Diabetes Sci Technol.* 2012;6(2):412–420.

CHAPTER 12

DIABETES MANAGEMENT: NONINSULIN THERAPIES

Sarah L. Anderson and Jennifer M. Trujillo

1. **What noninsulin medication classes are used to treat type 2 diabetes (T2D)?**

   First-line therapy for T2D, in the absence of contraindications or compelling indications, is metformin. Metformin is a biguanide and an oral agent that prevents the production of glucose in the liver, reduces the amount of glucose absorbed by the intestines, and improves the body's sensitivity to insulin. Metformin is recommended as a first-line agent because it is effective and has good evidence to support its use, including a reduced risk of macrovascular outcomes based on the United Kingdom Prospective Diabetes Study (UKPDS).

   If metformin monotherapy is not sufficient for getting a patient to their glycemic goal, if metformin therapy is contraindicated, or if patients have specific characteristics warranting the addition of an agent, regardless of glycosylated hemoglobin (A1c), there are a variety of noninsulin second-line drug therapies available. These include sulfonylureas, glucagon-like peptide-1 (GLP-1) receptor agonists, dipeptidyl peptidase-4 (DPP-4) inhibitors, sodium–glucose cotransporter 2 (SGLT-2) inhibitors, and thiazolidinediones (TZDs). The mechanisms and physiologic actions of each noninsulin drug category are summarized in Table 12.1.

2. **How do the noninsulin medication classes compare with respect to efficacy, safety, and ease of use?**

   Noninsulin medications vary considerably with respect to efficacy and safety. A patient-centered approach should be used when selecting an agent for a given patient. Specific consideration should be given to the A1c-lowering efficacy, the effect on weight, and the potential impact on cardiovascular (CV) events, heart failure (HF), and progression of chronic kidney disease (CKD). Safety considerations such as the risk of hypoglycemia and other adverse effects should also be considered, as should administration requirements and cost. Table 12.2 compares and contrasts the common noninsulin medications used to treat T2D. Most noninsulin medications result in similar A1c lowering, with meta-analysis data indicating that, in general, any second-line, noninsulin medication will lower A1c by approximately 0.7% to 1% when added to metformin. However, the DPP-4 inhibitors and SGLT-2 inhibitors tend to result in less A1c lowering than the other classes.

3. **How are noninsulin oral medications dosed?**

   Dosing information for oral medications commonly used to treat diabetes is summarized in Table 12.3. Dosing and administration information for GLP-1 receptor agonists is summarized in Table 12.4. Of note, all GLP-1 receptor agonists are administered subcutaneously, except for the newly approved oral semaglutide, which is an oral, once-daily medication. The GLP-1 receptor agonists can be categorized as short acting and long acting. Short-acting agents primarily target postprandial glucose (PPG) and are administered once or twice daily before meals. Long-acting agents target both fasting plasma glucose (FPG) and PPG and are administered once daily or once weekly. In general, many T2D medications are initiated at low doses and titrated to higher doses based on glucose-lowering response and tolerability. Because many patients may feel overburdened by treatment requirements and self-management expectations, it is reasonable to consider the dosing and administration requirements when making treatment decisions. However, clinicians should not automatically assume that patients are resistant to injectable therapy. Other drug characteristics, such as efficacy, impact on weight, and less frequent dosing, may be more highly valued by some patients. Many T2D medications also require renal dose adjustments or have renal thresholds, after which they can no longer be used. These renal use considerations are important because many patients with diabetes have renal dysfunction, and the use of certain agents in patients with renal impairment can increase the risk of adverse effects. Renal dosing is discussed in more detail in the response to question 7.

4. **How can the adverse effects of metformin be minimized?**

   The most common side effects of metformin are gastrointestinal (GI) in nature, including diarrhea, nausea, vomiting, and flatulence. In order to minimize these side effects, metformin should be initiated at a low dose and up-titrated in a stepwise fashion to the target dose of 2000 mg/day (usually given in two divided doses). Metformin should be initiated at 500 mg orally daily and up-titrated by 500 mg each week until a maximum tolerated dose or 2000 mg is achieved. If a patient's metformin doses are missed or held (e.g., during hospitalization), retitration may be required to avoid GI side effects when reinitiating metformin therapy. Other strategies for minimizing the GI-related side effects of metformin include taking metformin with food and using an extended-release (ER)

Table 12.1 Mechanisms and Physiologic Actions of Common Noninsulin Glucose-Lowering Agents to Treat Type 2 Diabetes

CLASS	COMPOUNDS	CELLULAR MECHANISM(S)	PRIMARY PHYSIOLOGIC ACTION(S)
Biguanides	• Metformin • Metformin ER	Activate AMP kinase, modulation of respiratory-chain complex 1 (? other)	↓ Hepatic glucose production
• Sulfonylureas; second generation	• Glyburide • Glipizide • Glimepiride	Close K_{ATP} channels on beta-cell plasma membranes	↑ Insulin secretion
• Thiazolidinediones (TZDs)	• Pioglitazone • Rosiglitazone	Activate the nuclear transcription factor PPAR-γ	↑ Insulin sensitivity
• Dipeptidyl peptidase-4 (DPP-4) inhibitors	• Sitagliptin • Saxagliptin • Linagliptin • Alogliptin	Inhibit DPP-4 activity, increasing postprandial incretin (GLP-1, GIP) concentrations	↑ Insulin secretion and ↓ glucagon secretion (both glucose dependent)
• Sodium-glucose cotransporter 2 (SGLT-2) inhibitors	• Canagliflozin • Dapagliflozin • Empagliflozin • Ertugliflozin	Inhibit SGLT-2 in the proximal nephron	Block glucose reabsorption by the kidney, increasing glucosuria
• Glucagon-like peptide-1 (GLP-1) receptor agonists	• Dulaglutide • Exenatide • Exenatide ER • Liraglutide • Lixisenatide • Semaglutide inj • Semaglutide oral	Activate GLP-1 receptors	↑ Insulin secretion (glucose dependent); ↓ glucagon secretion (glucose dependent); slows gastric emptying; ↑ satiety

Amp, Adenosine monophosphate; *ER,* extended release; *GIP,* glucose-dependent insulinotropic polypeptidase; *inj* = injectable; *PPAR-γ,* peroxisome proliferator-activated receptor gamma.

preparation; an important patient counseling point when using the ER preparations is that patients may see parts of the ER tablets in their stool.

Metformin also reduces intestinal absorption of vitamin B_{12} and may lower serum B_{12} concentrations. The longer the duration of metformin use, the more likely B_{12} deficiency is to occur. Because of the insidious onset of B_{12} deficiency, it is recommended to monitor serum B_{12} levels every 2 to 3 years and treat accordingly. Severe vitamin B_{12} deficiency may present as peripheral neuropathy (PN). If the symptoms of PN are present and the patient is taking metformin, a B_{12} level should be checked to determine whether the symptoms are attributable to B_{12} deficiency versus the progression of diabetes or another cause.

5. **What other noninsulin therapies are available to treat T2D?**
In addition to the first- and second-line agents listed in question 1, there are several other classes of oral diabetes medications that are used less frequently in practice. Meglitinides (nateglinide and repaglinide) enhance endogenous insulin secretion and reduce PPG, similar to sulfonylureas. These agents have a more rapid onset and are shorter acting than sulfonylureas and must be dosed within 30 minutes of eating a meal. Meglitinides may have a role in patients with a true allergy to sulfonylureas because they work similarly and have comparable A1c-lowering ability; however, they are more expensive.

Alpha-glucosidase inhibitors (acarbose and miglitol) have a modest ability to lower A1c (0.5%–0.8%) and work by slowing the absorption of dietary carbohydrates. Because of their mechanism, the hallmark side effect of these medications is GI intolerance, including flatulence and diarrhea, and many patients do not tolerate these effects.

Colesevelam, a bile acid sequestrant, modestly improves the A1c (0.5%) by decreasing bile acid reabsorption. It is unknown how this effect on resorption decreases blood glucose. An added benefit is that in addition to lowering blood glucose, it lowers low-density lipoprotein cholesterol (LDL-C).

Table 12.2 Comparison of Noninsulin Medication Classes for the Treatment of Type 2 Diabetes

	A1C EFFICACY	HYPOGLY- CEMIA RISK	EFFECT ON WEIGHT	ASCVD EFFECTS	HF EFFECTS	DKD EFFECTS	COST	ORAL/SC	ADVERSE EFFECTS AND SAFETY
Metformin	High	No	Neutral	Potential benefit	Neutral	Neutral	Low	Oral	GI (diarrhea), B_{12} deficiency
SGLT-2 inhibitors	Intermediate	No	Loss	Benefit (canagliflozin, empagliflozin)	Benefit	Benefit	High	Oral	GU infections, risk of volume depletion, hypotension, amputation, bone fractures, DKA, Fournier's gangrene
GLP-1 RAs	High	No	Loss	Benefit (dulaglutide, liraglutide, SC semaglutide)	Neutral	Benefit on secondary renal endpoints of CVOTs (dulaglutide, liraglutide, SC semaglutide)	High	SC (oral semaglutide)	GI (nausea, vomiting), injection-site reactions, risk of thyroid C-cell tumors, acute pancreatitis
DPP-4 inhibitors	Intermediate	No	Neutral	Neutral	Potential risk: saxagliptin	Neutral	High	Oral	Joint pain, risk of pancreatitis
TZDs	High	No	Gain	Potential benefit (pioglitazone)	Increased risk	Neutral	Low	Oral	Edema, weight gain, risk of heart failure, bone fractures, bladder cancer
SUs	High	Yes	Gain	Neutral	Neutral	Neutral	Low	Oral	Hypoglycemia, weight gain

ASCVD, Atherosclerotic cardiovascular disease; *CVOT*, cardiovascular outcomes trial; *DKA*, diabetic ketoacidosis; *DKD*, diabetic kidney disease; *DPP*, dipeptidyl peptidase; *GI*, gastrointestinal; *GLP*, glucagon-like peptide; *GU*, genitourinary; *HF*, heart failure; *RA*, receptor agonist; *SC*, subcutaneous; *SGLT*, sodium–glucose cotransporter; *SU*, sulfonylurea; *TZD*, thiazolidinecione.

Table 12.3 Dosing Recommendations for Common Oral Medications Used to Treat Type 2 Diabetes

GENERIC NAME	STARTING DOSE	USUAL RECOMMENDED DOSE	MAXIMUM DOSE (MG/DAY)	DOSING/USE IN RENAL INSUFFICIENCY[a]
Biguanides				
Metformin	500 mg once or twice daily or 850 mg once daily, titrate to target dose as tolerated	1000 mg twice daily	2550	Do not initiate if eGFR 30–45 Do not use if eGFR <30
Metformin XR	500–1000 mg once daily, titrate to target dose as tolerated	2000 mg once daily or 1000 mg twice daily	2500	Do not initiate if eGFR 30–45 Do not use if eGFR <30
Sulfonylureas (second generation)				
Glimepiride	1–2 mg once daily (1 mg once daily in older adults)	4 mg once daily	8	Initiate conservatively at 1 mg in renal insufficiency to avoid hypoglycemia
Glipizide	5 mg once daily (2.5 mg daily in older adults)	5–10 mg once daily	40	Initiate conservatively at 2.5 mg in renal insufficiency to avoid hypoglycemia
Glipizide XL	5 mg once daily (2.5 mg once daily in older adults)	5–10 mg once daily	20	Initiate conservatively at 2.5 mg in renal insufficiency to avoid hypoglycemia
Glyburide	2.5–5 mg once daily (1.25 mg once daily in older adults)	5–10 mg once daily	20	Consider alternative agent or initiate conservatively at 1.25 mg in renal insufficiency to avoid hypoglycemia
Glyburide micronized	1.5–3 mg once daily (0.75 mg once daily in older adults)	6 mg once daily	12	Consider alternative agent or initiate conservatively at 0.75 mg in renal insufficiency to avoid hypoglycemia
Thiazolidinediones				
Pioglitazone	15 mg once daily	15–30 mg once daily	45	No dose adjustment required
Rosiglitazone	4 mg once daily or in two divided doses	4 mg once daily or in two divided doses	8	No dose adjustment required
SGLT-2 Inhibitors				
Canagliflozin	100 mg once daily	100–300 mg once daily	300	100 mg once daily if eGFR 45–60[a] Avoid if eGFR <45
Dapagliflozin	5 mg once daily	5–10 mg once daily	10	Avoid if eGFR <60
Empagliflozin	10 mg once daily	10–25 mg once daily	25	Avoid if eGFR <30
Ertugliflozin	5 mg once daily	5–15 mg once daily	15	Avoid if eGFR <60

Continued

Table 12.3 Dosing Recommendations for Common Oral Medications Used to Treat Type 2 Diabetes—cont'd

GENERIC NAME	STARTING DOSE	USUAL RECOMMENDED DOSE	MAXIMUM DOSE (MG/DAY)	DOSING/USE IN RENAL INSUFFICIENCY[a]
DPP-4 inhibitors				
Alogliptin	25 mg once daily	25 mg once daily	25	12.5 mg once daily if CrCl 30–60; 6.25 mg once daily if CrCl <30
Linagliptin	5 mg once daily	5 mg once daily	5	No dose adjustment needed
Saxagliptin	2.5–5 mg once daily	5 mg once daily	5	2.5 mg once daily if eGFR ≤50
Sitagliptin	100 mg once daily	100 mg once daily	100	50 mg once daily if eGFR 30–50 25 mg once daily if eGFR <30

[a]Patients with albuminuria >300 mg/day may continue 100 mg once daily to reduce the risk of end-stage renal disease, doubling of serum creatinine, cardiovascular death, and hospitalization for heart failure.
DPP-4, Dipeptidyl peptidase-4; *eGFR*, estimated glomerular filtration rate; *SGLT-2*, sodium glucose cotransporter 2; *XL*, extended release; *XR*, extended release.

Lastly, the immediate-release dopaminergic agonist bromocriptine also has evidence to support its ability to lower blood glucose by activating central dopamine-2 receptors and increasing insulin sensitivity. Like colesevelam, its effect on A1c lowering is modest. It is not commonly used because of cost and its side-effect profile (dizziness, nausea, fatigue).

6. Which noninsulin medication classes are used to treat type 1 diabetes?
   Many noninsulin medications have been studied as adjuncts to insulin in the treatment of type 1 diabetes (T1D). Pramlintide is an amylin analog and is the only noninsulin agent that is approved by the U.S. Food and Drug Administration (FDA) as adjunctive therapy for T1D. Pramlintide regulates glucose by reducing glucagon secretion, slowing gastric emptying, and increasing satiety. It primarily targets PPG and must be administered before each meal. Randomized controlled trials show modest improvements in A1c, PPG, and weight when pramlintide is added to insulin. Because of the GI side effects (nausea, vomiting, abdominal pain), the potential risk of severe hypoglycemia, modest results, and administration requirements, pramlintide is not widely used. Metformin, GLP-1 receptor agonists, and SGLT-2 inhibitors have also been studied in T1D, with most showing small reductions in weight and A1c. SGLT-2 inhibitor use in T1D is associated with an increased risk of diabetic ketoacidosis (DKA), and therefore close monitoring and education are required. The risks and benefits of adjunctive therapy in T1D continue to be evaluated.

7. Which medications should not be used (or require dose adjustments) in patients with renal dysfunction?
   Metformin should not be initiated in a patient whose estimated glomerular filtration rate (eGFR) is <45 mL/min/1.73 m^2 and should not be used in patients with an eGFR of <30 mL/min/1.73 m^2 because of the increased risk of lactic acidosis. There is a discrepancy with what is recommended for patients currently taking metformin whose eGFR falls below 44 but remains above 30 mL/min/1.73 m^2; the metformin prescribing information states that the benefit of continuing therapy should be reassessed, whereas experts recommend that metformin should be dose-adjusted to a maximum of 500 mg twice daily. The DPP-4 inhibitors alogliptin, saxagliptin, and sitagliptin need to be dose-adjusted for patients with renal dysfunction. Linagliptin is the only DPP-4 inhibitor that does not require renal dose adjustments. These agents may play a role in patients with renal dysfunction–related contraindications to metformin. Glyburide is not recommended in patients with renal dysfunction because of its active metabolite that can accumulate and increase the risk of hypoglycemia. Finally, it is important to recognize that although certain SGLT-2 inhibitors may be used in patients down to an eGFR of 30 mL/min/1.73 m^2, their glucose-lowering ability is significantly diminished at an eGFR of 45 mL/min/1.73 m^2. The renal function of patients receiving exenatide twice daily with a creatinine clearance (CrCl) of 30 to 50 mL/min should be carefully monitored when increasing from 5 to 10 mcg. Exenatide should not be used in patients with a CrCl <30 mL/min. There is limited experience with using liraglutide or dulaglutide in patients with severe renal impairment (CrCl 15–29 mL/min). Patients should not receive lixisenatide with a CrCl of <15 mL/min. The prescribing information for dulaglutide, injectable semaglutide, and oral semaglutide does not make specific recommendations for renal

Table 12.4 Dosing and Administration of GLP-1 Receptor Agonists

	GENERIC NAME	DOSE	INTERVAL	RENAL DOSE/USE	AVAILABILITY, STORAGE, PREPARATION, ADMINISTRATION
Short acting	Exenatide	5–10 mcg	Twice daily (30–60 minutes before breakfast and dinner)	Avoid if eGFR <30	• Multidose pens (5 mcg/dose, 10 mcg/dose, 60 doses per pen) • Pen needles not supplied with pen • Keep refrigerated • After first use, store at room temperature • Discard 30 days after first use
	Lixisenatide	10–20 mcg	Once daily (1 hour before breakfast)	Limited experience in severe renal impairment; avoid if eGFR <15	• Multidose pen (10 mcg, 20 mcg, 14 doses per pen) • Pen needles not supplied with pen • Keep refrigerated • After first use, store at room temperature • Discard 14 days after first use.
Long acting	Dulaglutide	0.75–4.5 mg	Once weekly	Limited experience in severe renal impairment	• Single-dose pen (0.75 mg, 1.5 mg, 3 mg, 4.5 mg) • Pen needle attached • Keep refrigerated • May store at room temperature for 14 days
	Exenatide XR	2 mg	Once weekly	Avoid if eGFR <30	• Single-dose pen (2 mg) • Pen needle supplied with pen • Keep refrigerated; may store at room temperature for 4 weeks • Store flat in original packaging, protected from light • Remove from refrigerator 15 minutes prior to mixing • Requires reconstitution; administer dose immediately once reconstituted
	Liraglutide	0.6–1.8 mg	Once daily	Limited experience in severe renal impairment	• Multidose pen (6 mg/mL, 3 mL; each pen delivers doses of 0.6, 1.2, or 1.8 mg) • Pen needles not supplied with pen • Keep refrigerated • After first use, store at room temperature • Discard 30 days after first use
	Semaglutide	0.25–1 mg	Once weekly	No dose adjustment recommended	• Multidose pen (1.34 mg/mL; 1.5 mL, lower dose pen delivers 0.25 mg or 0.5 mg doses; high dose pen delivers 1 mg dose) • Pen needles supplied with pen • Keep refrigerated • After first use, store at room temperature • Discard 56 days after first use
	Oral semaglutide	3–14 mg	Once daily	No dose adjustment recommended	• Oral tablets (3 mg, 7 mg, 14 mg) • Must be taken 30 minutes before first food, beverage, or other oral medication of the day, with no more than 4 ounces of plain water • Swallow tablets whole; do not crush or chew

eGFR, Estimated glomerular filtration rate; *GLP-1*, glucagon-like peptide-1.

dose adjustment. TZDs do not require dose adjustments in renal dysfunction; however, the American Diabetes Association (ADA) Standards of Medical Care generally do not recommend the use of TZDs in patients with renal dysfunction because of the potential for fluid retention.

8. **What is the impact on weight of the different diabetes medications?**

The ADA Standards of Medical Care recommend that when choosing glucose-lowering medications for patients with T2D who are overweight or obese, the medication's impact on weight should be considered. Medication classes that are known to cause weight loss include GLP-1 receptor agonists and SGLT-2 inhibitors. GLP-1 receptor agonists appear to produce more weight loss than SGLT-2 inhibitors, but both are considered preferred in patients with a compelling need to promote weight loss or minimize weight gain. Within the GLP-1 receptor agonist class, there is significant heterogeneity, with injectable semaglutide offering the greatest weight loss, followed by liraglutide, dulaglutide, exenatide, and lixisenatide. Metformin is considered to be weight neutral, although some studies have shown a small average loss of 2 to 3 kg. DPP-4 inhibitors are weight neutral. Sulfonylureas and TZDs cause weight gain. The average weight gain with sulfonylureas is 1 to 2 kg and 3 to 4 kg with TZDs, but this increases when they are used in combination with insulin. It is important to note that there is also significant heterogeneity in individual patient response. Current practice guidelines point out that patients can gain as much as 10 kg in the first 3 to 6 months of therapy with sulfonylureas, TZDs, or insulin. Conversely, some patients may achieve no weight loss with GLP-1 receptor agonists or SGLT-2 inhibitors, whereas others may lose as much as 25 kg. Most weight loss occurs in the first 3 to 6 months and is sustained over time.

9. **Which medications confer the highest risk of hypoglycemia?**

The noninsulin medications that confer the highest risk of hypoglycemia are the sulfonylureas and meglitinides, both of which are considered insulin "secretagogues." They increase insulin secretion from pancreatic beta cells in a glucose-independent manner, meaning they cause insulin secretion regardless of blood glucose concentrations. Thus, they have a high risk of inadvertently leading to hypoglycemia. All sulfonylureas are capable of producing hypoglycemia. The second-generation sulfonylureas (glyburide, glipizide, and glimepiride) have a lower risk of hypoglycemia than first-generation sulfonylureas; therefore, first-generation agents are rarely used and should be avoided. Within the second-generation agents, glyburide has the highest risk of hypoglycemia, particularly in patients with renal dysfunction, because of its active metabolite that is renally eliminated. Glyburide is identified in the Beers Criteria as a potentially inappropriate medication in patients 65 and older because of the risk of hypoglycemia. Appropriate patient selection, dosage, and patient education are important to minimize hypoglycemic episodes. Hypoglycemia is more likely to occur when calorie intake is deficient, after strenuous or prolonged exercise, when alcohol is ingested, or when sulfonylureas are used in combination with insulin. Patients taking sulfonylureas should be instructed to eat at consistent times and should be educated on the prevention, detection, and treatment of hypoglycemia.

10. **Which agents have evidence of CV benefit in patients with T2D?**

In 2008, the FDA set a requirement that all new drugs developed and studied for the treatment of T2D must undergo CV safety testing. These trials uniformly included patients with existing atherosclerotic CV disease (ASCVD) or indicators of high ASCVD risk and studied a three-point major adverse cardiovascular events (MACE) endpoint, including a composite of CV death, nonfatal myocardial infarction, and nonfatal stroke. In these cardiovascular outcomes trials (CVOTs), dulaglutide, liraglutide, semaglutide injectable, canagliflozin, and empagliflozin have demonstrated beneficial effects on CV outcomes, as demonstrated in Dulaglutide and Cardiovascular Outcomes in Type 2 Diabetes (REWIND), a double-blind, randomized, placebo-controlled trial; Liraglutide Effect and Action in Diabetes: Evaluation of Cardiovascular Outcome Results (LEADER); Trial to Evaluate Cardiovascular and Other Long-Term Outcomes With Semaglutide in Subjects With Type 2 Diabetes (SUSTAIN-6); the Canagliflozin Cardiovascular Assessment Study (CANVAS); and the Empagliflozin Cardiovascular Outcome Event Trial in Type 2 Diabetes Mellitus Patients (EMPA-REG OUTCOME), respectively.

The current ADA Standards of Medical Care endorse the use of a GLP-1 receptor agonist or SGLT-2 inhibitor with proven CV benefit when the patient has established ASCVD or indicators of high ASCVD risk, independent of baseline A1c. The current American Association of Clinical Endocrinologists (AACE) guidelines also advocate for the use of SGLT-2 inhibitors and/or GLP-1 receptor agonists independent of glycemic control if the patient has established ASCVD or high ASCVD risk.

11. **Which agents have evidence of renal benefit in patients with T2D?**

Both SGLT-2 inhibitors and GLP-1 receptor agonists have demonstrated renal benefits in patients with T2D. Mechanistically, SGLT-2 inhibitors decrease intraglomerular pressure and filtration, glucose reabsorption in the renal tubules, weight, blood pressure, albuminuria, oxidative stress, and blunt increases in angiotensinogen and other inflammatory activity. Empagliflozin, canagliflozin, and dapagliflozin are the SGLT-2 inhibitors that have demonstrated renal benefit. Evidence from the Canagliflozin and Renal Outcomes in type 2 Diabetes and Nephropathy (CREDENCE) trial demonstrated that based on beneficial renal effects, canagliflozin may be used in patients with an eGFR down to 30 mL/min/1.73 m^2 when the primary goal is renal protection (not glucose lowering).

The Dapagliflozin in Patients with Chronic Kidney Disease (DAPA-CKD) trial demonstrated renal benefit in patients with CKD, both with and without T2D, who received dapagliflozin.

Because of the stronger primary outcome evidence with SGLT-2 inhibitors, the ADA Standards of Medical Care favor the use of an SGLT-2 inhibitor with proven benefit for patients with T2D and CKD over a GLP-1 receptor agonist. The AACE guidelines further recognize that canagliflozin is preferred for patients with stage 3 CKD. A GLP-1 receptor agonist may be used if additional glucose lowering is needed or if the patient does not tolerate or has a contraindication to an SGLT-2 inhibitor. Dulaglutide, liraglutide, and semaglutide all have demonstrated renal benefit in clinical trials. An advantage of using a GLP-1 receptor agonist over an SGLT-2 inhibitor in patients with T2D and CKD is that they can be administered in patients with more severe renal dysfunction where the use of an SGLT-2 inhibitor may not be as effective for glucose lowering.

12. Which agents have evidence of heart failure benefit in patients with T2D?

There are several SGLT-2 inhibitors with demonstrated benefit in patients with heart failure with reduced ejection fraction (HFrEF). Both empagliflozin and canagliflozin demonstrated in their respective CVOTs that each agent reduced hospitalization for heart failure. The Dapagliflozin in Patients With Heart Failure and Reduced Ejection Fraction (DAPA-HF) trial demonstrated that the use of dapagliflozin in patients with HFrEF, with or without T2D, decreased worsening HF and death from CV causes. Because of these positive data, dapagliflozin is FDA approved in patients with and without T2D who have HFrEF to reduce the risk of CV death and hospitalization from HF. Empagliflozin recently demonstrated similar benefit of reduced hospitalizations for HF and CV death in patients with HFrEF with or without T2D in the Cardiovascular and Renal Outcomes with Empagliflozin in Heart Failure (EMPEROR-Reduced) trial. There are numerous ongoing studies of SGLT-2 inhibitors in patients with and without T2D and comorbid heart failure with preserved ejection fraction (HFpEF).

Both the ADA Standards of Medical Care and the AACE guidelines endorse the use of an SGLT-2 inhibitor with a proven reduction in HF outcomes in patients with T2D and HF. The AACE guidelines further recognize that dapagliflozin is preferred for patients with HFrEF. A GLP-1 receptor agonist may be used if additional glucose lowering is needed or if the patient does not tolerate or has a contraindication to an SGLT-2 inhibitor.

13. Which medication classes should not be used in combination?

Because of their overlapping mechanisms of action, GLP-1 receptor agonists and DPP-4 inhibitors should not be used in combination. Both promote increased circulating GLP-1 and are not likely to demonstrate increased efficacy when used in combination. Similarly, sulfonylureas and meglitinides should not be used in combination. Both are insulin secretagogues and would potentially increase the risk of severe hypoglycemia if used in combination. Consider stopping or decreasing the dose of sulfonylureas and TZDs when starting insulin to minimize the risk of hypoglycemia and weight gain. Although SGLT-2 inhibitors can be used in combination with insulin, special attention should be paid to the increased risk of DKA when using that combination. Patient education and monitoring are needed. Finally, there is a lack of data to support using GLP-1 receptor agonists in combination with rapid-acting insulin. Short-acting GLP-1 receptor agonists, such as twice-daily exenatide and lixisenatide, have a pronounced prandial effect that may be duplicated with the use of rapid-acting insulin or sulfonylureas. If a GLP-1 receptor agonist is initiated in a patient who is on >30 units of rapid-acting insulin, it is recommended that the rapid-acting insulin dose be decreased by approximately 50%. If a patient is on a lower dose of rapid-acting insulin, consideration should be given to stopping it when a GLP-1 receptor agonist is added.

14. What are the relative costs of noninsulin therapies for diabetes?

In general, older oral medications are less expensive than newer oral medications and those that are injectable. The costs of metformin, sulfonylureas, and TZDs are low, whereas the costs of DPP-4 inhibitors, SGLT-2 inhibitors, and GLP-1 receptor agonists (injectable and oral) are high. Alpha-glucosidase inhibitors and meglitinides are also low cost, with the exception of miglitol, which is priced similarly to a DPP-4 inhibitor. Bile acid sequestrants (tablets and powder for suspension) and bromocriptine are also high cost. Cost can be a significant barrier to achieving glucose control. Strategies to overcome cost-related barriers are discussed in more detail in Chapter 27.

KEY POINTS

1. Noninsulin options for the treatment of T2D include metformin, sulfonylureas, thiazolidinediones, GLP-1 receptor agonists, DPP-4 inhibitors, and SGLT-2 inhibitors. The decision of which to add should depend on whether the patient has ASCVD, CKD, or HF, in addition to other patient and drug considerations, such as glycemic efficacy, risk of hypoglycemia, effect on weight, ease of use, mechanism of delivery, cost, and side effects.
2. The most common side effect of metformin is diarrhea. This side effect is usually transient and can be minimized by starting at a low dose (500 mg once daily) and titrating the dose slowly over time to target dose of 2000 mg per day (usually 1000 mg twice daily), taking the medication with food, and using the extended-release formulation.
3. Certain SGLT-2 inhibitors and GLP-1 receptor agonists have beneficial effects in patients with T2D and ASCVD or ASCVD risk. Empagliflozin, canagliflozin, dulaglutide, liraglutide, and semaglutide have demonstrated a reduction in MACE (a composite of CV death, nonfatal myocardial infarction, and nonfatal stroke) in CV outcome trials.
4. Certain SGLT-2 inhibitors and GLP-1 receptor agonists have beneficial effects in patients with T2D and CKD. Both classes can delay the onset of CKD and delay its progression.

5. Certain SGLT-2 inhibitors have beneficial effects in patients with T2D and HF; SGLT-2 inhibitor use in this population may decrease hospitalizations for heart failure and CV death.
6. Many noninsulin therapies for T2D work synergistically when used in combination. However, combinations that duplicate mechanisms of action or increase the risk of hypoglycemia should be avoided.

BIBLIOGRAPHY

American Diabetes Association. 9. Pharmacologic approaches to glycemic treatment: standards of medical care in diabetes – 2021. *Diabetes Care.* 2021;44(Suppl 1):S111–S124.

American Diabetes Association. 8. Obesity management for the treatment of type 2 diabetes: standards of medical care in diabetes – 2021. *Diabetes Care.* 2021;44(Suppl 1):S100–S110.

Apovian CM, Aronne LJ, Bessesen DH, et al. Pharmacological management of obesity: an Endocrine Society clinical practice guideline. *Journal of Clinical Endocrinology & Metabolism.* 2015;100(2):342–362.

Garber AJ, Handelsman Y, Grunberger G, et al. Consensus Statement by the American Association Of Clinical Endocrinologists and American College Of Endocrinology on the Comprehensive Type 2 Diabetes Management Algorithm - 2020 Executive Summary. *Endocr Pract.* 2020;26(1):107–139.

Gerstein HC, Colhoun HM, Dagenais GR, et al. Dulaglutide and cardiovascular outcomes in type 2 diabetes (REWIND): a double-blind, randomised, placebo-controlled trial. *Lancet.* 2019;394(10193):121–130.

Heerspink HJL, Stefansson BV, Correa-Rotter R, et al. Dapagliflozin in patients with chronic kidney disease. *N Engl J Med.* 2020;383(15):1436–1446.

Mann JFE, Brown-Frandsen K, Marso SP, et al. Liraglutide and renal outcomes in type 2 diabetes. *N Engl J Med.* 2017;31:839–848.

Marso SP, Bain SC, Consoli A, et al. Semaglutide and cardiovascular outcomes in patients with type 2 diabetes. *N Engl J Med.* 2016;375:1834–1844.

Marso SP, Daniels GH, Brown-Frandsen K, et al. Liraglutide and cardiovascular outcomes in type 2 diabetes. *N Engl J Med.* 2016;375:311–322.

McMurray JJV, Solomon SD, Inzucchi SE, et al. Dapagliflozin in patients with heart failure and reduced ejection fraction. *N Engl J Med.* 2019;381:1995–2008.

Nauck MA, Meier JJ. Are all GLP-1 agonists equal in the treatment of type 2 diabetes? *European Journal of Endocrinology.* 2019;181(6):R211–R234.

Neal B, Perkovic V, Mahaffey KW, et al. Canagliflozin and cardiovascular and renal events in type 2 diabetes. *N Engl J Med.* 2017;377(7):644–657.

Packer M, Anker SD, Butler J, et al. Cardiovascular and renal outcomes with empagliflozin in heart failure. *N Engl J Med.* 2020;383(15):1413–1424.

Perkovic V, Jardine MJ, Neal B, et al. Canagliflozin and renal outcomes in type 2 diabetes and nephropathy. *N Engl J Med.* 2019;380(24):2295–2306.

Tuttle KR, Lakshmanan MC, Rayner B, et al. Dulaglutide versus insulin glargine in patients with type 2 diabetes and moderate-to-severe chronic kidney disease (AWARD-7): a multicentre, open-label, randomised trial. *Lancet Diabetes Endocrinol.* 2018;6(8):605–617.

UK Prospective Diabetes Study (UKPDS) Group. Effect of intensive blood-glucose control with metformin on complications in overweight patients with type 2 diabetes (UKPDS 34). *Lancet.* 1998;352:854–865.

UK Prospective Diabetes Study (UKPDS) Group. Intensive blood-glucose control with sulfonylureas or insulin compared with conventional treatment and risk of complications in patients with type 2 diabetes (UKPDS 33). *Lancet.* 1998;352:837–853.

Wanner C, Inzucchi SE, Lachin JM, et al. Empagliflozin and progression of kidney disease in type 2 diabetes. *N Engl J Med.* 2016 Jul 28;375(4):323–334.

Wiviott SD, Raz I, Bonaca MP, et al. Dapagliflozin and cardiovascular outcomes in type 2 diabetes. *N Engl J Med.* 2018;380:347–357.

Zinman B, Wanner C, Lachin JM, et al. Empagliflozin, cardiovascular outcomes, and mortality in type 2 diabetes. *N Engl J Med.* 2015;373:2117–2128.

CARBOHYDRATE COUNTING AND PRECISE INSULIN DOSING

Michael T. McDermott, MD

1. **Define and explain the carbohydrate-to-insulin (C:I) ratio**
   The C:I ratio is an estimate of the grams of carbohydrate that will be covered by each 1 unit of insulin. A C:I ratio of X:1 means that 1 unit of insulin should be given for each X grams of carbohydrate to be consumed. The initial C:I ratio for each person is usually calculated as follows: 500/Total daily dose (TDD) of insulin. The C:I ratio must then be evaluated and adjusted to achieve optimal preprandial to postprandial blood glucose (BG) excursions (optimal: 30- to 50-mg/dL rise from premeal to 2 hours postmeal).

2. **How do you determine if the current C:I ratio is correct?**
   We test the accuracy of each person's C:I ratio with the following protocol:
   A. Preparation for the test meal: consume something that is easily covered at the meal prior to the test meal so that the glucose level immediately before the test meal is in the target range and does not require a correction dose. If glucose prior to the test meal is <70 mg/dL or >140 mg/dL, don't proceed with the test.
   B. If the glucose just before the test meal is in the desired range (70–140 mg/dL), eat a meal that has a well-known carbohydrate content and less than 20 g of fat.
   C. Test your glucose level just before the test meal, take the insulin dose calculated from your C:I ratio, and recheck your glucose 2 hours after the test meal; calculate the prepost glucose excursion. The glucose excursion from premeal to 2 hours postmeal should be about 30 to 50 mg/dL.
   D. If the rise is >50 mg/dL, the C:I ratio should be strengthened; if the rise is <30 mg/dL, the C:I ratio should be weakened.

3. **What is a high-BG correction factor (CF)?**
   A CF is an estimate of the BG drop expected for each 1 unit of insulin given when BG is elevated above the goal. A CF of N:1 means that 1 unit of insulin will drop the BG N mg/dL; therefore, a person will give 1 unit of insulin for every N mg/dL the current BG level is above the BG target. We calculate an initial CF as 1650/TDD (some providers use 1800/TDD, 1700/TDD, or 1500/TDD). The initial CF must then be evaluated and adjusted to achieve appropriate reductions of high BG to the target range by 4 hours after the dose is given.

4. **How do you calculate and use the insulin bolus on board (BOB) and duration of insulin action (DIA) estimates?**
   BOB and *IOB* are similar terms used to indicate how much insulin is still active after the last rapid-acting insulin bolus; I will use the term *BOB* here. *Duration of insulin action (DIA)* and *active insulin time (AIT)* are similar terms used to indicate how long an insulin bolus lasts for an individual; I will use the term *DIA* here. DIA is often ~4 hours, but some people consider their DIA to be shorter (~3 hours) or longer (~5 hours) based on their own experience.
   To calculate the BOB, use the previous bolus dose and subtract from that the same dose multiplied by the time elapsed since that bolus, divided by the DIA. The formula is therefore: BOB = Bolus – Bolus × (Elapsed time since bolus/DIA). Example: If a 6-unit bolus was taken 2 hours ago and the DIA is 4 hours, the BOB is 3 units (6 – 6 × [2/4] = 3). When a person plans to take a high-BG correction dose, the BOB should be subtracted from the planned correction dose.

5. **Do people who take basal-bolus insulin need to do these calculations before every meal and correction dose?**
   People who administer insulin by multiple daily injections (MDIs) should be very familiar with their C:I ratio and CF and use them to calculate every meal bolus and correction bolus. Insulin pumps automatically calculate the necessary insulin dose for the carbohydrate content, the correction dose, and the BOB and display the recommended dose of insulin. In either case, accurate carbohydrate counting is essential.

6. **Explain what additional information is provided by a continuous glucose monitor (CGM)**
   A CGM is a subcutaneous device that measures interstitial glucose every 3 to 5 minutes and displays it real time or intermittently. A person sees the current glucose value along with a trend arrow to indicate the direction glucose is going (trend). CGM will be discussed in more depth in a subsequent chapter.

7. **What basic carbohydrate-counting skills should every patient with diabetes and their providers know?**

   Carbohydrate counting is usually taught by a Certified Diabetes Care and Education Specialist (CDCES). However, all providers involved in managing people with diabetes on insulin regimens should be familiar with the basics of carbohydrate counting. Table 13.1 is useful as an introduction to the basics of carbohydrate counting and for the practice cases presented later in this chapter.

8. **Practice with carbohydrate counting and precise insulin dosing**

   Let's work through some cases. Table 13.1 lists the estimated carbohydrate contents for the common meals presented here. Note that in these cases, people taking MDI injections will round their insulin doses to the nearest whole digit, whereas those using insulin pump therapy can give fractional doses if needed.

Table 13.1 Carbohydrate-Counting Basics

15-Gram (g) Carbohydrate Servings (60 kcal of carbohydrate)
1 slice of bread = 15 g carbohydrate
1 small roll = 15 g carbohydrate
1 small potato (3 oz) = 15 g carbohydrate
½ cup of mashed potatoes = 15 g carbohydrate
½ cup of corn = 15 g carbohydrate
½ cup of peas = 15 g carbohydrate
⅓ cup of cooked rice = 15 g carbohydrate
⅓ cup of cooked pasta = 15 g carbohydrate
1 medium apple = 15 g carbohydrate
½ of a 6-inch banana = 15 g carbohydrate
2 Oreos = 15 g carbohydrate
2 × 2-inch unfrosted cake = 15 g carbohydrate
½ cup (4 oz) of fruit juice = 15 g carbohydrate
1.25 cup (10 oz) of milk = 15 g carbohydrate
1.5 cup (12 oz) regular beer or nonalcoholic beer = 15 g carbohydrate

30-Gram (g) Carbohydrate Servings (120 kcal of carbohydrate)
1 medium potato (6 oz) = 30 g carbohydrate
1 cup of mashed potatoes = 30 g carbohydrate
1 cup of corn = 30 g carbohydrate
1 cup of peas = 30 g carbohydrate
⅔ cup of cooked rice = 30 g carbohydrate
⅔ cup of cooked pasta = 30 g carbohydrate
1 6-inch banana = 30 g carbohydrate
4 Oreos = 30 g carbohydrate
1 cup (8 oz) wine cooler = 30 g carbohydrate
1.5 cup (12 oz) microbrew beer = 30 g carbohydrate
½ cup (4 oz) margarita = 30 g carbohydrate
½ cup (4 oz) daiquiri = 30 g carbohydrate

45-Gram (g) Carbohydrate Servings (180 kcal of carbohydrate)
1 cup of cooked rice = 45 g carbohydrate
1 cup of cooked pasta = 45 g carbohydrate
6 Oreos = 45 g carbohydrate

Other Gram (g) Carbohydrate Servings (1 g carbohydrate = 4 kcal)
1 small corn tortilla = 10 g carbohydrate
1 cup (8 oz) milk = 12 g carbohydrate
1 can (12 oz) regular soda = 40 g carbohydrate
1 bottle (20 oz) regular soda = 75 g carbohydrate
1 teaspoon sugar (5 mL) = 4 g carbohydrate
1 tablespoon sugar (15 mL) = 12 g carbohydrate
1 teaspoon honey (5 mL) = 5 g carbohydrate
1 tablespoon honey (15 mL) = 15 g carbohydrate

CASE 1

Victor has type 1 diabetes mellitus and manages this with MDIs as follows:
    Basal insulin: 32 units daily
    Bolus insulin: C:I ratio = 10:1, CF = 40:1, BG target = 100 mg/dL
    Premeal BG = 180 mg/dL

Planned meal:
Ham sandwich
Medium apple
Oreo cookies—2
Milk—1 cup

How many grams of carbohydrate does this meal contain?	_____ grams
How much insulin will be needed to cover the carbohydrates?	_____ units
How much insulin will be needed to correct the premeal glucose?	_____ units
What total dose of insulin should be taken?	_____ units

CASE 2

Hayley has type 1 diabetes mellitus and manages this with an insulin pump as follows:
    Basal insulin: 28 units daily
    Bolus insulin: C:I ratio = 12:1, CF = 45:1, BG target = 100 mg/dL
    Premeal BG = 235 mg/dL

Planned meal:
Small corn tortilla
Cooked rice—⅓ cup
Fruit juice—1 cup
Banana—6-inch portion

How many grams of carbohydrate does this meal contain?	_____ grams
How much insulin will be needed to cover the carbohydrates?	_____ units
How much insulin will be needed to correct the premeal glucose?	_____ units
What total dose of insulin should be taken?	_____ units

CASE 3

Chloe has type 1 diabetes mellitus and manages this with MDIs as follows:
    Basal insulin: 18 units daily
    Bolus insulin: C:I ratio = 15:1, CF = 50:1, BG target = 120 mg/dL
    Premeal BG = 220 mg/dL

Planned meal:
Cooked pasta—1 cup
Peas—½ cup
Small roll
Wine cooler

How many grams of carbohydrate does this meal contain?	_____ grams
How much insulin will be needed to cover the carbohydrates?	_____ units
How much insulin will be needed to correct the premeal glucose?	_____ units
What total dose of insulin should be taken?	_____ units

CASE 4

Mac has type 2 diabetes mellitus and manages this with MDIs as follows:
    Basal insulin: 36 units daily
    Bolus insulin: C:I ratio = 8:1, CF = 25:1, BG target = 100 mg/dL
    Premeal BG = 175 mg/dL

Planned meal:
Eggs, scrambled—2
Toast—2 slices
Honey—1 teaspoon on each piece of toast
Fruit juice—1 cup

How many grams of carbohydrate does this meal contain?   _____ grams
How much insulin will be needed to cover the carbohydrates?   _____ units
How much insulin will be needed to correct the premeal glucose? _____ units
What total dose of insulin should be taken?   _____ units

CASE 5

Gene has type 1 diabetes mellitus and manages this with an insulin pump as follows:
    Basal insulin: 32 units daily
    Bolus insulin: C:I ratio = 10:1, CF = 35:1, BG target = 110 mg/dL
    Premeal BG = 180 mg/dL

    Planned meal:
    Beef—6 oz.
    Baked potato—medium
    Corn—½ cup
    Microbrew beer—one
    Regular beer—one

How many grams of carbohydrate does this meal contain?   _____ grams
How much insulin will be needed to cover the carbohydrates?   _____ units
How much insulin will be needed to correct the premeal glucose? _____ units
What total dose of insulin should be taken?   _____ units

CASE 6

Katy has type 1 diabetes mellitus and manages this with an insulin pump as follows:
    Basal insulin: 22 units daily
    Bolus insulin: C:I ratio = 15:1, CF = 50:1, BG target = 120 mg/dL
    Premeal BG = 195 mg/dL

    Planned meal:
    Grilled cheese sandwich
    Mashed potatoes—1 cup
    Banana—6-inch portion
    Regular soda—12 oz

How many grams of carbohydrate does this meal contain?   _____ grams
How much insulin will be needed to cover the carbohydrates?   _____ units
How much insulin will be needed to correct the premeal glucose? _____ units
What total dose of insulin should be taken?   _____ units

CASE 7

Emily has type 2 diabetes mellitus and manages this with MDIs as follows:
    Basal insulin: 38 units daily
    Bolus insulin: C:I ratio = 8:1, CF = 25:1, BG target = 110 mg/dL
    Premeal BG = 210 mg/dL

    Planned meal:
    Eggs, fried—2
    Bacon—2 slices
    French toast—2 slices
    Banana, sliced—3-inch portion
    Powdered sugar—1 teaspoon
    Tea with honey—1 teaspoon

How many grams of carbohydrate does this meal contain?   _____ grams
How much insulin will be needed to cover the carbohydrates?   _____ units
How much insulin will be needed to correct the premeal glucose? _____ units
What total dose of insulin should be taken?   _____ units

CASE 8

Leonard has type 1 diabetes mellitus and manages this with an insulin pump as follows:
    Basal insulin: 26 units daily
    Bolus insulin: C:I ratio = 12:1, CF = 40:1, BG target = 100 mg/dL
    Premeal BG = 200 mg/dL

    Planned meal:
    Baked chicken— 2 pieces
    Mashed potatoes—1 cup
    Peas—1 cup
    Milk—1 cup

How many grams of carbohydrate does this meal contain?	_____ grams
How much insulin will be needed to cover the carbohydrates?	_____ units
How much insulin will be needed to correct the premeal glucose?	_____ units
What total dose of insulin should be taken?	_____ units

CASE 9

Sonja has type 1 diabetes mellitus and manages this with an insulin pump as follows:
    Basal insulin: 24 units daily
    Bolus insulin: C:I ratio = 15:1, CF = 60:1, BG target = 110 mg/dL
    Premeal BG = 200 mg/dL

    Planned meal (Friday night):
    Beef—8 oz
    Corn tortillas, small—3
    Rice—⅔ cup
    Margarita—8 oz

How many grams of carbohydrate does this meal contain?	_____ grams
How much insulin will be needed to cover the carbohydrates?	_____ units
How much insulin will be needed to correct the premeal glucose?	_____ units
What total dose of insulin should be taken?	_____ units

CASE 10

Henry has type 2 diabetes mellitus and manages this with MDIs as follows:
    Basal insulin: 42 units daily
    Bolus insulin: C:I ratio = 8:1, CF = 30:1, BG target = 120 mg/dL
    Presnack BG = 210 mg/dL (4 hours after lunch)

    Planned snack:
    Oreo cookies—4
    Milk—1 cup

How many grams of carbohydrate does this meal contain?	_____ grams
How much insulin will be needed to cover the carbohydrates?	_____ units
How much insulin will be needed to correct the premeal glucose?	_____ units
What total dose of insulin should be taken?	_____ units

9. Here are my answers. Yours may be slightly different if you disagree with the carbohydrate contents I have listed. This is OK as long as you follow sound principles of carbohydrate counting and do accurate math

CASE 1

Victor has type 1 diabetes mellitus and manages this with MDIs as follows:
    Basal insulin: 32 units daily
    Bolus insulin: C:I ratio = 10:1, CF = 40:1, BG target = 100 mg/dL
    Premeal BG = 180 mg/dL

Planned meal:
Ham sandwich (30 g)
Medium apple (15 g)
Oreo cookies—2 (15 g)
Milk—1 cup (12 g)

How many grams of carbohydrate does this meal contain?	72 grams
How much insulin will be needed to cover the carbohydrates?	7 units
How much insulin will be needed to correct the premeal glucose?	2 units
What total dose of insulin should be taken?	9 units

CASE 2

Hayley has type 1 diabetes mellitus and manages this with an insulin pump as follows:
Basal insulin: 28 units daily
Bolus insulin: C:I ratio = 12:1, CF = 45:1, BG target = 100 mg/dL
Premeal BG = 235 mg/dL

Planned meal:
Small corn tortilla (10 g)
Cooked rice—⅓ cup (15 g)
Fruit juice—1 cup (30 g)
Banana—6-inch portion (30 g)

How many grams of carbohydrate does this meal contain?	85 grams
How much insulin will be needed to cover the carbohydrates?	7.1 units
How much insulin will be needed to correct the premeal glucose?	3 units
What total dose of insulin should be taken?	10.1 units

CASE 3

Chloe has type 1 diabetes mellitus and manages this with MDIs as follows:
Basal insulin: 18 units daily
Bolus insulin: C:I ratio = 15:1, CF = 50:1, BG target = 120 mg/dL
Premeal BG = 220 mg/dL

Planned meal:
Cooked pasta—1 cup (45 g)
Peas—½ cup (15 g)
Small roll (15 g)
Wine cooler (30 g)

How many grams of carbohydrate does this meal contain?	105 grams
How much insulin will be needed to cover the carbohydrates?	7 units
How much insulin will be needed to correct the premeal glucose?	2 units
What total dose of insulin should be taken?	9 units

CASE 4

Mac has type 2 diabetes mellitus and manages this with MDIs as follows:
Basal insulin: 36 units daily
Bolus insulin: C:I ratio = 8:1, CF = 25:1, BG target = 100 mg/dL
Premeal BG = 175 mg/dL

Planned meal:
Eggs, scrambled—2 (0 g)
Toast—2 slices (30 g)
Honey—1 teaspoon on each piece of toast (10 g)
Fruit juice —1 cup (30 g)

How many grams of carbohydrate does this meal contain?	70 grams
How much insulin will be needed to cover the carbohydrates?	9 units
How much insulin will be needed to correct the premeal glucose?	3 units
What total dose of insulin should be taken?	<u>12 units</u>

CASE 5

Gene has type 1 diabetes mellitus and manages this with an insulin pump as follows:
    Basal insulin: 32 units daily
    Bolus insulin: C:I ratio = 10:1, CF = 35:1, BG target = 110 mg/dL
    Premeal BG = 180 mg/dL

    <u>Planned meal:</u>
    Beef—6 oz. (0 g)
    Baked potato—medium (30 g)
    Corn—½ cup (15 grams)
    Microbrew beer—one (30 g)
    Regular beer—one (15 g)

How many grams of carbohydrate does this meal contain?	90 grams
How much insulin will be needed to cover the carbohydrates?	9 units
How much insulin will be needed to correct the premeal glucose?	2 units
What total dose of insulin should be taken?	<u>11 units</u>

CASE 6

Katy has type 1 diabetes mellitus and manages this with an insulin pump as follows:
    Basal insulin: 22 units daily Bolus insulin: C:I ratio = 15:1, CF = 50:1, BG Target = 120 mg/dL
    Premeal BG = 195 mg/dL

    <u>Planned meal:</u>
    Grilled cheese sandwich (30 g)
    Mashed potatoes—1 cup (30 g)
    Banana—6-inch portion (30 g)
    Regular soda—12 oz (40 g)

How many grams of carbohydrate does this meal contain?	130 grams
How much insulin will be needed to cover the carbohydrates?	8.7 units
How much insulin will be needed to correct the premeal glucose?	1.5 units
What total dose of insulin should be taken?	<u>10.2 units</u>

CASE 7

Emily has type 2 diabetes mellitus and manages this with MDIs as follows:
    Basal insulin: 38 units daily
    Bolus insulin: C:I ratio = 8:1, CF = 25:1, BG target = 110 mg/dL
    Premeal BG = 210 mg/dL

    <u>Planned Meal:</u>
    Eggs, fried—2 (0 g)
    Bacon—2 slices (0 g)
    French toast—2 slices (30 g)
    Banana, sliced—3-inch portion (15 g)
    Powdered sugar—1 teaspoon (4 g)
    Tea with honey—1 teaspoon (5 g)

How many grams of carbohydrate does this meal contain?	54 grams
How much insulin will be needed to cover the carbohydrates?	7 units
How much insulin will be needed to correct the premeal glucose?	4 units
What total dose of insulin should be taken?	<u>11 units</u>

CASE 8

Leonard has type 1 diabetes mellitus and manages this with an insulin pump as follows:
    Basal insulin: 26 units daily
    Bolus insulin: C:I ratio = 12:1, CF = 40:1, BG target = 100 mg/dL
    Premeal BG = 200 mg/dL

    Planned meal:
    Baked chicken—2 pieces (0 g)
    Mashed potatoes—1 cup (30 g)
    Peas—1 cup (30 g)
    Milk—1 cup (12 g)

How many grams of carbohydrate does this meal contain?	72 grams
How much insulin will be needed to cover the carbohydrates?	6 units
How much insulin will be needed to correct the premeal glucose?	2.5 units
What total dose of insulin should be taken?	8.5 units

CASE 9

Sonja has type 1 diabetes mellitus and manages this with an insulin pump as follows:
    Basal insulin: 24 units daily
    Bolus insulin: C:I ratio = 15:1, CF = 60:1, BG target = 110 mg/dL
    Premeal BG = 200 mg/dL

    Planned meal (Friday night):
    Beef—8 oz. (0 g)
    Corn tortillas, small—3 (30 g)
    Rice—⅔ cup (30 g)
    Margarita—8 oz (60 g)

How many grams of carbohydrate does this meal contain?	120 grams
How much insulin will be needed to cover the carbohydrates?	8 units
How much insulin will be needed to correct the premeal glucose?	1.5 units
What total dose of insulin should be taken?	9.5 units

CASE 10

Henry has type 2 diabetes mellitus and manages this with MDIs as follows:
    Basal insulin: 42 units daily
    Bolus insulin: C:I ratio = 8:1, CF = 30:1, BG target = 120 mg/dL
    Presnack BG = 210 mg/dL (4 hours after lunch)

    Planned snack:
    Oreo cookies—4 (30 g)
    Milk—1 cup (12 g)

How many grams of carbohydrate does this meal contain?	42 grams
How much insulin will be needed to cover the carbohydrates?	5 units
How much insulin will be needed to correct the premeal glucose?	3 units
What total dose of insulin should be taken?	8 units

10. **How do you assess if your patients are counting their carbohydrates accurately?**
There are numerous carbohydrate-counting quizzes and other assessment tools available on the Internet that patients and providers can use to assess and improve their carbohydrate-counting skills. The following quiz is adapted from one used at the Cleveland Clinic. Try it.

University of Colorado Hospital Carbohydrate Counting Quiz

NAME: _____   DATE: _____

FOOD	DOES THIS FOOD CONTAIN CARBOHYDRATES? (CIRCLE ONLY ONE ANSWER)		
1. Bread	Yes	No	Don't Know
2. Breakfast Sausages	Yes	No	Don't Know
3. Baked Potato	Yes	No	Don't Know
4. Maple Syrup, Regular	Yes	No	Don't Know
5. American Cheese	Yes	No	Don't Know
6. Low-Fat Milk	Yes	No	Don't Know
7. Apple Juice	Yes	No	Don't Know
8. Soda Pop (not diet)	Yes	No	Don't Know
9. Apple	Yes	No	Don't Know
10. Cooked Dried Beans (Lentils, Navy Beans)	Yes	No	Don't Know

FOOD	HOW MANY GRAMS OF CARBOHYDRATE DOES THIS PORTION CONTAIN? (CIRCLE ONE.)						
11. 1 cup milk	0 g	15 g	30 g	45 g	60 g	75 g	Don't Know
12. 1 cup pasta	0 g	15 g	30 g	45 g	60 g	75 g	Don't Know
13. 1 cup Cooked Rice	0 g	15 g	30 g	45 g	60 g	75 g	Don't Know
14. 1 cup Juice	0 g	15 g	30 g	45 g	60 g	75 g	Don't Know
15. 1 cup Hot Cereal	0 g	15 g	30 g	45 g	60 g	75 g	Don't Know
16. 1 cup Cooked Dried Beans	0 g	15 g	30 g	45 g	60 g	75 g	Don't Know
17. 1 cup Mashed Potatoes	0 g	15 g	30 g	45 g	60 g	75 g	Don't Know

For each question circle the best answer below.

18. Read the Nutrition Facts label to the right. What is the serving size?

Don't know   1 cup   2 cups   4 cups

19. How many grams of carbohydrate would you consume if you ate 1 serving?

Don't know   228 g   5 g   31 g

20. How many grams of carbohydrate would you consume if you ate the whole package?

Don't know   456 g   10 g   62 g

Number of correct answers: _____

Percent correct answers: _____% (Number correct/20 × 100)

Answers:

1. Yes	2. No	3. Yes	4. Yes	5. No
6. Yes	7. Yes	8. Yes	9. Yes	10. Yes
11. 15g	12. 30g	13. 45g	14. 30g	15. 30g
16. 30g	17. 30g	18. 1 cup	19. 31g	20. 62g

Nutrition Facts

Serving Size cup (228g)

Serving Per Container 2

Amount Per serving

Calories 260 Calories fromFat 120

	% Daily Value*
Total Fat 13g	20%
Saturated Fat 5g	25%
Cholesterol 30mg	10%
Sodium 660mg	28%
Total Carbohydrate 31g	10%
Dietary Fiber 0g	0%
Sugar 5g	
Protein 5g	

Vitamin A 4%	•	Vitamin C 2%	
Calcium 15%	•	Iron 4%	

* Percent daily values are based on a 2,000 calorie diet. Your daily values may be higher or lower depending on your calorie needs:

		Calories:	2,000	2,500
Total Fat	Less than		65g	80g
Sat Fat	Less than		20g	25g
Cholesterol	Less than		300mg	300mg
Sodium	Less than		2400mg	2400mg
Total Carbohydrate			300g	375g
Dietary Fiber			25g	30g

Caloies per gram:

Fat 9 • Carbohydrate 4 • Protein 4

KEY POINTS

1. Precise mealtime insulin dosing requires accurate carbohydrate counting and an appropriate C:I ratio that produces a premeal to 2-hour postmeal BG excursion of 30 to 50 mg/dL.
2. The C:I ratio is an estimate of the grams of carbohydrate that each 1 unit of insulin will cover; a C:I ratio of X:1 means that 1 unit of insulin should be given for each X grams of carbohydrate to be consumed. The initial C:I ratio for each person is often calculated as follows: 500/TDD of insulin.
3. A CF is the amount of insulin that should be added to the mealtime dose when the premeal BG is above the target range or that is taken between meals to correct high-BG values. The CF is an estimate of the expected BG drop for each 1 unit of insulin given when the BG is elevated above the goal; a CF of N:1 means that a person should take 1 unit of insulin for every N mg/dL the current BG level is above the individualized target. We calculate an initial CF for each person as 1650/TDD.

BIBLIOGRAPHY

Aleppo G, Laffel LM, Ahmann AJ, et al. A practical approach to using trend arrows on the Dexcom G5 CGM System for the management of adults with diabetes. *J Endocr Soc.* 2017 Nov 20;1(12):1445–1460.

Bell KJ, Fio CZ, Twigg S, et al. Amount and type of dietary fat, postprandial glycemia, and insulin requirements in Type 1 Diabetes: a randomized, within-subject trial. *Diabetes Care.* 2020;43:59–66.

Elleri D, Allen JM, Harris J, et al. Absorption patterns of meals containing complex carbohydrates in type 1 diabetes. *Diabetologia.* 2013 May;56(5):1108–1117.

Kudva YC, Ahmann AJ, Bergenstal RM, et al. Approach to using trend arrows in the FreeStyle Libre flash glucose monitoring systems in adults. *J Endocr Soc.* 2018 Nov 14;2(12):1320–1337.

Laffel LM, Aleppo G, Buckingham BA, et al. A practical approach to using trend arrows on the Dexcom G5 CGM System to manage children and adolescents with diabetes. *J Endocr Soc.* 2017 Nov 20;1(12):1461–1476.

Smart CEM, King BR, Lopez PE. Insulin dosing for fat and protein: it is time? *Diabetes Care.* 2020;43:13–15.

Walsh J., Roberts R. *Pumping Insulin* 3rd Ed, Torrey Pines Press, San Diego 2000.

The Diabetes Carbohydrate and Fat Gram Guide. 4th Edition. Publisher, American Diabetes Association.

Warshaw HS, Bolderman KM. Practical carbohydrate counting: a how-to-teach guide for health professionals. American Diabetes Association, Arlington, VA, 2008.

APPS

Calorie Count: www.caloriecount.com/apps
Calorie King: www.calorieking.com/foods
Dbees: www.dbees.com
Diabetes App:
https://itunes.apple.com/us/app/diabetes-app-blood-sugar-control/id387128141?mt=8
Diabetes Pilot: http://www.diabetespilot.com/
Diabetic Connect: http://www.diabeticconnect.com/
Figwee: https://itunes.apple.com/us/app/figwee-portion-explorer/id435839234?mt=8
Fit Day: www.fitday.com
Fooducate: https://play.google.com/store/apps/details?id=com.fooducate.nutritionapp&hl=en
Glooko: https://www.glooko.com/
Glucool Diabetes: https://play.google.com/store/apps/details?id=com.michaelfester.glucool.lite
Glucose Buddy: www.glucosebuddy.com
GoMeals: www.gomeals.com
My Fitness Pal: www.myfitnesspal.com/
OnTrack Diabetes: https://play.google.com/store/apps/details?id=com.gexperts.ontrack
Spark People: www.sparkpeople.com
WaveSense Diabetes Manager: http://wavesense-diabetes-manager.appsios.net/

TYPE 2 DIABETES MANAGEMENT: SELECTING GLYCEMIC TARGETS AND CHOOSING THE RIGHT THERAPY

CHAPTER 14

Joshua J. Neumiller, PharmD, CDCES, FADCES, FASCP

1. **What are the general glycemic targets for people with type 2 diabetes?**
   Generally recommended glycemic targets for people with type 2 diabetes vary slightly by organization. In terms of hemoglobin A1c recommendations, the American Association of Clinical Endocrinologists (AACE)/American College of Endocrinology (ACE) recommend an optimal A1c goal of ≤6.5% if it can be achieved safely and without undue financial burden. The American Diabetes Association (ADA) is a bit more conservative, with a recommended general A1c goal of <7.0% for many nonpregnant adults. Table 14.1 provides a summary of glycemic targets recommended by the ADA. Although the AACE/ACE and ADA recommend general glycemic targets for people with diabetes, both organizations stress the importance of individualizing glycemic targets based on patient-specific considerations.

2. **When is it appropriate to set less stringent glycemic targets?**
   Both the ADA and AACE/ACE stress the importance of individualizing glycemic targets based on patient-specific considerations that may affect the risks and benefits of intensified therapy. Table 14.2 outlines key factors that may support the establishment of less stringent glycemic goals in people with type 2 diabetes. Notably, a severe hypoglycemic episode and/or frequent hypoglycemia should trigger reevaluation of current glycemic targets and the current treatment strategy. Depending on the situation, targeting a higher A1c or switching to glucose-lowering medications with a lower hypoglycemia risk may be appropriate.

3. **What is the recommended first-line treatment for people with type 2 diabetes?**
   The ADA recommends metformin and comprehensive lifestyle management (including interventions to manage weight and increase physical activity) as first-line therapy for people with type 2 diabetes. Metformin does require dose up-titration to minimize gastrointestinal adverse events, and the response to therapy should be reassessed every 3 to 6 months to avoid clinical inertia. For patients who cannot tolerate metformin or have a contraindication to use, an agent from another class of medications can be chosen based on patient- and medication-specific considerations.

4. **How long should metformin be used in people with type 2 diabetes?**
   Metformin is generally continued in patients with type 2 diabetes as long as they tolerate the medication and do not develop a contraindication (e.g., the development of chronic kidney disease with an estimated glomerular filtration rate [eGFR] of <30 mL/min/1.73 m^2). Metformin can be continued in combination with all other glucose-lowering medications, including insulin.

5. **Is initial combination therapy ever appropriate in people with type 2 diabetes?**
   The ADA states that initial combination therapy can be considered to extend the time to treatment failure in select patients with type 2 diabetes, with many patients requiring dual combination therapy to achieve glycemic goals when A1c is ≥1.5% above their individualized goal. The AACE/ACE guidance gives strong support to initial combination therapy, with initial dual combination therapy generally recommended for patients presenting with an A1c of ≥7.5% to 9.0%. The decision to start a patient on initial combination therapy or not, and which medications will be used, is dependent on a variety of factors, including the presence of vascular comorbidities, cost, and other patient-specific considerations.

6. **When is the early use of insulin therapy appropriate for people with type 2 diabetes?**
   Early use of insulin should be considered in any patients with type 2 diabetes who have severe hyperglycemia or when barriers to the use of alternative glucose-lowering agents are present. The ADA recommends initiating insulin in patients with type 2 diabetes presenting with a blood glucose of ≥300 mg/dL, an A1c of >10%, and/or if the patient is experiencing symptoms of overt hyperglycemia (e.g., polyuria and/or polydipsia) or recent weight loss. After glycemia is better controlled with insulin, the regimen can often be simplified once glucose toxicity resolves. Regimen simplification can include simplification of the insulin regimen or full conversion to an oral glucose-lowering regimen in some patients.

Table 14.1 Recommended Glycemic Targets for Many Nonpregnant Adults With Diabetes	
A1c	<7.0%[a]
Preprandial (premeal) glucose	80–130 mg/dL[a]
Postprandial (1–2 hours after the meal) glucose	<180 mg/dL[a]

[a]Goals should be individualized based on patient-specific considerations.
Adapted from American Diabetes Association. 6. Glycemic targets: Standards of Medical Care in Diabetes—2021. *Diabetes Care.* 2021;44(Suppl 1):S73–S84.

Table 14.2 Factors That May Support Setting Less Stringent Glycemic Targets in People With Type 2 Diabetes
• High risk or concern for hypoglycemia or other drug side effects
• Long duration of diabetes
• Short life expectancy (long-term benefits of a more intensive goal will likely not be realized)
• High comorbidity/complications burden
• Patient preference for a less intensive/burdensome treatment approach
• Limited resources and/or support systems

Adapted from American Diabetes Association. 6. Glycemic targets: Standards of Medical Care in Diabetes—2021. *Diabetes Care.* 2021;44(Suppl 1):S73–S84.

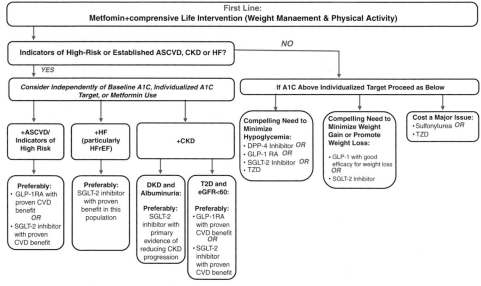

Fig. 14.1 American Diabetes Association recommendations for overall approach to use of glucose-lowering medications in type 2 diabetes. *A1c,* hemoglobin A1c; *ASCVD,* atherosclerotic cardiovascular disease; *CKD,* chronic kidney disease; *CVD,* cardiovascular disease; *eGFR,* estimated glomerular filtration rate; *HF,* heart failure; *TZD,* thiazolidinedione. (Adapted from American Diabetes Association. 9. Pharmacologic approaches to glycemic treatment: Standards of Medical Care in Diabetes—2021. *Diabetes Care.* 2021;44[Suppl 1]:S111–S124.)

7. **Are additional glucose-lowering medications only added to metformin in response to an elevated A1c?**

   No, guidelines now recommend the addition of specific glucose-lowering medications to manage comorbidities even when the A1c is at or below goal. Based on findings from recent large cardiovascular and kidney outcome studies, the use of glucagon-like peptide-1 (GLP-1) receptor agonists and sodium–glucose cotransporter 2 (SGLT-2) inhibitors with proven cardiovascular and/or kidney benefits is recommended in high-risk patients with type 2 diabetes. The addition of these medications to mitigate cardiovascular and kidney risk is recommended in appropriate patients irrespective of their current A1c or individualized A1c target (Fig. 14.1).

Table 14.3 Potential Considerations When Selecting a GLP-1 Receptor Agonist or an SGLT-2 Inhibitor for Cardiovascular Benefit

	GLP-1 RECEPTOR AGONISTS	SGLT-2 INHIBITORS
MACE prevention	+++	+++
HF prevention		+++
Weight loss	+++	+
Considerations that may prompt the use of a medication from an alternative class	• Persistent nausea • History of gastroparesis • Active gallbladder disease • History of MEN2 or medullary thyroid cancer • History of proliferative retinopathy (caution with semaglutide or dulaglutide)	• History of amputation, severe peripheral arterial disease, or active diabetic foot ulcers (caution with canagliflozin) • History of recurrent genital candidiasis • History of diabetic ketoacidosis • History of fracture (caution with canagliflozin)

GLP-1, Glucagon-like peptide-1; *HF*, heart failure; *MACE*, major adverse cardiovascular events; *MEN2*, multiple endocrine neoplasia type 2; *SGLT-2*, sodium–glucose cotransporter 2.
Adapted from Das SR, Everett BM, Birtcher KK, et al. 2020 expert consensus decision pathway on novel therapies for cardiovascular risk reduction in patients with type 2 diabetes: A report of the American College of Cardiology Solution Set Oversight Committee. *J Am Coll Cardiol.* 2020;76(9):1117–1145.

8. **What glucose-lowering medications are preferred in people with predominant atherosclerotic cardiovascular disease (ASCVD)?**

    As shown in Fig. 14.1, an agent with proven cardiovascular benefit from either the GLP-1 receptor agonist or SGLT-2 inhibitor class is preferred in patients with established ASCVD or indicators of high ASCVD risk. The ADA defines indicators of high ASCVD risk as follows: age ≥55 years with >50% coronary, carotid, or lower-extremity artery stenoses, or the presence of left ventricular hypertrophy. Table 14.3 provides a framework proposed by the American College of Cardiology (ACC) when deciding between a GLP-1 receptor agonist or SGLT-2 inhibitor for cardiovascular benefit.

9. **Which glucose-lowering medications are preferred in patients with comorbid heart failure?**

    SGLT-2 inhibitors have consistently demonstrated benefits on heart failure outcomes in large cardiovascular outcome trials—even in people without diabetes. SGLT-2 inhibitors are therefore preferentially recommended for use in patients with type 2 diabetes with comorbid heart failure, provided they do not have a contraindication to SGLT-2 inhibitor therapy.

10. **Are there any glucose-lowering medications that should be avoided in people with heart failure?**

    There are several glucose-lowering medications that should be avoided in patients with heart failure. The thiazolidinediones—pioglitazone and rosiglitazone—both carry a black-box warning for causing or exacerbating heart failure. Both agents are formally contraindicated for use in patients with New York Heart Association (NYHA) Class III or IV heart failure. Nonetheless, thiazolidinediones are generally avoided in patients with any degree of heart failure. The dipeptidyl peptidase-4 (DPP-4) inhibitor saxagliptin is also typically recommended to be avoided in patients with heart failure because of an observed increased risk for heart failure hospitalization in a large cardiovascular outcome trial with this medication. An increased risk for heart failure hospitalization was not noted, however, in large cardiovascular outcome trials with other agents from the DPP-4 inhibitor class.

11. **Are any glucose-lowering therapies specifically recommended in people with type 2 diabetes and chronic kidney disease (CKD)?**

    SGLT-2 inhibitors have been shown in several studies to slow the progression of CKD in patients with type 2 diabetes. The ADA preferentially recommends the use of an SGLT-2 inhibitor with evidence of improving CKD outcomes in patients with type 2 diabetes who have CKD and albuminuria (see Fig. 14.1). Similarly, the Kidney Disease Improving Global Outcomes (KDIGO) 2020 guideline for diabetes management in CKD recommends first-line treatment with metformin and an SGLT-2 inhibitor in patients with type 2 diabetes who have comorbid CKD. If a patient cannot tolerate or has a contraindication to SGLT-2 inhibitor treatment, the ADA recommends the use of a GLP-1 receptor agonist with proven cardiovascular benefit as an alternative.

Table 14.4 Hypoglycemia Risk of Glucose-Lowering Medications

High Risk
- Insulin (mealtime insulin > basal insulin)
- Sulfonylureas (glimepiride, glipizide, glyburide)
- Meglitinides (nateglinide, repaglinide)

Low Risk
- Metformin
- DPP-4 inhibitors (alogliptin, linagliptin, saxagliptin, sitagliptin)
- GLP-1 receptor agonists (exenatide, dulaglutide, liraglutide, lixisenatide, semaglutide)
- SGLT-2 inhibitors (canagliflozin, dapagliflozin, empagliflozin, ertugliflozin)
- Thiazolidinediones (pioglitazone, rosiglitazone)

DDP-4, dipeptidyl peptidase-4; *GLP-1*, glucagon-like peptide-1; *SGLT-2*, sodium–glucose cotransporter 2.
Adapted from American Diabetes Association. 9. Pharmacological approaches to glycemic treatment: Standards of Medical Care in Diabetes—2021. *Diabetes Care.* 2021;44(Suppl 1):S111-S124.

12. **Which glucose-lowering medications are recommended where there is a compelling need to minimize hypoglycemia?**
    When intensifying therapy in patients with type 2 diabetes to lower A1c, one major consideration recommended by the ADA is hypoglycemia risk. When there is a compelling need to minimize hypoglycemia, the following medication classes are preferred: DPP-4 inhibitors, GLP-1 receptor agonists, SGLT-2 inhibitors, and thiazolidinediones. Table 14.4 provides a summary of major glucose-lowering medication classes and their risk of contributing to hypoglycemia. Although these medications have a low inherent risk of contributing to hypoglycemia, patients should still be monitored closely for hypoglycemia when these medications are added to background insulin or sulfonylurea therapy.

13. **Are there any glucose-lowering medications that can help with weight loss?**
    Treatment with both GLP-1 receptor agonists and SGLT-2 inhibitors can result in weight loss. For this reason, the ADA preferably recommends the addition of an agent from one of these classes when there is a compelling need to minimize weight gain or promote weight loss. Of note, agents from the GLP-1 receptor agonist class have variable effects on weight. The ADA provides the following ranking of GLP-1 receptor agonists based on their observed efficacy for weight loss: semaglutide > liraglutide > dulaglutide > exenatide > lixisenatide. Although only indicated for use in patients with type 2 diabetes who use mealtime insulin, treatment with the noninsulin injectable agent pramlintide can also result in weight loss.

14. **Which glucose-lowering medications are recommended for use when cost is a major barrier?**
    Metformin, sulfonylureas, and thiazolidinediones are currently the most affordable glucose-lowering agents in the United States. For patients for whom cost is a major issue, the ADA recommends the use of a sulfonylurea or a thiazolidinedione as an add-on to metformin in patients requiring dual therapy. If there is a compelling reason to use an agent from a more expensive medication class (e.g., the presence of ASCVD, heart failure, or CKD), the utilization of available patient assistance programs may be an option.

15. **Are there any glucose-lowering combinations that should be avoided?**
    The GLP-1 receptor agonist and DPP-4 inhibitor classes lower glucose through augmenting the incretin effect, with GLP-1 receptor agonists being more potent glucose-lowering agents. The ADA recommends avoiding the use of this combination. If it is decided to initiate a GLP-1 receptor agonist in a patient on background DPP-4 inhibitor therapy, it is recommended that the DPP-4 inhibitor be discontinued.

16. **If a person with type 2 diabetes requires the greater efficacy of an injectable glucose-lowering agent, which class of medications is recommended by the ADA for initial consideration?**
    The ADA recommends that a GLP-1 receptor agonist be *considered* as the first injectable agent. This recommendation is based on good efficacy, low risk of hypoglycemia, and favorable effects on weight that can be achieved with a long-acting GLP-1 receptor agonist compared with the addition of basal insulin in many patients.

17. **How is basal insulin typically initiated and titrated in a person with type 2 diabetes?**
    There is no one correct approach to the initiation and titration of basal insulin in a patient with type 2 diabetes. The ADA recommends starting with either 10 units once daily or calculating a weight-based initial dose of

0.1 to 0.2 units/kg per day. For patients likely to require larger insulin doses (e.g., those with notable obesity and/or insulin resistance), using a weight-based starting dose may help expedite the basal insulin titration and improvement in fasting glucose. Any evidence-based titration algorithm can be used to titrate the basal insulin to the patient's individualized fasting blood glucose target. An example approach recommended by the ADA is to increase the basal insulin dose by 2 units every 3 days until the fasting glucose target is achieved. The basal insulin can be decreased by 10% to 20% with the occurrence of any unexplained hypoglycemia.

18. **If the fasting blood glucose is at goal but the A1c remains elevated after titrating a patient's basal insulin, what is recommended next?**
As illustrated in Fig. 14.2, if a patient with type 2 diabetes has an A1c above target despite adequately titrated basal insulin, the next recommended step for many patients is to add mealtime insulin. The ADA recommends initially adding a single dose of mealtime insulin to the largest meal or the meal where the patient experiences the most pronounced postprandial glucose spike. A reasonable starting dose is four units or a dose equal to 10% of the current basal insulin dose, which can be titrated by 1 to 2 units or 10% to 15% twice weekly. If the A1c remains elevated after careful titration of the single mealtime insulin dose, a second injection can be added to the next largest meal. The insulin regimen can then be intensified stepwise as needed to meet the individualized needs of the patient. Of note, for patients on basal insulin who are not already being treated with a GLP-1 receptor agonist, another approach is to consider the addition of a GLP-1 receptor agonist to assist with postprandial control (see Fig. 14.2).

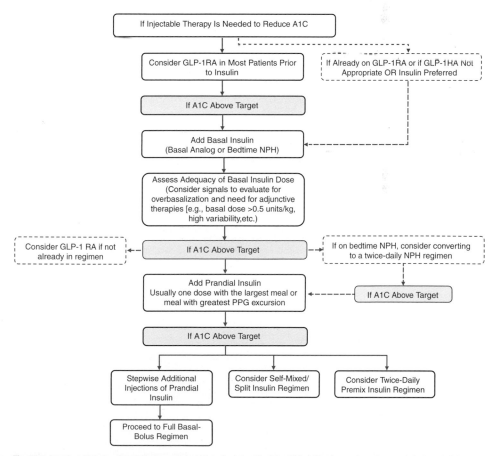

Fig. 14.2 American Diabetes Association recommendations for intensification of injectable glucose-lowering agents in type 2 diabetes. *A1c*, hemoglobin A1c; *FPG*, fasting plasma glucose; *kg*, kilograms; *NPH*, neutral protamine Hagedorn; *PPG*, postprandial glucose. Adapted from American Diabetes Association. 9. Pharmacologic approaches to glycemic treatment: Standards of Medical Care in Diabetes—2021. *Diabetes Care.* 2021;44[Suppl 1]:S111–S124.

KEY POINTS

1. The ADA recommends a general A1c goal of <7.0% for many nonpregnant adults with diabetes, whereas the AACE/ACE guidelines recommend an optimal goal of ≤6.5% if it can be achieved safely and affordably.

2. Although general glycemic goals are recommended for people with type 2 diabetes, goals should always be individualized based on patient-specific considerations that may affect the risks and/or benefits of intensive treatment. Factors that may warrant less stringent glycemic goals include the following: high risk for hypoglycemia or other drug side effects, long duration of diabetes, limited life expectancy (the long-term benefits of a more intensive goal will likely not be realized), high comorbidity/complications burden, and patient preferences.

3. The ADA recommends metformin and comprehensive lifestyle management as first-line therapy in patients with type 2 diabetes. Metformin should be continued for as long as it is tolerated.

4. Initial combination therapy can be considered to extend the time to treatment failure or when more than one glucose-lowering agent is needed to achieve glycemic targets.

5. Early initiation of insulin therapy is recommended in patients presenting with a blood glucose of ≥300 mg/dL, an A1c of >10%, and/or if the patient is experiencing symptoms of overt hyperglycemia or catabolism.

6. GLP-1 receptor agonists and SGLT-2 inhibitors with proven cardiovascular and kidney benefit are recommended for use in patients with comorbid atherosclerotic cardiovascular disease, heart failure, and/or CKD. SGLT-2 inhibitors are preferred in the setting of heart failure and albuminuric CKD. The addition of these agents to mitigate cardiovascular and kidney risk is recommended irrespective of the patient's A1c or A1c goal.

7. Thiazolidinediones and the DPP-4 inhibitor saxagliptin should be avoided in patients with heart failure.

8. When intensifying therapy to improve A1c, major considerations for the selection of glucose-lowering agents include the following: (1) avoidance of hypoglycemia, (2) minimization of weight gain or promotion of weight loss, and (3) cost considerations.

9. GLP-1 receptor agonists and DPP-4 inhibitors are not recommended for use in combination.

10. The ADA recommends consideration of a GLP-1 receptor agonist as the first injectable agent in patients with type 2 diabetes because of its good efficacy, low risk of hypoglycemia, and beneficial effects on weight. For patients requiring insulin therapy to meet individualized goals, the stepwise addition of basal insulin followed by mealtime insulin is recommended.

BIBLIOGRAPHY

Alicic RZ, Neumiller JJ, Johnson EJ, et al. Sodium-glucose cotransporter 2 inhibition and diabetic kidney disease. *Diabetes.* 2019;68(2):248–257.

American Diabetes Association. 6. Glycemic targets: Standards of Medical Care in Diabetes – 2021. *Diabetes Care.* 2021;44(Suppl 1):S73–S84.

American Diabetes Association. 9. Pharmacologic approaches to glycemic treatment: Standards of Medical Care in Diabetes – 2021. *Diabetes Care.* 2021;44(Suppl 1):S111–S124.

American Diabetes Association. Standards of Medical Care in Diabetes – 2021 Abridged for Primary Care Providers. *Clin Diabetes.* 2021;39(1):14–43.

Buse JB, Wexler DJ, Tsapas A, et al. 2019 update to: Management of hyperglycemia in type 2 diabetes, 2018. A consensus report by the American Diabetes Association (ADA) and the European Association for the Study of Diabetes (EASD). *Diabetes Care.* 2020;43(2):487–493.

Das SR, Everett BM, Birtcher KK, et al. 2020 expert consensus decision pathway on novel therapies for cardiovascular risk reduction in patients with type 2 diabetes: A report of the American College of Cardiology Solution Set Oversight Committee. *J Am Coll Cardiol.* 2020;76(9):1117–1145.

Davies MJ, D'Alessio DA, Fradkin J, et al. Management of hyperglycemia in type 2 diabetes, 2018. A consensus report by the American Diabetes Association (ADA) and the European Association for the Study of Diabetes (EASD). *Diabetes Care.* 2018;41(12):2669–2701.

de Boer IH, Caramori ML, Chan JCN, et al. Executive summary of the 2020 KDIGO diabetes management in CKD guideline: evidence-based advances in monitoring and treatment. *Kidney Int.* 2020;98(4):839–848.

Garber AJ, Handelsman Y, Grunberger G, et al. Consensus statement by the American Association of Clinical Endocrinologists and American College of Endocrinology on the comprehensive type 2 diabetes management algorithm – 2020 executive summary. *Endocr Pract.* 2020;26(1):107–139.

CHAPTER 15

DIABETES PREVENTION

Kayce M. Shealy, PharmD, BCPS, CDCES

1. **What is prediabetes?**
   Prediabetes is defined as a condition of increased risk of future type 2 diabetes (T2D), as a result of either impaired fasting glucose or impaired glucose tolerance. People with prediabetes are an intermediate group of people who have blood glucose levels that are higher than the defined normal level but not high enough to meet the diagnostic criteria for diabetes. Based on the American Diabetes Association (ADA) Standards of Medical Care, prediabetes is diagnosed by a fasting plasma glucose (FPG) level, a plasma glucose level 2 hours after an oral glucose tolerance test (OGTT), or a glycosylated hemoglobin (A1c) level. Table 15.1 includes the diagnostic criteria for prediabetes and T2D.

2. **Why is the prevention of T2D important?**
   The development of T2D is relatively slow and progressive. The decline in beta-cell function has been estimated to begin more than 10 years prior to the diagnosis of diabetes; this leads to prolonged hyperglycemia and higher risks of developing costly complications. Diabetes is associated with microvascular complications such as nephropathy, retinopathy, and neuropathy and with macrovascular complications such as ischemic heart disease. These complications necessitate more complex and costly treatment and medical care. The total costs related to a diagnosis of diabetes equated to approximately $327 billion in 2017 in the United States, and excess medical costs per person with diabetes per year increased from $8417 in 2012 to $9601 in 2017. Additionally, T2D is the leading cause of adult-onset blindness and the seventh-leading cause of death in the United States. Thus early detection of those at risk for the development of T2D and implementation of strategies to prevent T2D are vital in slowing the progression of the disease and ultimately lowering the risk of complications.

   Although there are currently no strategies that are 100% effective in preventing T2D, focused interventions that include dietary and activity modifications with or without medications have delayed or reduced the prevalence of microvascular complications, as demonstrated in the Diabetes Prevention Program Outcomes Study (DPPOS), even in those patients who progressed to overt diabetes. Evidence-based strategies to prevent diabetes, such as intensive lifestyle modifications with weight loss, are cost effective compared with treating complications associated with long-standing T2D.

3. **What are the risk factors for developing T2D in adults?**
   - Overweight or obesity
   - First-degree family relative with diabetes
   - African American, Latino, Native American, Asian American, Pacific Islander ethnicities
   - History of cardiovascular disease
   - Hypertension
   - Low high-density lipoprotein cholesterol (HDL-C; <35 mg/dL or 0.9 mmol/L) or elevated triglyceride (>250 mg/dL or 2.82 mmol/L)
   - History of polycystic ovarian syndrome (PCOS)
   - Physical inactivity
   - Conditions associated with insulin resistance (e.g., acanthosis nigricans)

4. **What are the risk factors for developing T2D in children and adolescents?**
   - Maternal history of gestational diabetes mellitus during the child's gestation
   - Family history in first- or second-degree relative
   - African American, Latino, Native American, Asian American, Pacific Islander ethnicities
   - Signs of insulin resistance or conditions associated with insulin resistance (e.g., acanthosis nigricans)

5. **Should asymptomatic people be screened for T2D?**
   Asymptomatic adults who are overweight or obese with one additional risk factor identified from the previous lists should be screened for T2D at a minimum of every 3 years, or more frequently depending on initial results and risks. Others who should be screened include the following:
   - All asymptomatic adults beginning at age 45 years at least every 3 years, or more frequently depending on initial results and risks
   - Women with a history of gestational diabetes at least every 3 years, or more frequently depending on initial results
   - Children who are overweight or obese (≥85th percentile) with an additional risk factor identified from the previous lists beginning at age 10 or puberty at a minimum of every 3 years, or more frequently depending on initial results and if body mass index (BMI) increases

Table 15.1 American Diabetes Association Standards of Medical Care Diagnostic Criteria

PARAMETER/TEST	NORMAL	PREDIABETES	T2D
A1c	<5.7%	5.7%–6.4%	≥6.5%
FPG	<100 mg/dL	100–125 mg/dL	≥126 mg/dL
2-hour plasma glucose after 75-gram OGTT	<140 mg/dL	140–199 mg/dL	≥200 mg/dL

A1c, Glycosylated hemoglobin; *FPG*, fasting plasma glucose; *OGTT*, oral glucose tolerance test; *T2D*, type 2 diabetes.

6. **How should people be screened for T2D?**
   Assessment of asymptomatic adults can be done using a validated screening tool, the Diabetes Risk Test (https://www.diabetes.org/risk-test) from the ADA. This screening tool asks seven questions to identify individual risk factors such as family history, physical inactivity, and increased body weight. Those people who score 5 or higher on this screening tool, as well as those who are overweight with at least one additional risk factor, should have further diagnostic testing. Blood tests that are used for diagnostic purposes include FPG, OGTT, and A1c. The use of A1c as a diagnostic tool in people with conditions that alter hemoglobin glycation, such as pregnancy and hemoglobinopathies, should be done cautiously, and this test is more costly. However, the use of A1c is the only diagnostic method that does not require fasting.

7. **Describe lifestyle interventions to prevent diabetes**
   Preventing diabetes, and treating prediabetes (those identified as at risk), includes intensive behavioral and lifestyle interventions in addition to medications. Sustained weight loss of at least 7% and moderate-intensity physical activity for at least 150 minutes per week are effective in the long-term prevention of T2D, as demonstrated in the Diabetes Prevention Program (DPP) trial. Participants in the DPP set caloric intake goals that included an overall deficit of 500 to 1000 calories per day based on initial body weight and no more than 25% of calories from fat, in addition to increasing physical activity to lose approximately 1 to 2 pounds per week over a 6-month time period. These intensive lifestyle interventions and weight loss have been effective in preventing the development of T2D for at least 15 years, based on evidence in the DPP Outcomes Study. Because other weight-loss strategies have been shown to be effective and patient preference must be considered, the ADA Standards of Medical Care suggest that a variety of eating patterns can be considered to prevent T2D in people with prediabetes. Other lifestyle strategies to consider include increasing the consumption of high-fiber foods and omega-3 fatty acids and reducing the intake of sweetened beverages.

8. **What medications have been studied to prevent diabetes?**
   Several medications have been studied for diabetes prevention, as shown in the following list. However, no medications are currently approved by the U.S. Food and Drug Administration (FDA) for diabetes prevention, and medications are less effective than lifestyle modifications, according to results from the DPP. Of the medications studied, metformin has the strongest evidence for preventing diabetes, with demonstrated long-term durability, and is cost effective. The use of other medications is limited because of cost, adverse effects, and a lack of evidence of sustained prevention.
   - Metformin 850 mg twice daily
   - Acarbose 100 mg three times daily
   - Rosiglitazone 8 mg daily
   - Pioglitazone 30 to 45 mg daily
   - Orlistat 120 mg three times daily
   - Liraglutide 3 mg daily
   - Phentermine 7.5 to 15 mg/topiramate 46 to 92 mg once daily

9. **What is the preferred treatment for prediabetes?**
   Intensive lifestyle interventions with or without metformin have demonstrated long-term prevention. Intensive lifestyle interventions were generally more effective than metformin in preventing T2D in the DPP, but this difference was minimized near the end of the 15-year follow-up period. Metformin has been demonstrated to be just as effective as intensive lifestyle interventions specifically in patients with a BMI of ≥35 kg/m², those <60 years of age, or those who have a history of gestational diabetes (GDM). Additionally, both interventions have demonstrated long-term cost-efficacy and were similar in reducing the prevalence of microvascular complications at 15 years. The ADA Standards of Medical Care recommend that all patients with prediabetes should initiate lifestyle modifications with the goal of at least 7% weight loss, and metformin should be considered in people with prediabetes, especially for those patients with a BMI of ≥35 kg/m², those under the age of 60, and women with a history of GDM. Metformin may also be considered in those patients unable to sustain 7% weight loss.

KEY POINTS

1. Prediabetes is a metabolic condition of increased risk of developing T2D in the future.
2. Identification of those at risk of developing diabetes is important to delay the progression of the diabetes disease process and prevent potential long-term complications.
3. Intense lifestyle interventions that result in a sustained weight loss of at least 7% and include at least 150 minutes of moderate-intensity physical activity per week are effective in long-term prevention.
4. Metformin should be considered for people with prediabetes for the prevention of T2D, especially for people with a BMI of $\geq$35 kg/m^2, those aged <60 years, or those with a history of GDM.

BIBLIOGRAPHY

1. Aguiar EJ, Morgan PJ, Collins CE, Plotnikoff RC, Young MD, Callister R. Efficacy of the type 2 diabetes prevention using lifestyle education program RCT. *Am J Prev Med.* 2016;50(3):353–364. https://doi.org/10.1016/j.amepre.2015.08.020.
2. American Diabetes Association. Classification and Diagnosis of Diabetes: Standards of Medical Care in Diabetes—2021. *Diabetes Care.* 2021;44(Suppl 1):S15–S33. https://doi.org/10.2337/dc21-S002.
3. American Diabetes Association. Prevention or Delay of Type 2 Diabetes: Standards of Medical Care in Diabetes—2021. *Diabetes Care.* 2021;44(Suppl 1):S34–S39. https://doi.org/10.2337/dc21-S003.
4. Centers for Disease Control and Prevention. *Diabetes Report Card 2019.* Atlanta, GA: Centers for Disease Control and Prevention, US Dept of Health and Human Services; 2020.
5. Chiasson JL, Josse RG, Gomis R, et al. Acarbose for prevention of type 2 diabetes mellitus: the STOP-NIDDM randomised trial for The STOP-NIDDM Trial Research Group Members. *Lancet.* 2002;359(9323):2072–2077. https://doi.org/10.1016/S0140-6736(02)08905-5.
6. DeFronzo RA, Tripathy D, Schwenke DC, et al. Pioglitazone for diabetes prevention in impaired glucose tolerance. *N Engl J Med.* 2011;364:1104–1115. https://doi.org/10.1056/NEJM1010949.
7. Fonseca VA. Defining and characterizing the progression of type 2 diabetes. *Diabetes Care.* 2009;32(Suppl 2):S151–S156. https://doi.org/10.2337/dc09-S301.
8. Garvey WT, Ryan DH, Henry R, et al. Prevention of type 2 diabetes in subjects with prediabetes and metabolic syndrome treated with phentermine and topiramate extended release. *Diabetes Care.* 2014;37:912–921. https://doi.org/10.2337/dc13-1518.
9. Gerstein HC, Yusuf S, Bosch J, et al. DREAM (Diabetes REduction Assessment with ramipril and rosiglitazone Medication) Trial Investigators. Effect of rosiglitazone on the frequency of diabetes in patients with impaired glucose tolerance or impaired fasting glucose: a randomised controlled trial. *Lancet.* 2006;368:1096–1105. https://doi.org/10.1016/S0140-6736(06)69420-8.
10. Knowles WC, Fowler SE, Hamman RF, et al. 10-year follow-up of diabetes incidence and weight loss in the Diabetes Prevention Program Outcomes Study for the Diabetes Prevention Program Research Group. *Lancet.* 2009;374(9702):1677–1686. https://doi.org/10.1016/S0140-6736(09)61457-4.
11. le Roux CW, Astrup A, Fujioka K, et al. 3 years of liraglutide versus placebo for type 2 diabetes risk reduction and weight management in individuals with prediabetes: a randomised, double-blind trial SCALE Obesity Prediabetes NN8022-1839 Study Group. *Lancet.* 2017;389:1399–1409. https://doi.org/10.1016/S0140-6736(17)30069-7.
12. Nathan DM, Barrett-Connor E, Crandall JP, et al. Long-term effects of lifestyle intervention or metformin on diabetes development and microvascular complications: the DPP Outcomes Study for the Diabetes Prevention Program Research Group. *Lancet Diabetes Endocrinol.* 2015;3(11):866–875. https://doi.org/10.1016/S2213-8587(15)00291-0.
13. Torgerson JS, Hauptman J, Boldrin MN, Sjöström L. XENical in the prevention of diabetes in obese subjects (XENDOS) study: a randomized study of orlistat as an adjunct to lifestyle changes for the prevention of type 2 diabetes in obese patients. *Diabetes Care.* 2004;27:155–161. https://doi.org/10.2337/diacare.27.1.155.
14. Vermunt PW, Milder IE, Wielaard F, de Vries JH, Baan CA, van Oers JA, Westert GP. A lifestyle intervention to reduce type 2 diabetes risk in Dutch primary care: 2.5-year results of a randomized controlled trial. *Diabet Med.* 2012;29(8):e223–e231. https://doi.org/10.1111/j.1464-5491.2012.03648.x.

CHAPTER 16

DIABETES AND PREGNANCY

Layla A. Abushamat, MD, MPH, and Linda A. Barbour, MD, MSPH

1. **Why is preconception counseling important in women with diabetes who desire pregnancy?**

   Women with poorly controlled diabetes mellitus (DM) have a higher risk of poor maternal and fetal outcomes, including diabetic ketoacidosis (DKA), preeclampsia, miscarriages, major malformations (especially heart, spine, and kidney), macrosomia, stillbirth, newborn respiratory distress syndrome (RDS), cardiomegaly, and hypoglycemia. These poor outcomes correlate with the degree of dysglycemia and its timing during gestation and other DM-associated comorbidities, especially maternal obesity, hypertension, and chronic kidney disease. There is a relatively linear relationship between fetal anomalies and hemoglobin A1c prior to organogenesis, which occurs at 5 to 8 weeks of gestation. Additionally, maternal DM complications such as proliferative retinopathy and diabetic nephropathy can worsen during pregnancy. Preconception counseling and care have a positive effect; they improve maternal and obstetric outcomes, improve perinatal morbidity and mortality, and reduce the risk of congenital malformations. Because many pregnancies in women with DM are unplanned, it is important to involve a multidisciplinary team in counseling women with DM frequently and regularly regarding the importance of preconception care and management.

2. **What are key preconception counseling recommendations in women with DM who desire pregnancy?**

   Women of childbearing age with DM should be advised to safely achieve and maintain an A1c of <6.5% prior to conception because this is associated with the least risk of congenital malformations (2%–3%, similar to the general population). The risk of adverse outcomes is reduced by approximately 50% with each 1% drop in A1c. Discussion of family planning is key, and effective contraception, preferably with long-acting reversible contraception (LARC), should be prescribed and used until adequate disease control is achieved. Focus should also be placed on current nutritional status (including body weight and vitamin deficiencies) and screening for and optimal management of complications (particularly nephropathy and retinopathy) and comorbidities (mood, obesity, sleep apnea, thyroid and occult cardiovascular disease). Given the much higher risk of stillbirth with the combination of diabetes and obesity, weight loss prior to pregnancy can also significantly improve pregnancy outcomes. Additionally, untreated sleep apnea, common in ~{1/3} of obese pregnant patients, worsens maternal insulin resistance and poses a significant threat of hypoxemia to the fetus, especially if severe. Medication and supplement reconciliation should also be completed. This review includes the implementation of medication substitutions that are safe in pregnancy, including the cessation of angiotensin-converting enzyme inhibitors (ACEis), angiotensin II receptor blockers (ARBs), and statins, all of which are associated with poor fetal outcomes if continued during pregnancy, although probably not with major malformations if used in the first trimester. Additionally, recommendations should be made for a multivitamin that includes adequate folic acid (0.8–1 mg daily) and baby aspirin (81–162 mg) because these can reduce the risk of neural tube defects and preeclampsia, respectively. There should also be a discussion about the risks of substance use (tobacco, alcohol, marijuana) and a plan created to aid with cessation.

3. **What is the optimal contraception for a woman with DM?**

   A combined oral contraceptive pill (OCP) with 20 to 30 ug estradiol is safe for nearly all women with DM unless they have a history of venous thromboembolism, uncontrolled hypertension, or severe hypertriglyceridemia. Otherwise, all methods of contraception have been found to be safe and efficacious in women with DM and far outweigh the risk of an unintended pregnancy. LARC, such as an intrauterine device (IUD) or Nexplanon implant, carries no metabolic or thrombotic risk and is especially effective.

4. **Define the White Classification of Diabetes in Pregnancy**

   This classification system was developed as a perinatal risk tool for type 1 DM (T1DM) and is still sometimes used. It has been modified to include gestational diabetes (GDM) and aids with the prediction of pregnancy complications based on age of T1DM onset, DM duration, and the presence of different vascular complications (Table 16.1).

5. **Is T1DM or type 2 DM (T2DM) associated with worse pregnancy outcomes?**

   Adverse pregnancy outcomes with T2DM are at least as high as those in T1DM. Because of the concomitant risk factors often associated with T2DM, including obesity, hypertension, insulin resistance, hypertriglyceridemia (also a risk factor for fetal overgrowth), and sleep apnea, the perinatal death rate is higher in T2DM, likely from the fetus sometimes outgrowing its placental blood supply and developing ischemia. In fact, the combination of class 3 obesity and preexisting DM increases the stillbirth risk near term by 30-fold.

Table 16.1 Modified White Classification System

CLASS	AGE OF ONSET (YEARS)	DURATION (YEARS)	VASCULAR DISEASE	MEDICATION
Gestational Diabetes				
A1	Any	N/A	No	No
A2	Any	N/A	No	Yes
Pregestational Diabetes				
B	>20	<10	No	Yes
C	10–19	10–19	No	Yes
D	<10	>20	Benign retinopathy	Yes
F	Any	Any	Nephropathy	Yes
R	Any	Any	Proliferative retinopathy	Yes
T	Any	Any	Renal transplant	Yes
H	Any	Any	CAD	Yes

CAD, Coronary artery disease; *N/A*, not applicable.

6. How does the intrauterine environment during the gestation of a mother with DM differ from that of a mother without DM, and what are potential long-term effects on the offspring?

The offspring of mothers with pregestational DM or GDM are, on average, heavier at every gestational age and at birth compared with offspring of mothers without DM, as long as there is not placental insufficiency. This increased fat mass is also associated with an increased risk of childhood obesity, metabolic syndrome, and T2DM. These long-term effects are thought to be attributable to the intrauterine metabolic environment in mothers with DM, and concurrent maternal obesity appreciably adds to this risk. This environment includes maternal hyperglycemia, hyperlipidemia, insulin resistance, and increased oxidative stress. Glucose is transferred across the placenta to the fetus down a concentration gradient and is a major teratogen. The fetus responds with hyperinsulinemia as early as 14 weeks, contributing to organomegaly, excess growth, fat accumulation, and multiple adverse outcomes. Additionally, this environment is thought to promote epigenetic changes in utero that may also alter fetal mitochondrial function and appetite regulation; this is currently under intense investigation.

7. What is the role of exercise in pregnant women with DM?

Exercise is safe for most pregnant women with DM and can be used therapeutically to reduce fasting and postprandial hyperglycemia, prevent excessive weight gain (risk factor for fetal overgrowth), and improve placental function. Contraindications to exercise in pregnancy include vaginal bleeding, active premature labor, heart or lung disease, and severe anemia or preeclampsia. Moderate prenatal exercise is beneficial, provided adequate hydration is maintained and overheating does not occur; this has been shown to reduce the likelihood of cesarean birth by 55%. The American College of Obstetrics and Gynecology (ACOG) recommends that pregnant women should engage in an exercise plan with a goal of 20 to 30 minutes of moderate physical activity at least 5 days a week.

8. What metabolic changes occur in the first trimester of pregnancy, and how do these changes drive DM management?

The first trimester of pregnancy is an anabolic state promoting nutrient storage to prepare for the duration of gestation. Leptin, cortisol, and insulin secretion rise and promote lipoprotein lipase activation and fatty acid generation in adipose tissue, increased lipogenesis, and decreased fatty acid oxidation, all in an effort to stimulate maternal fat storage. An increase in adiponectin enhances insulin sensitivity in some women. These changes are variable based on baseline insulin sensitivity, with normal-weight women favoring lipogenesis during this period and obese women favoring net lipolysis that persists throughout all of gestation. In women with T1DM, this early rise in insulin sensitivity predisposes mothers to hypoglycemia, particularly at night when there is prolonged fasting. During the first trimester, the focus should be on improving glucose control while minimizing hypoglycemia. Hypoglycemia is especially common if women develop pregnancy-related nausea and vomiting; this may require aggressive antiemetic treatment to prevent hypoglycemia from insulin taken for food that is later vomited.

9. **Describe the metabolic changes characteristic of the second and third trimesters of pregnancy**

   Whereas the first trimester is a period of relative insulin sensitivity, the second and third trimesters are characterized by an exponential rise in insulin resistance driven by human placental growth hormone (hPGH), human placental lactogen (HPL), and tumor necrosis factor-alpha (TNF-α). There are increased fetal and placental glucose demands during the second and third trimesters as a result of the limited ability of the fetus to oxidize fat for energy. These demands lead to rapid depletion of maternal glycogen stores. To reserve carbohydrates for increasing fetal-placental glucose demands, which are likely to exceed 150 g in the third trimester, there is a rise in skeletal muscle, adipose tissue, and liver insulin resistance and hepatic gluconeogenesis. Increased insulin resistance leads to diminished inhibition of maternal lipolysis by insulin. These changes lead to maternal use of fatty acids as an alternative energy source earlier in the fasting state, characterizing pregnancy as a ketogenic state. There is a marked rise in triglycerides (TGs) and free fatty acids throughout gestation, further promoting the insulin resistance of pregnancy. TGs increase up to threefold in pregnancy as a result of estrogen; women with severe hypertriglyceridemia (fasting TG > 400 mg/dL) may need to be treated with high doses of omega-3 fatty acids or a fibrate (Gemfibrozil preferred) to prevent TG-induced pancreatitis. With these changes, women with DM may require two- to fivefold higher doses of insulin compared with prepregnancy requirements.

10. **How does the postpartum period affect DM management?**

    Upon placental delivery, insulin sensitivity is rapidly restored to below prepregnancy levels as a result of the immediate fall of insulin-resistance–promoting placental hormones, rapid weight loss, and the increased energy demands of lactation. Postpartum insulin requirements are usually 35% to 40% of those during the third trimester and 10% to 20% less than prepregnancy requirements; thus, glycemic goals need to be immediately relaxed because of the risks of severe maternal hypoglycemia with the demands of a newborn at home. If insulin requirements decrease >10% to 20% prior to delivery, concern for the development of placental insufficiency or autoimmune adrenal insufficiency in mothers with T1DM should be high; the former often manifests as preeclampsia and increases the risk of stillbirth, especially in an already-overgrown fetus.

11. **Identify glycemic goals during pregnancy**

    Although increasing A1c is associated with worse maternal-fetal outcomes and is a useful collective measure, A1c does not capture the full picture of glycemic control or variability, especially given that A1c declines by approximately 0.8% in pregnancy as a result of increased red blood cell turnover. Fasting glucose levels fall appreciably in normal pregnancy to ~75 mg/dL, but trying to achieve these goals in women, especially those with T1DM, is likely to result in hypoglycemic unawareness and neonatal hypoglycemia, a significant risk to the mother and fetus because the fetus has no capacity for gluconeogenesis. Both the ADA and ACOG recommend the following glucose targets:
    - Fasting plasma glucose <95 mg/dL
    - 1-hour postprandial glucose <140 mg/dL
    - 2-hour postprandial glucose <120 mg/dL

    These levels have been identified as leading to a reduction in adverse fetal outcomes. Women with DM who have hypoglycemia unawareness may need slightly higher goals.

12. **Discuss the role of real-time continuous glucose monitoring (RT-CGM) in pregnancy**

    RT-CGM during pregnancy in women with T1DM has been associated with increased time in the pregnancy glucose target ranges, less glucose variability, and overall improvement in neonatal outcomes (lower risk of large for gestational age [LGA], neonatal hypoglycemia, neonatal intensive care unit [NICU] admission). A time in range (TIR) of 63 to 140 mg/dL is recommended for pregnancy and is likely a better indicator of overall glycemic control than A1c. However, for women with T1DM, a TIR of 70 to 140 mg/dL may be safer due to the increased risk of maternal hypoglycemia. Evidence from RCTs and cohort studies supporting CGM in pregnancy, especially for T1DM, is building, and recently Medicaid has agreed to reimburse its use for Type 1 DM in pregnancy, as has the UK.

13. **What is the role of the insulin pump during pregnancy?**

    The use of continuous subcutaneous insulin infusion (CSII) by insulin pumps and sensor-integrated insulin delivery systems (hybrid closed-loop pumps) in pregnancy is an ongoing area of research. Studies have shown no difference in maternal or fetal outcomes in participants on CSII versus multiple daily injection (MDI) therapy in T1DM, although CSII has been associated with earlier (second-trimester) control without an increase in hypoglycemia. It is particularly useful when subtle insulin dosage changes are needed, especially in women with T1DM who need variable basal insulin dosing during the night. Hybrid closed-loop therapy has been shown to result in greater time spent in pregnancy glucose target ranges and lower overnight mean glucose levels but without a difference in adverse pregnancy outcomes, although data is limited. Pregnancy data with the Medtronic 670G and Tandem Control IQ pumps should be forthcoming, but "looping" is not recommended either in or out of pregnancy at this time. There are significant differences among the available pumps and sensors in regard to their algorithms and their ability to target optimal glucose levels, provide microboluses, and prevent hypoglycemia. Pump failures, often resulting from insertion problems or kinked tubing, increase the risk of DKA because they contain rapid-acting insulin. Therefore, pumps are best used in women who are already skilled in carbohydrate counting, using correction factors, and successful pump use prior to conception.

14. **What is the role of noninsulin agents in periconception and pregnancy?**
Few data are available on the use of many agents during pregnancy, particularly dipeptidyl peptidase-4 (DPP-4) inhibitors, glucagon-like peptide-1 (GLP-1) agonists, sodium–glucose cotransporter 2 (SGLT-2) inhibitors, and thiazolidinediones (TZDs). Some of the available data are concerning, especially for SGLT-2 inhibitors and TZDs. Glyburide (sulfonylurea) and metformin (biguanide) are the most commonly used oral agents, but they are highly likely to fail in women with preexisting DM. The American Diabetes Association (ADA) and ACOG both recommend insulin as a first-line agent, even in those with GDM. Metformin and glyburide have been shown to cross the placenta, metformin more so than glyburide. Glyburide has been associated with a higher risk of macrosomia than insulin in GDM, possibly as a result of not being dosed appropriately 1 hour prior to meals or from crossing the placenta and stimulating fetal hyperinsulinemia. Metformin is concentrated in fetal mitochondria and may decrease cell-cycle proliferation and have growth-restrictive properties, especially in the placenta. In two large GDM and polycystic ovary syndrome (PCOS) randomized controlled trials (RCTs), the 5- to 10-year-old offspring of women who took metformin were heavier, possibly as a result of mild nutrient restriction in utero followed by an obesogenic postnatal environment. Metformin was recently studied in an RCT as an adjunct to insulin therapy in T2DM in Canada and Australia (MiTY trial). Although there was no difference in the primary composite fetal outcome, adding metformin did result in a slight decrease in A1c (6.1% vs. 5.9%), insulin dose, weight gain (1.8 kg), and LGA and macrosomia rates; however, there was also nearly a twofold increase in small-for-gestational-age (SGA) infants, another risk factor for childhood metabolic disease. Therefore, the long-term safety of these medications for the offspring needs further study. However, women with pregestational DM who are on metformin or glyburide prior to pregnancy can continue these agents until a safe transition is made to insulin therapy because these agents are not teratogens, unlike hyperglycemia.

15. **How are glargine, detemir, and neutral protamine Hagedorn (NPH) used during pregnancy?**
NPH can be useful for women with fasting hyperglycemia from hepatic insulin resistance, which is very common in Latin American women, if it is given immediately before bedtime because it usually peaks in 5 to 8 hours. Both glargine and detemir have been shown to be safe and efficacious as long-acting insulin analogs in pregnancy. They are usually given at ~40% of the total daily dose of insulin; they may be particularly beneficial in pregnant women with DM who experience recurrent hypoglycemia. There are few data on degludec in pregnancy, but all insulins are too large to cross the placenta.

16. **Discuss the role of short-acting or rapid-acting insulin analogs during pregnancy**
Regular insulin requires administration 30 minutes prior to meals, peaks at 3 to 4 hours, and lasts up to 8 hours. Rapid-acting insulin analogs are given 15 minutes prior to meals, peak at 1 hour, and last 3 to 4 hours. Given this difference in pharmacokinetics, rapid-acting insulin analogs (aspart, lispro, glulisine) may reduce hypoglycemia and postprandial hyperglycemia compared with regular insulin. Rapid-acting insulins are especially beneficial in achieving good control when women are willing to learn how to count carbohydrates, use a correction factor, and dose their insulin using an intensive, flexible regimen, which is especially critical to the optimal treatment of women with T1DM. Ultra-rapid-acting insulins (Fiasp and Lyumjev) have not been studied extensively in pregnant women but would not be expected to cross the placenta and may potentially be useful in patients who need to pre-bolus for a significant time before meals due to their more rapid onset. Their use in insulin pumps has not yet been adequately studied.

17. **How does pregnancy affect coronary artery disease (CAD) morbidity and mortality in women with DM?**
Pregnant women with DM have higher morbidity and mortality rates from CAD as a result of the increased cardiovascular (CV) stress associated with increased plasma volume, cardiac output, oxygen consumption, and left ventricular size. In women with preexisting CAD, this stress can lead to decreased myocardial perfusion. Therefore, the cardiac status of all women with DM and CV risk factors (hypertension, smoking, hyperlipidemia, autonomic neuropathy, strong family history, severe microvascular disease) should be functionally tested prior to conception. Asymptomatic women over age 35 years or with long-standing DM, hypertension, or CV risk factors should have a resting electrocardiogram (ECG). Testing with an echocardiogram is also recommended in women with long-standing DM, hypertension, vascular disease, or concerns for sleep apnea, which can cause pulmonary hypertension, a major risk factor for maternal and fetal morbidity.

18. **What is the relationship between pregnancy and diabetic nephropathy or hypertension?**
Pregnancy leads to a ~50% increase in the glomerular filtration rate (GFR) and an increase in proteinuria that can sometimes become nephrotic-range proteinuria; however, it is not associated with a decline in kidney function unless women have moderate to severe renal impairment (creatinine $\geq$ 1.4 mg/dL). Women with more

severe renal disease (creatinine $\geq$ 2.0 mg/dL) have a 30% to 50% chance of a permanent GFR decline that may lead to dialysis during pregnancy. Furthermore, women with elevated serum creatinine, severe hypertension, or nephrotic-range proteinuria have an extremely high risk of developing preeclampsia, preterm delivery, and fetal growth restriction. Baby aspirin therapy is recommended for all women with preexisting DM, hypertension, or any degree of renal disease. Women who have had a successful renal transplant 1 to 2 years prior to pregnancy and are on stable immunosuppressive therapy have a much better risk profile than women with severe renal disease without transplant. Severe hypertension alone (blood pressure $\geq$ 160/110 mm Hg on no medications) carries an approximately 50% risk of preeclampsia; although treating blood pressure is important to prevent maternal hypertensive complications, it does not prevent preeclampsia, a disease characterized by abnormal early placentation, angiogenesis, and placental insufficiency. Furthermore, overtreatment of maternal blood pressure can actually decrease placental perfusion, and therefore aggressive treatment to a goal of <130/80 mm Hg in pregnancy is not recommended.

19. **Discuss the effects of pregnancy on diabetic retinopathy**
Pregnancy can lead to the progression of proliferative retinopathy. This is primarily attributable to its hypercoagulable state, increase in growth factors, and relative anemia. Therefore all women with DM should be screened for retinopathy prior to conception and be treated for proliferative retinopathy if indicated. An ophthalmologic exam is recommended in the first trimester, with the frequency of follow-up based on this visit. Dilated retinal exams and laser therapy can be safely achieved in pregnancy. Although data are limited, topical anti–vascular endothelial growth factor (anti-VEGF) therapy is likely to be safe if necessary.

20. **Define the risk of DKA in pregnancy, and explain how it affects the fetus**
DKA occurs in pregnancy at lower blood glucose levels (<250 mg/dL), just as it does in patients using SGLT-2 inhibitors, termed *euglycemic DKA*. Given the early transition from carbohydrate to lipid metabolism within 12 hours, pregnancy is a ketogenic state, coined the "accelerated starvation of pregnancy." The high progesterone levels in pregnancy cause a primary respiratory alkalosis with a compensatory metabolic acidosis, leading to decreased buffering capacity. Coupled with an increase in plasma volume, hyperfiltration leading to glycosuria, and maternal glucose freely diffusing across the placenta, these factors predispose pregnant women to DKA at much lower glucose levels. Women with T1DM are especially predisposed; however, in the setting of infections, prolonged fasting, or steroids to promote fetal lung maturity, women with T2DM and GDM can also develop DKA. There is a particularly high risk in women with nausea and oral nutrition intolerance, as often occurs early in pregnancy or in hyperemesis gravidarum. Although the fetal mortality rate attributable to DKA has been on the decline, it continues to remain high, especially in the late second and third trimesters because of fetal acid–base and electrolyte abnormalities and ischemia. There is also an increased risk of preterm birth and NICU admission. Therefore any suspicion for DKA should be treated as an emergency, and women should have ketone strips at home to ensure ketone levels are decreasing with appropriate insulin treatment and adequate oral intake. The treatment of DKA in pregnant women requires an additional 100 to 150 g of carbohydrate per day to meet placental and fetal demands in order to resolve starvation ketosis.

21. **What fetal surveillance measures are recommended in pregnant women with DM?**
An early ultrasound is recommended in women with DM to confirm viability and date the pregnancy. At 18 to 22 weeks of gestation, a formal anatomy scan should be done to evaluate for fetal anomalies. Echocardiography is considered at 20 to 24 weeks if the A1c is >6.5% (some experts use >7.5%), if a four-chamber view of the heart is inadequately visualized on ultrasound, or if cardiac anomalies are in question. Because neonates delivered to women with pregestational DM are at risk of macrosomia (poor glycemic control) and fetal growth restriction (placental insufficiency), fetal growth scans are usually offered at 28 to 32 weeks of gestation and prior to delivery. Antenatal fetal monitoring with nonstress tests, biophysical profiles, or modified biophysical profiles should be offered at 32 weeks of gestation because of the increased risk of stillbirth, or earlier in women with poor control, with pregestational DM, or with GDM requiring insulin. Delivery should be planned at 37 to 38 weeks with poorly controlled or complicated pregestational DM, especially in those who are obese, given its significant contribution to perinatal deaths. Women with well-controlled or uncomplicated DM and reassuring antenatal testing may be delivered near 39 weeks, a time when induction in normal, healthy women was shown to have the most favorable newborn outcomes and not increase the risk of cesarean delivery. Obstetric complications, severe growth restriction, or severe preeclampsia warrant delivery earlier than 37 weeks (term), and the optimal timing of delivery should be determined with the expertise of a maternal-fetal medicine specialist (perinatologist) or obstetrician experienced in diabetes in pregnancy management.

22. **What is GDM, and how is it diagnosed?**
GDM results from an inability of women to increase insulin secretion sufficiently to overcome the increased insulin demands and insulin resistance of pregnancy. Historically, it has been difficult to distinguish between GDM and undiagnosed T2DM in pregnancy, but now the same diagnostic criteria for DM outside of pregnancy (A1c $\geq$ 6.5%, fasting blood glucose [FBG] $\geq$ 126 mg/dL, or random glucose $\geq$ 200 mg/dL) at any time during pregnancy are

Table 16.2 Oral Glucose Tolerance Test Diagnostic Criteria (in mg/dL) for Diabetes Mellitus (DM) Complicating Pregnancy and Gestational Diabetes Mellitus (GDM)

CRITERIA	DM COMPLICATING PREGNANCY	GDM	
	WHO	IADPSG	CARPENTER AND COUSTAN
Glucose administered (g)	75	75	100
Plasma Glucose Thresholds (mg/dL, positive if ≥)			
Fasting	≥126	≥92	≥95
1 hour	—	≥180	≥180
2 hour	≥200	≥153	≥155
3 hour	—	—	≥140

IADPSG, International Association of Diabetes and Pregnancy Study Group; *WHO*, World Health Organization.

used to distinguish preexisting DM (usually T2DM but occasionally maturity-onset diabetes of the young [MODY]) from GDM. Women with risk factors for T2DM (overweight/obese adults with PCOS, metabolic syndrome, prior history of GDM or a macrosomic infant, etc.) should be screened for DM at their first prenatal visit using standard diagnostic criteria. The ACOG also recommends an early screen for GDM in women at high risk if preexisting DM has been excluded. If an oral glucose tolerance test (OGTT) is done and they meet the criteria for GDM, they would be managed as GDM (early GDM); many of these women have prediabetes. All other women without risk factors are usually universally screened at 24 to 28 weeks of gestation. There is currently no consensus on the best diagnostic test to use to diagnose GDM. Two strategies are currently used for diagnosis:

1. **"One-Step" Approach:** A 75-g OGTT with plasma glucose measurements when fasting (after 8 hours overnight), at 1 hour, and at 2 hours. The diagnosis is made if a single plasma glucose value is greater than or equal to the thresholds determined by the International Association of Diabetes and Pregnancy Study Group (IADPSG; Table 16.2). These values have been associated with a 1.75-fold increased risk of LGA. Approximately 20% of pregnant women would meet the criteria for GDM with this method (compared with 6%–7% using the criteria in the "two-step" approach). Given the added expense of treatment, there is a debate about whether this larger population would clearly benefit from treatment. RCTs are currently ongoing to compare outcomes from this approach versus the "two-step" approach.

2. **"Two-Step" Approach:** A 50-g oral glucose loading test (nonfasting) with plasma glucose measurement at 1 hour. If the glucose level is ≥130 to 140 mg/dL (threshold selected by differences in positive and negative predictive values desired), a 100-g OGTT is performed with measurements of plasma glucose levels when fasting and at 1, 2, and 3 hours. The diagnosis is made if 2 out of 4 plasma glucose values are abnormal by the Carpenter–Coustan criteria (Table 16.2).

23. **What poor maternal-fetal outcomes are associated with GDM?**
    Women with GDM are at increased risk of developing preeclampsia, having a cesarean section, experiencing preterm labor as a result of polyhydramnios, and developing T2DM later in life (70% within 22–28 years and up to 50% within 5–10 years after pregnancy). In Latin American women, 60% of those with GDM will develop T2DM within 5 years after pregnancy, and up to 80% will develop T2DM if they have evidence of prediabetes on a 75-g 2-hour OGTT postpartum. Poor fetal outcomes with GDM include macrosomia, LGA, hyperbilirubinemia, cardiac septal hypertrophy, RDS, shoulder dystocia/birth trauma, neonatal hypoglycemia, and very rarely, stillbirth, especially in those requiring insulin and who have more severe hyperglycemia and those with Class 3 obesity. Additionally, offspring of mothers with GDM are more likely to develop obesity and DM later in life.

24. **Discuss diet therapy and pharmacologic therapy in GDM**
    Most women with GDM can use lifestyle (nutritional modifications and physical activity) to meet postprandial glucose targets. Glycemic control can be improved with the intake of complex carbohydrates and the avoidance of saturated fat and simple carbohydrates, along with the ingestion of good-quality fat and protein across the day. A total of 175 g of complex carbohydrates is recommended in the late second and third trimesters in all pregnant women because of the increased fetal and placental glucose requirements. Low-carbohydrate diets are ketogenic and not recommended. Lifestyle modifications alone are less effective if fasting hyperglycemia is present. If fasting and 1- to 2-hour postprandial goals are not achieved ~70% of the time (question 9) or if there is evidence of LGA on a growth ultrasound, pharmacologic therapy should be instituted. As with pregnant women

with pregestational DM, insulin is the preferred therapeutic agent; glyburide and metformin can be used cautiously because they do cross the placenta and may pose a risk as a result of fetal exposure leading to intrauterine programming and long-term health effects (question 12).

25. **Describe the relationship between maternal DM and lactation**
All women with DM should be encouraged to breastfeed, given the benefits from maternal immunoglobulins and the human oligosaccharides that reduce the risk of necrotizing enterocolitis. Furthermore, breastfeeding has been shown to decrease the risk of the development of T2DM in mothers with GDM and obesity in the offspring. Mothers with GDM and DM have a higher risk of delayed onset of lactogenesis and breastfeeding difficulties; a lactation consultant can be extremely valuable. Women with T1DM are at risk of hypoglycemia with breastfeeding, necessitating a decrease in pregestational insulin dosing by 10% to 20% and an increase in caloric intake of ~200 kcal per day if they are not trying to lose weight. Glyburide and metformin are compatible with breastfeeding, but continuing to treat T2DM with a sulfonylurea long term is less desirable given that unloading the pancreas may be better for long-term beta cell function.

26. **What is the role of glucose monitoring postpartum?**
Blood glucose should be monitored closely postpartum in women with DM and GDM because of the expected drastic decrease in insulin requirements upon placental delivery. Most women with GDM do not require treatment. However, at 6 to 12 weeks postdelivery, a 75-g OGTT should be performed to assess for DM (FBG $\geq$ 126 mg/dL; 2-hr $\geq$ 200 mg/dL) or prediabetes (FBG 100–125 mg/dL; 2-hr 140–199 mg/dL). Primary DM prevention should be implemented in women with GDM, especially if they manifest prediabetes. A1c is not an effective marker of glycemic control at 6 weeks postdelivery and should not be used for diagnosis. Rescreening for DM should be performed every 1 to 3 years because many women with a history of GDM enter their next pregnancy with undiagnosed T2DM, resulting in an increased risk of major malformations. As noted, it is especially important to prescribe effective contraception until another pregnancy, if desired, can be optimally planned.

27. **What are the risks of COVID-19 in pregnant women with diabetes and should vaccines be recommended?**
Pregnant women are at higher risk for more severe COVID-19 infections, hospitalizations, the need for respiratory support, and death compared to nonpregnant women, and their infants are at higher risk for preterm delivery, growth restriction, and admission to the NICU. Preexisting diabetes, obesity, and hypertension further increase the risk for maternal ICU admissions and NICU stays. Given that COVID-19 vaccinations have been given in ~90,000 pregnant women with no evidence of increased maternal or newborn risks and may protect the newborn with antibodies, the American College of Obstetrics and Gynecology recommends COVID-19 vaccines for all pregnant women, and the Society of Maternal-Fetal Medicine recommends vaccines especially for women with underlying medical conditions including diabetes, obesity, or hypertension.

KEY POINTS 1: PRECONCEPTION COUNSELING IN DIABETES

1. Preconception counseling and care have been shown to improve maternal outcomes, improve perinatal morbidity and mortality, and reduce the risk of congenital malformations. Associated comorbidities should also be diagnosed and optimally controlled.
2. In the absence of major contraindications, all forms of contraception are safe and efficacious in women with diabetes and safer than unintended pregnancies.

KEY POINTS 2: PREGESTATIONAL DIABETES IN PREGNANCY

1. The risk for congenital abnormalities can be reduced to the baseline population risk if A1c is $\leq$6.5% prior to conception (before 5–8 weeks' gestation).
2. T2DM poses at least as high of a risk as T1DM because of the associated comorbidities of obesity, hypertension, hyperlipidemia, and sleep apnea and is associated with a higher stillbirth rate, especially when complicated by maternal obesity, and should be optimally treated preconception.
3. Insulin requirements decrease in the first trimester but double to quadruple in the second and third trimesters as a result of pregnancy-induced insulin resistance. Adding metformin to insulin in T2DM to decrease insulin requirements is controversial and may be associated with an increased risk of SGA and potentially childhood obesity risk.
4. Proteinuria, diabetic retinopathy, autonomic neuropathy, and severe diabetic nephropathy may worsen with pregnancy. ACEis and ARBs should be discontinued in women actively trying to conceive or in the early first trimester, as soon as pregnancy is confirmed.
5. Pregnancy is a ketogenic state, and women with diabetes can go into diabetic ketoacidosis at lower glucose levels (even <200 mg/dL) in pregnancy.

KEY POINTS 3: GDM

1. There is no current consensus between major societies on the diagnostic criteria for GDM and the role of early screening for GDM, but there is evidence that women with prediabetes in the first trimester have a similar risk of adverse pregnancy outcomes as women with T2DM.
2. The use of oral agents to manage GDM in pregnancy is controversial because of the ability of glyburide and metformin to cross the placenta, leading to unknown long-term effects on the fetus.
3. Women with GDM are at increased risk of developing T2DM in later life. They should be screened for T2DM at 6 weeks postpartum and then every 1 to 3 years thereafter.

KEY POINTS 4: POSTPARTUM CARE IN DIABETES

1. Insulin requirements drastically drop upon placental delivery, and women with DM are at high risk of hypoglycemia postpartum, requiring less insulin than prepregnancy.
2. Women with DM often have a delay in milk production and difficulties in breastfeeding, but breastfeeding should be encouraged, with close monitoring for hypoglycemia.
3. Effective contraception is critical postpartum, even in breastfeeding mothers, to prevent undesired pregnancies and so that appropriate preconception counseling can be readdressed.

BIBLIOGRAPHY

1. ACOG Practice Bulletin No. 201 Pregestational Diabetes Mellitus. *Obstet Gynecol*. 2018;132(6):e228–e248.
1a. American College of Obstetrics and Gynecology. COVID-19 vaccines in pregnancy: conversation guide for clinicians. https://www.acog.org/-/media/project/acog/acogorg/files/pdfs/clinical-guidance/practice-advisory/covid19vaccine-conversation-guide-121520-v2.pdf?la=en&hash=439FFEC1991B7DD3925352A5308C7C42.
2. Physical Activity and Exercise During Pregnancy and the Postpartum Period, ACOG Committee Opinion, Number 804. *Obstet Gynecol*. 2020;135(4):e178–e188.
3. American Diabetes A 2. Classification and diagnosis of diabetes: standards of medical care in diabetes-2020. *Diabetes Care*. 2020;43(Suppl 1):S14–S31.
4. American Diabetes A 14. Management of diabetes in pregnancy: standards of medical care in diabetes-2020. *Diabetes Care*. 2020;43(Suppl 1):S183–S192.
5. Barbour LA. Metabolic culprits in obese pregnancies and gestational diabetes mellitus: big babies, big twists, big picture: the 2018 Norbert Freinkel Award Lecture. *Diabetes Care*. 2019;42(5):718–726.
6. Barbour LA, Feig DS. Metformin for gestational diabetes mellitus: progeny, perspective, and a personalized approach. *Diabetes Care*. 2019;42(3):396–399.
7. Browne K, Park BY, Goetzinger KR, Caughey AB, Yao R. The joint effects of obesity and pregestational diabetes on the risk of stillbirth. *J Matern Fetal Neonatal Med*. 2019;1–7.
8. Buschur E, Stetson B, Barbour LA. Diabetes in pregnancy. In: Carr B, ed. *Endotext.org*. 2018.
9. Committee on Practice B-O ACOG Practice Bulletin No. 190: Gestational Diabetes Mellitus. *Obstet Gynecol*. 2018;131(2):e49–e64.
10. Dutton H, Borengasser SJ, Gaudet LM, Barbour LA, Keely EJ. Obesity in pregnancy: optimizing outcomes for mom and baby. *Med Clin North Am*. 2018;102(1):87–106.
11. Egan AM, Dow ML, Vella A. A review of the pathophysiology and management of diabetes in pregnancy. *Mayo Clin Proc*. 2020
12. Feghali MN, Scifres CM. Novel therapies for diabetes mellitus in pregnancy. *BMJ*. 2018;362:k2034.
13. Feig DS, Donovan LE, Corcoy R, et al. Continuous glucose monitoring in pregnant women with type 1 diabetes (CONCEPTT): a multicentre international randomised controlled trial. *Lancet*. 2017;390(10110):2347–2359.
14. Feig DS, Donovan LE, Zinman B, et al. Metformin in women with type 2 diabetes in pregnancy (MiTy): a multicentre, international, randomised, placebo-controlled trial. *Lancet Diabetes Endocrinol*. 2020;8(10):834–844.
15. McIntyre HD, Catalano P, Zhang C, Desoye G, Mathiesen ER, Damm P. Gestational diabetes mellitus. *Nat Rev Dis Primers*. 2019;5(1):47.
16. Napoli A. Insulin therapy and diabetic pregnancy. *Am J Ther*. 2020;27(1):e91–e105.
17. Yamamoto JM, Murphy HR. Benefits of real-time continuous glucose monitoring in pregnancy. *Diab Technol Ther*. 2021;23(Supp 1):S8–S14.

CHAPTER 17

DIABETES MANAGEMENT IN PATIENTS WITH CANCER

Elizabeth Tupta, NP-C

1. **Is diabetes associated with cancer risk?**

   Yes. People with diabetes have a 20% to 25% increased risk for developing cancer compared with those without diabetes. Most studies have evaluated cancer risk and type 2 diabetes (T2DM) and found T2DM to be associated with a 2-fold higher risk for liver, pancreatic, and endometrial cancers and a 1.5-fold increased risk for colon, rectal, ovarian, and bladder cancers. The relationship between cancer risk and type 1 diabetes (T1DM) has been less well studied, but it also appears to be associated with an increased malignancy risk, especially for liver, pancreatic, and endometrial cancers and also for thyroid, stomach, kidney, and lung cancers.

   Whether the relationship between diabetes and cancer is causal or correlational is unclear. Possible direct mechanisms for increased cancer risk include hyperglycemia, hyperinsulinemia, high levels of IGF-1, increased inflammatory cytokines, and alterations of insulin signaling pathways. Indirect links include common underlying risk factors such as age, obesity, alcohol, physical activity, and smoking. More rigorous studies are needed to determine whether there is a direct causal relationship between diabetes and cancer.

2. **Do people with diabetes and cancer have a worse prognosis?**

   Studies support that adults with diabetes also have a higher risk of cancer mortality compared with individuals without diabetes (hazard ratio = 1.25). The strongest mortality risk has been associated with liver, colorectal, ovarian, lung, bladder, and breast cancers. This risk was significantly reduced after adjusting for fasting glucose and hemoglobin A1c levels, supporting that poor glycemic control negatively affects cancer outcomes.

3. **What factors may contribute to the increased cancer mortality risk in people with diabetes?**
   1. Hyperglycemia:
      - Promotes tumor-cell metabolism and growth through increased glucose uptake
      - Stimulates IGF-1 signaling pathways, promoting angiogenesis and metastases
      - Increases levels of reactive oxygen species (ROS), which may promote DNA mutations and tumor-cell progression
   2. Hyperinsulinemia:
      - Stimulates insulin and IGF-1 receptors, which are expressed by cancer cells and are responsible for tumor growth, invasion, and metastases
      - Increases free estrogen and testosterone levels in women and men through decreased hepatic synthesis of sex-hormone–binding globulin and increased androgen production by the ovaries, increasing the risk of breast and endometrial cancers
   3. Inflammatory cytokines:
      - Insulin resistance and associated obesity cause an increase in free fatty acids and proinflammatory cytokines such as tumor necrosis factor-α and interleukin-6, all of which may play a role in malignancy and cancer progression.
   4. Compromised immune system:
      - Impaired innate immunity may decrease the efficacy of cancer therapies.
   5. Comorbid conditions:
      - Individuals with diabetes are at higher risk of having other underlying comorbidities, such as cardiovascular disease, kidney disease, and peripheral neuropathy, which may limit the ability to provide aggressive therapy and increases the risk for dose-limiting toxicities.

4. **Why is glycemic control important in the cancer population?**

   Hyperglycemia has been associated with an increased risk for infection, hospitalization with increased length of stay, cancer progression, and overall mortality. Hyperglycemia may also contribute to malnutrition and weight loss and exacerbate fatigue and diabetic complications such as neuropathy. Therefore effectively treating hyperglycemia may improve cancer outcomes while enhancing quality of life.

5. **What are appropriate glycemic targets for cancer patients?**

   Currently, there are no guidelines that establish glycemic targets for patients with cancer and diabetes. Clarification of treatment goals requires a collaborative discussion between patients, families, and providers. When determining A1c targets, providers should consider similar factors as in the general diabetes population,

Table 17.1 Antidiabetic Therapy and Special Considerations for the Oncology Population

DRUG	SPECIAL CONSIDERATIONS
Biguanides	• Considered drug of choice for patients with cancer and diabetes • Antitumor effects • Avoid if nausea, vomiting, or malnutrition • Available in liquid form if difficulty swallowing • Consider alternative if frequent need for CT imaging with contrast and eGFR < 60 • Contraindicated if eGFR < 30 or active liver disease
Sulfonylureas	• Avoid if high hypoglycemia risk • Avoid if irregular eating patterns • Avoid if decreased PO intake, nausea, or vomiting • Alternative to insulin for treatment of steroid-induced hyperglycemia
Meglitinides	• Avoid if high hypoglycemia risk • Avoid if decreased PO intake, nausea, or vomiting • May consider "as needed" if irregular eating patterns
Thiazolidinediones	• Avoid if history of bladder cancer • Contraindicated if active bladder cancer or heart failure
DPP-4 inhibitors	• Avoid if pancreatitis risk • Renal dosing for sitagliptin, saxagliptin, alogliptin
GLP-1 agonists	• Avoid if pancreatitis risk • Avoid if weight loss, decreased PO intake, nausea, or vomiting • Contraindicated if personal or family history of medullary thyroid cancer
SGLT-2 inhibitors	• Avoid if weight loss, decreased PO intake, nausea, or vomiting • Avoid with eGFR < 45, contraindicated with eGFR < 30 • Consider DKA risk • Canagliflozin associated with increase renal-cell carcinoma risk
Insulin	• Drug of choice if severe hyperglycemia, symptomatic hyperglycemia, or CIADM • Best option if anorexia, weight loss, or muscle wasting • Choose rapid-acting insulin if erratic eating patterns • Consider NPH with steroid-induced hyperglycemia

CIADM, Checkpoint inhibitor-associated autoimmune diabetes mellitus; *CT*, computed tomography; *DDP-4*, dipeptidyl peptidase-4; *DKA*, diabetic ketoacidosis; *eGFR*, estimated glomerular filtration rate; *GLP-1*, glucagon-like peptide-1; *NPH*, neutral protamine Hagedorn; *SGLT-2*, sodium–glucose cotransporter 2.

including hypoglycemia risk, life expectancy, financial limitations, available support, and patient preferences. Additional unique considerations include cancer therapy side effects that increase the risk for hypoglycemia, such as nausea, vomiting, and malnutrition.

It is important to educate patients and families early regarding the potential shift in glycemic targets based on the course of the cancer trajectory. In general, the goal A1c is 7% to 8%, with a higher target closer to 8.5% in those with increased frailty and hypoglycemia risk. For patients who are terminally ill, glycemic goals should shift from focusing on the A1c to the prevention of hypoglycemia and symptomatic hyperglycemia, with suggested blood glucose (BG) targets of 108 to 270 mg/dL for a prognosis of months to years and 180 to 360 mg/dL for a prognosis of days to weeks.

6. **List available antidiabetic therapies for oncology patients and special considerations when selecting an optimal therapy**
When selecting appropriate diabetes therapies, the American Diabetes Association (ADA) guidelines for pharmacologic management should be followed. Table 17.1 lists the available therapies and unique factors to consider within the cancer population.

7. **Explain how metformin may improve cancer outcomes.**
Metformin is considered the first-line antidiabetic drug of choice for individuals with cancer because of its efficacy, safety, and antitumor effects. There are multiple proposed mechanisms that may contribute to metformin's

anticancer effects: (1) decreased protein synthesis and cell growth through adenosine monophosphate kinase (AMPK) activation and mechanistic target of rapamycin (mTOR) inhibition, (2) the induction of tumor-cell apoptosis, (3) decreased circulating insulin levels, (4) immune system activation, and (5) destruction of cancer stem cells. Research supports that metformin may work adjunctively with chemotherapy to reduce tumor size and metastasis risk and is associated with a lower risk of relapse and mortality. Metformin has also been shown to enhance the effect of radiotherapy by increasing ROS, leading to increased DNA damage.

8. **What cancer therapies are associated with an increased risk for hyperglycemia in patients with cancer with or without underlying diabetes?**
   Because many cancer therapies affect pathways that regulate glucose and insulin metabolism, individuals receiving cancer therapies, with or without underlying diabetes, are at high risk for developing hyperglycemia during cancer treatment. Hyperglycemia is one of the most common toxicities for phosphoinositide 3-kinase (PI3K)/Akt pathway inhibitors used for the treatment of breast cancer, with up to 65% of patients who receive alpelisib experiencing high BG levels. mTOR inhibitors, which work within the PI3K signaling pathway, are also used in breast cancer therapy and similarly cause a high incidence of hyperglycemia, ranging from 13% to 50%. Tyrosine kinase inhibitors (TKIs) are a broad class of targeted therapies that include epidermal growth factor receptor (EGFR) (erlotinib) and *BCR-ABL1* (imatinib) inhibitors. TKIs are used for the treatment of certain lung cancers and chronic myelogenous leukemia (CML) and have been linked to both hypoglycemia and hyperglycemia. The immune checkpoint inhibitors (ICIs), which are used in numerous malignancies, such as metastatic melanoma, lymphoma, and lung cancer, have caused a novel type of autoimmune diabetes referred to as *checkpoint inhibitor-associated autoimmune diabetes mellitus* (CIADM). Additionally, treatment with glucocorticoids is associated with an incidence of hyperglycemia ranging from 30% to 50% in hospitalized patients without a prior history of diabetes. Please refer to Table 17.2 for a complete list of cancer therapies associated with hyperglycemia, along with recommended monitoring and treatments.

9. **Explain how ICIs work and how they cause autoimmune diabetes**
   Programmed cell death protein 1 (PD-1) and cytotoxic T lymphocyte–associated antigen-4 (CTLA-4) are regulatory proteins that promote self-tolerance by preventing T-cell activation and inducing T-cell apoptosis. Tumor cells evade the immune system by expressing ligands that activate these inhibitory pathways, allowing the tumor cells to survive. ICIs are monoclonal antibodies that target PD-1, its ligand (programmed cell death protein 1 ligand [PDL-1]), or CTLA-4 to promote T-cell activation and tumor cell death. PD-1 and PDL-1 inhibitors have been associated with CIADM.
   We know that T1DM is caused by autoimmune destruction of insulin-producing beta cells. There is also evidence to support the involvement of the PD-1 pathway in the development and progression of autoimmune diabetes. PDL-1 is expressed on inflamed pancreatic islet cells, allowing for the inhibition of autoreactive T-cells and preventing the destruction of beta cells. Studies investigating the development of autoimmune diabetes with the nonobese diabetic mouse model have shown that PD-1 blockade precipitates the rapid development of autoimmune diabetes. Furthermore, there is evidence that humans with T1DM have a significantly lower expression of PD-1 in CD4+ T cells compared with the general healthy population. Therefore it is proposed that treatment with a PD-1/PDL-1 inhibitor blocks this inhibition and allows for the activation of autoreactive T-cells, leading to beta-cell destruction.

10. **Have CTLA-4 inhibitors been associated with CIADM?**
    There have been very few case reports of CIADM associated with CTLA-4 inhibitor monotherapy, with most cases having received previous PD-1 inhibitor therapy. It is proposed that CTLA-4 affects naïve T cells, whereas the PD-1 pathway seems to play a role in regulating autoreactive T cells throughout the life span.

11. **What is the incidence of CIADM?**
    CIADM is very rare, with incidence rates of between 0.1% and 1% reported.

12. **How do people with CIADM typically present?**
    Affected individuals often present with an acute onset of hyperglycemia and diabetic ketoacidosis (DKA). The A1c level is usually only moderately elevated (median 7.6%), with a typically low or undetectable C-peptide, supporting a short duration of hyperglycemia and rapid beta-cell destruction. Approximately 50% of people with CIADM do not have diabetes-associated autoantibodies. All those reported to have positive antibodies have had positive anti–glutamine acid decarboxylase (GAD) antibodies.

13. **What are risk factors for the development of CIADM?**
    Underlying autoimmune disease and other autoimmune adverse effects secondary to ICIs are associated with a higher risk of developing CIADM. Patients who develop CIADM often experience other autoimmune adverse effects, such as thyroiditis, pancreatitis, and colitis, either before, during, or after developing autoimmune diabetes. Studies that have investigated the presence of high-risk human leukocyte antigen (HLA) haplotypes

Table 17.2 Cancer Therapies Associated With Hyperglycemia

DRUG	MECHANISM OF HYPERGLYCEMIA	ONSET	MONITORING	INTERVENTIONS
ICIs (PD-1/PDL-1 inhibitors (pembrolizumab) as monotherapy or combined with CTLA-4 inhibitors (ipilimumab)	PD-1 blockade allows for beta-cell destruction by autoreactive T cells	1–52 weeks	BG at baseline and prior to each infusion × 12 weeks, then every 3–6 weeks	• If DKA, treat per institution guidelines • Initiate insulin therapy if FBG > 160 mg/dL and concern for T1DM **If BG > 250 mg/dL:** • Hold therapy and evaluate for DKA • Evaluate for T1DM • Initiate insulin therapy
TKIs-EGFR/*BCR-ABL* inhibitors (nilotinib, sunitinib)	• Unknown • Some TKIs associated with hypoglycemia (imatinib and dasatinib)	1–3 weeks	• FBG at baseline and days 1, 8, and 15 of each cycle • Start home monitoring BID if FBG > 160 mg/dL or any random BG > 200 mg/dL	• Start metformin 500 mg BID if 2 BG > 160 mg/dL in 1 week • Hold therapy if FBG > 500 mg/dL, restart when FBG < 250 mg/dL and consider dose reduction
PI3K-Akt-mTOR inhibitors (alpelisib, idelalisib, everoliums)	• ↑ Insulin resistance, ↓ insulin secretion, ↓ glycogen synthesis, ↓ glucose utilization	1–2 cycles	• FBG and A1c at baseline • FBG prior to each cycle • Start home BG monitoring once FBG > 160 mg/dL or any random BG > 200 mg/dL	• See Fig. 17.1 • Ketogenic diet and SGLT-2 inhibitors may increase treatment effectiveness • Insulin may decrease treatment effectiveness
Anti-CD30 drug conjugate (Brentuximab)	• Unknown Proposed mechanisms: • Cytokine release syndrome • Type B insulin resistance syndrome	1–4 weeks	• Monitor BG levels prior to each treatment • Home monitoring for 1–2 weeks after infusion • Ensure home monitoring with existing DM	• Insulin therapy initially, usually requiring intravenous insulin therapy • Insulin therapy often not needed after initial hyperglycemic episode • Dose reduction with subsequent cycles
Platinum analogs (cisplatin)	Unknown	1–2 weeks	Monitor BG weekly after infusion	• Initiate antidiabetic therapy if BG > 180 mg/dL × 2 or A1c > 7% • Treat DKA/HHS per institution guidelines

Continued

Table 17.2 Cancer Therapies Associated With Hyperglycemia—cont'd

DRUG	MECHANISM OF HYPERGLYCEMIA	ONSET	MONITORING	INTERVENTIONS
Corticosteroids	• ↑ Insulin resistance • ↓ Insulin release	• Usually within 48 hours • May occur later with longer steroid duration/exposure	• Monitor BG ACHS × 48 hours if no preexisting DM • Increase BG monitoring to ACHS if preexisting DM	• Initiate NPH at the same time as steroid dose or basal (30%)/bolus (70%) therapy if BG > 180 mg/dL × 2 OR if preexisting DM with A1c > 7.5% • May consider sulfonylurea in place of insulin
Calcineurin inhibitors	• ↑ insulin resistance • ↑ beta cell apoptosis	• Days to weeks • Risk decreases with dose decrease	• Routine lab monitoring per transplant protocol • Initiate home BG monitoring with serum BG > 180 mg/dL	• Initiate antidiabetic therapy if BG > 180 mg/dL × 2 or A1c ≥ 7%
Hormone-based therapies	• ↓ Insulin secretion • ↑ Insulin resistance	• Risk increases > 2 yr on SERM and > 6 mo on ADT	• Initiate home BG monitoring if serum BG > 180 mg/dL	• Initiate antidiabetic therapy if BG > 180 mg/dL × 2 or A1c ≥ 7%

ACHS, before meals and bedtime; *ADT*, androgen deprivation therapy; *BG*, blood glucose; *CTLA-4*, cytotoxic T lymphocyte–associated antigen-4; *DKA*, diabetic ketoacidosis; *DM*, diabetes mellitus; *eGFR*, estimated glomerular filtration rate; *FBG*, fasting blood glucose; *HHS*, hyperglycemic hyperosmolar syndrome; *ICI*, immune checkpoint inhibitor; *mTOR*, mechanistic target of rapamycin; *PI3K*, phosphoinositide 3-kinase; *NPH*, neutral protamine Hagedorn; *PD-1*, programmed cell death protein 1; *PDL-1*, programmed cell death protein 1; *SGLT-2*, sodium–glucose cotransporter 2; *T1DM*, type 1 diabetes mellitus; *SERM*, selective estrogen receptor modulator; *SGLT-2*, sodium–glucose cotransporter 2; *TKI*, tyrosine kinase inhibitor.

associated with T1DM (DR3-DQB1*02:01 and/or DR4-DQB1*03:02) have reported conflicting data; therefore more evidence is needed to determine the genetic risk associated with high-risk HLA haplotypes. Furthermore, individuals still may develop CIADM despite HLA haplotypes normally associated with protection from T1DM.

14. **How is CIADM different from T1DM?**
In contrast to the younger age of onset usually associated with T1DM, the median age of onset for CIADM is 63 years. Whereas people with T1DM often go through a "honeymoon period," those with CIADM have a rapid decline in C-peptide levels and no apparent honeymoon phase. Unlike T1DM, CIADM has a lower association with insulin autoantibodies. Although the risk for developing T1DM has been associated with high-risk HLA haplotypes that are present in over 90% of individuals with T1DM, these haplotypes have not been associated with genetic risk for CIADM. When comparing CGM data from people with CIADM to those with T1DM, there were no apparent differences in glycemic variability.

15. **How do you monitor for CIADM?**
Please refer to Table 17.2 for specific monitoring guidelines. Providers should educate people on the signs and symptoms of hyperglycemia and DKA prior to the initiation of ICIs and consider providing those with a history of autoimmune disease and/or autoimmune adverse ICIs effects with a glucometer for closer monitoring. Currently, it is not recommended that HLA or autoantibody screening be performed.

16. **What is the recommended treatment for CIADM?**
Treatment includes evaluation and treatment for DKA and initiation of insulin therapy. Treatment with corticosteroids is not recommended because there is no evidence of clinical efficacy, and these agents will contribute to worsening glycemic control. Please refer to Table 17.2.

17. **Explain how PI3K-Akt-mTOR inhibitors cause hyperglycemia.**
    The PI3K-Akt pathway regulates glucose metabolism through insulin signaling, whereas mTOR complex 1 regulates beta-cell function. Inhibiting this pathway reduces glucose uptake in adipose tissue and skeletal muscle, reduces glycogenesis, promotes glycogenolysis, and may impair insulin secretion.

18. **What is the recommended diabetes therapy for hyperglycemia secondary to PI3K-Akt-mTOR inhibitors?**
    Please refer to Fig. 17.1.

19. **Describe how certain diabetes therapies may affect the efficacy of PI3K pathway inhibitors**
    Insulin stimulates the PI3K pathway. Hyperglycemia caused by PI3K inhibitor therapy results in compensatory hyperinsulinemia that reactivates the PI3K pathway and may decrease the efficacy of treatment. Recent evidence supports that sodium–glucose cotransporter 2 (SGLT-2) inhibitors effectively reduce BG and subsequent hyperinsulinemia after treatment with PI3K pathway inhibitors and reduce tumor signaling. Therefore SGLT-2 inhibitors may increase PI3K inhibitor treatment effectiveness. Ketogenetic diets have also been demonstrated to reduce tumor signaling secondary to hyperinsulinemia; however, carbohydrate restriction should not be enforced for patients who struggle with nausea, vomiting, weight loss, and/or malnutrition. Furthermore, ketogenic diets should be avoided with SGLT-2 inhibitor therapy because of the increased risk for DKA associated with this medication class. Insulin administration has been demonstrated to increase tumor signaling and therefore may reduce the antitumor efficacy of PI3K therapy. Insulin therapy may still need to be considered when there is difficulty achieving glycemic control or with high-grade hyperglycemia.

20. **How do you monitor for steroid-induced hyperglycemia?**
    For prednisone dose equivalents of ≥ 10 mg daily:
    • No preexisting diabetes: Monitor BG levels three to four times daily before meals for 48 hours and stop if BG values are consistently <180 mg/dL.
    • Preexisting diabetes: Increase the frequency of home glucose monitoring to include before meals and at bedtime.
    　　Prednisone tends to have less effect on fasting BG but often causes large postprandial BG excursions and peak BG levels after lunch and dinner. Therefore it is important to monitor afternoon and evening BG when people are taking high doses of prednisone. However, the duration of hyperglycemia depends on the type and dosing of the steroid. For example, BG tends to be elevated for 12 hours after prednisone dosing, followed by an overnight BG drop; in contrast, dexamethasone may cause hyperglycemia for 24 to 72 hours after each dose.

21. **When should you initiate additional antidiabetic therapies for steroid-induced hyperglycemia?**
    • No preexisting diabetes: BG > 180 mg/dL × 2.
    • Preexisting diabetes: On insulin, A1c > 7.5% on noninsulin meds *or* receiving >20 units of correction insulin/24 hours.

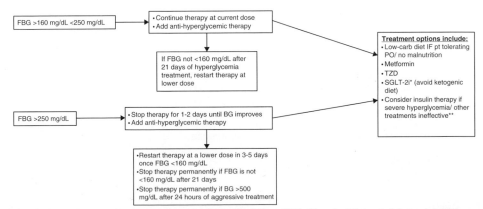

Fig. 17.1 Treatment of hyperglycemia secondary to phosphoinositide 3-kinase (PI3K)-Akt-mechanistic target of rapamycin (mTOR) inhibitor therapy.

Table 17.3 End-of-Life Diabetes Management

	TYPE 2 DM	TYPE 1 DM
BG monitoring frequency*	−No insulin: stop −On insulin: once daily −Continuous glucose monitor: continue per individual/ family preference	−Once daily −Continuous glucose monitor: continue per individual/ family preference
BG targets*	−Avoid symptomatic hyperglycemia and hypoglycemia −Consider target of 180-360 mg/dL**	−Avoid ketoacidosis/ symptomatic hyperglycemia and hypoglycemia −Consider target of 180-360 mg/dL**
Orals/ GLP-1 agonists	Stop	−N/A
Insulin therapy***	−Stop prandial insulin −Consider stopping basal if lower dose −Continue insulin pump if individual/ family preference −Reduce insulin dose by 25%	−Stop prandial insulin −Continue basal insulin therapy −Continue insulin pump if individual/ family preference −Reduce insulin dose by 25%

*Frequency of BG monitoring and BG targets should be determined in coordination with patient and family.
**Recommended BG targets vary based on guidelines.
***Insulin regimen should be determined in coordination with patient and family preference. Recommend discussing goals of care with patient and family at the time of diagnosis.

22. **Discuss treatment strategies for steroid-induced hyperglycemia**
    Intermediate-acting human insulin (neutral protamine Hagedorn [NPH]) dosed at the same time as prednisone works well for treating steroid-induced hyperglycemia with this agent (see Chapter 20 "Diabetes Management in the Hospital"). When dexamethasone is used, long-acting basal insulins may also be considered, given the longer duration of hyperglycemia with this agent; however, basal insulin alone may be ineffective at controlling postprandial hyperglycemia. If a person is already on basal insulin, one may consider increasing the insulin dose on dexamethasone treatment days. Treatment with basal-bolus therapy may also be necessary, with 30% of the total daily dose distributed as basal insulin and 70% as bolus insulin. For people who wish to avoid injections, a sulfonylurea such as glipizide may be needed to control postprandial BG excursions.

23. **How do you manage hyperglycemia in terminal illness?**
    There are limited guidelines available that provide recommendations regarding diabetes management during the end of life. The goal of diabetes management is to reduce symptomatic hyperglycemia while avoiding hypoglycemia. Diabetes regimens should be simplified and the number of fingerstick BG tests reduced. The Diabetes UK recommendations for end-of-life diabetes care adopted a four-stage Gold Standards Framework (ABCD) to assist providers with tailoring diabetes therapies according to the stage of terminal illness:
    A—"All": Upon diagnosis, stable, prognosis of a year plus
      a. Review appropriateness of current regimen.
      b. Adjust medications as needed based on weight loss, reduced oral intake, and kidney and liver function.
      c. Consider the use of a continuous/flash glucose monitoring system to reduce fingerstick burden.
    B—"Benefits": Unstable, advanced disease, months prognosis
      a. Goal is to simplify regimen and reduce side effects, with consideration of caregiver availability.
      b. Consider replacing multiple pills with once-daily long-acting insulin.
      c. Consider changing from twice-daily to once-daily long-acting insulin (glargine or degludec).
        i. Reduce total daily insulin dose by 25%.
    C—"Continuing Care": Deteriorating, weeks prognosis
      a. Adjust frequency of BG monitoring based on patient/caregiver preference.
      b. Continue to monitor for symptoms and signs of hyperglycemia.
      c. Insulin may require frequent adjustments.
    D—"Days": Final days, days prognosis
      a. The goal is to minimize symptoms and reduce the need for invasive testing.
      b. See Table 17.3 for a management algorithm.

KEY POINTS

1. Diabetes is associated with an increased cancer risk and increased cancer mortality risk.
2. Uncontrolled hyperglycemia is associated with increased infection risk, higher symptom burden, malnutrition, and worse cancer outcomes.

3. There are numerous cancer therapies that cause hyperglycemia, including ICIs, TKIs, mTOR inhibitors, PI3K pathway inhibitors, and steroids.
4. CIADM is distinct from T1DM, with rapid C-peptide decline and low association with diabetic-associated antibodies.
5. End-of-life care should focus on reducing hypoglycemia and symptoms of hyperglycemia.

BIBLIOGRAPHY

Ansari M, Salama AD, Chitnis T, Smith RN, et al. The programmed death-1 pathway regulates autoimmune diabetes in nonobese diabetic mice. *J Exp Med*. 2003;198(1):63–69.

Brahmer JR, Lacchetti C, Schneider BJ, et al. Management of immune-related adverse events in patients treated with immune checkpoint inhibitor therapy: American Society of Clinical Oncology clinical practice guideline. *J Clin Oncol*. 2018;36(17):1714–1768.

Clotman K, Janssens K, Specenier P, Weets I, De Block CEM. Programmed cell death-1 inhibitor-induced type 1 diabetes mellitus. *J Clin Endocrinol Metab*. 2018;103(9):3144–3154.

Duan W, Shen X, Lei J, et al. Hyperglycemia, a neglected factor during cancer progression. *Biomed Res Int*. 2014;2014:461917.

Emerging Risk Factors Collaboration. Diabetes mellitus, fasting glucose, and risk of cause-specific death. *N Engl J Med*. 2011;364(9):829.

Gadi S, Neel B, LeRoith D, Gallagher EJ. Type 2 diabetes mellitus and cancer: the role of pharmacotherapy. *J Clin Oncol*. 2016;34(35):4261–4269.

Giovannuci E, Harlan DM, Archer MC, et al. Diabetes and cancer: a consensus report. *CA- Cancer J Clin*. 2010;60(4):1674–1685.

Hopkins BD, Pauli C, Du X, et al. Suppression of insulin feedback enhances the efficacy of PI3K inhibitors. *Nature*. 2018;560(23):499–503.

Huang CU, Lin YS, Liu YH, Lin SC, Kang BH. Hyperglycemia crisis in head and neck cancer patients with platinum-based chemotherapy. 2018;81(12):1060-1064.

Mathioudakis N, Dungan K, Baldwin D, et al. Steroid-associated hyperglycemia. In: Draznin B, ed. *Managing Diabetes and Hyperglycemia in the Hospital Setting: A Clinician's Guide*. American Diabetes Association; 2016:99–114.

Nunnery SE, Mayer IA. Management of toxicity to isoform α-specific PI3K inhibitors. *Ann Onc*. 2019;30(Supplement 10):x21–x26.

Saraei P, Asadi I, Kakar MA, Moradi-Kor N. The beneficial effects of metformin on cancer prevention and therapy: a comprehensive review of recent advances. *Cancer Manag Res*. 2019;11:3295–3313.

Sona MF, Myung SK, Park K, Jargalsaikhan G. Type 1 diabetes mellitus and risk for cancer: a meta-analysis of observational studies. *Jpn J Clin Oncol*. 2018;48(5):426–433.

Venessa H, Tsang M, McGrath RT, et al. Checkpoint inhibitor-associated autoimmune diabetes is distinct from type 1 diabetes. *J Clin Endocrinol Metab*. 2019;104(11):5499–5506.

Villadolid J, Ersek, JL, Fong MK, Sirianno L, Story ES. Management of hyperglycemia from epidermal growth receptor (EGFR) tyrosine kinase inhibitors (TKIs) targeting T790M mediated resistance. 2015;4(5):576-583.

UK Diabetes. *End of life diabetes care: clinical care recommendations*, 3rd ed. Available at https://www.diabetes.org.uk/resources-s3/2018-03/EoL_Guidance_2018_Final.pdf. Published 2018. Accessed September 7, 2020.

CHAPTER 18

DIABETES IN OLDER ADULTS

Scott M. Pearson, PharmD, BCACP

1. **What are the recommended glycemic targets in older adults?**
   Glycemic targets for older adults are slightly different compared with those for the general adult population and are dependent on factors such as cognition and overall medical status. Several organizations have published recommendations on glycemic targets for older adults, including the American Diabetes Association (ADA; Table 18.1).

2. **Why are glycemic targets often relaxed in older adults?**
   Glycemic targets are relaxed in older adults based on a lack of demonstrated benefit of targeting more intensive glycosylated hemoglobin (A1c) goals. Stringent glycemic control is typically targeted in younger patients to prevent microvascular complications. However, microvascular complications typically take years to develop, and the risks of serious adverse events resulting from hypoglycemia with some medications outweigh the benefits of more intensive glycemic control in many older patients.

3. **Why is hypoglycemia concerning in older adults?**
   Hypoglycemia can contribute to cognitive impairment, falls, and fractures and has been associated with increased rates of cardiovascular events and mortality. Therefore treatment regimens in older adults should prioritize the avoidance of hypoglycemia.

4. **Can diabetes complications contribute to functional impairment in older adults?**
   Complications, such as neuropathy and retinopathy, can hinder older adults' ability to engage in activities of daily living and can also contribute to an increased risk of falls. Therefore, although glycemic targets may be less stringent in older adults, it is still important to ensure patients maintain adequate glycemic control and achieve these targets to prevent the development of complications while also minimizing the risk of hypoglycemia.

5. **How can cognitive impairment affect diabetes management?**
   Older adults with cognitive impairment may have difficulty managing complicated treatment regimens, particularly those involving insulin and regular monitoring of blood glucose. Patients with cognitive impairment may have more difficulty recognizing the symptoms of hypoglycemia and appropriately treating low blood glucose. It may also be more difficult for patients with cognitive impairment to adhere to regular mealtimes and consistent carbohydrate intake in meals. Older adults should be screened routinely for cognitive impairment and referred for further neuropsychological evaluation when appropriate.

6. **Should older adults with diabetes exercise?**
   Exercise that includes aerobic and resistance training is recommended for older adults and can preserve muscle mass and prevent frailty while improving insulin sensitivity and reducing cardiovascular risk. Exercise routines should be individualized depending on the patient's abilities and overall health.

7. **What is first-line medication therapy for type 2 diabetes in older adults?**
   Metformin is recommended as initial drug therapy in all adults with type 2 diabetes (without contraindications), regardless of age. Because renal function often worsens with aging, it is important to ensure that metformin not be used in patients with an estimated glomerular filtration rate of <30 mL/min/1.73 m^2 to minimize the risk of lactic acidosis. In patients with an estimated glomerular filtration rate of 30 to 44 mL/min/1.73 m^2, a maximum dose of metformin of 1000 mg/day is recommended.

8. **Should sliding-scale insulin be used in older adults?**
   The 2019 American Geriatrics Society (AGS) Beers Criteria recommend avoiding sliding-scale insulin in the absence of basal insulin in older adults in all care settings because of the elevated risk of hypoglycemia and lack of improvement in blood glucose management. If bolus insulin is necessary for patients in hospitals or long-term care settings who are not already receiving basal insulin, fixed or one-time doses of bolus insulin should be used initially instead of a sliding scale, and basal insulin should subsequently be initiated if warranted. Additionally, although sliding-scale insulin may be appropriate as part of a basal/bolus regimen in some patients, many older adults may have difficulty managing the complexity of a sliding scale and are at an elevated risk of hypoglycemia. Therefore sliding-scale insulin should also be initiated with caution in the outpatient setting.

Table 18.1 Glycemic Targets for Older Adults With Diabetes

PATIENT CHARACTERISTICS AND HEALTH STATUS	REASONABLE A1C GOAL	FASTING GLUCOSE	BEDTIME GLUCOSE
Healthy (few coexisting chronic illnesses, intact cognitive and functional status)	<7.0%–7.5%	80–130 mg/dL	80–180 mg/dL
Complex/intermediate (multiple coexisting chronic illnesses or multiple impairments in activities of daily living or mild to moderate cognitive impairment)	<8.0%	90–150 mg/dL	100–180 mg/dL
Very complex/poor health (long-term care or end-stage chronic illnesses or moderate to severe cognitive impairment or multiple dependencies in activities of daily living)	Avoid reliance on A1c; avoid hypoglycemia and symptomatic hyperglycemia	100–180 mg/dL	110–200 mg/dL

Modified from American Diabetes Association. 12. Older adults: Standards of medical care in diabetes-2021. *Diabetes Care.* 2021;44(Suppl 1):S168–S179.

9. **Are any other diabetes medications listed in the AGS Beers Criteria?**
   The 2019 AGS Beers Criteria recommend avoiding long-acting sulfonylureas (i.e., chlorpropamide, glimepiride, and glyburide) because of their prolonged half-lives in older adults and higher risk of prolonged hypoglycemia. If a sulfonylurea is used, glipizide is the preferred agent. Glipizide and all forms of insulin can also cause hypoglycemia in older adults but may still be appropriate in many cases.

10. **Name two diabetes medication classes that may worsen bone health**
    Thiazolidinediones and sodium–glucose cotransporter 2 (SGLT-2) inhibitors may have detrimental effects on bone mineral density and have each been associated with an increased risk of bone fractures in clinical trials. For the SGLT-2 inhibitors, these effects have primarily been seen with the medication canagliflozin and have not been seen with other agents. Therefore, although it is not clear whether this is a medication class effect for all SGLT-2 inhibitors or not, caution is advised when considering the use of either thiazolidinediones or SGLT-2 inhibitors in older adults with osteopenia or osteoporosis.

11. **Can SGLT-2 inhibitors be used safely in older adults?**
    SGLT-2 inhibitors have demonstrated cardiovascular benefits in both patients with atherosclerotic cardiovascular disease (ASCVD) and heart failure, in addition to renal benefits in patients with chronic kidney disease. Oral medication administration may also be advantageous to many patients. However, SGLT-2 inhibitors can cause hypotension, dehydration, and volume depletion, and older adults may be more sensitive to these side effects. Older patients are also more likely to develop urinary tract infections and genital mycotic infections than younger patients, and these side effects can occur with the use of SGLT-2 inhibitors. The possible increased risk of fractures may also be of concern to some older patients. Additionally, SGLT-2 inhibitor use is not recommended in patients with end-stage renal disease. These factors should all be considered when identifying appropriate patients for these medications.

12. **Is weight loss recommended in older adults with diabetes?**
    Weight loss can be desirable in older adults with diabetes who are overweight or obese. However, some older adults experience unintentional weight loss and undernutrition as a result of swallowing difficulties and lack of appetite from age-related changes. In patients who have limited oral intake and lack of appetite, agents that promote weight loss and satiety, such as glucagon-like peptide-1 (GLP-1) receptor agonists, should generally be avoided.

13. **What types of functional abnormalities in older adults might affect medication choice?**
    Some older adults may have reduced dexterity as a result of age-related changes to the musculoskeletal and nervous systems. Other comorbidities, such as osteoarthritis, osteoporosis, and Parkinson's disease, can also contribute to reduced dexterity. These functional limitations can hinder the ability of some patients to administer injectable medications and monitor blood glucose. If an injectable medication is warranted, the use of GLP-1 receptor agonists with simple administration techniques and/or insulin pens (instead of vials and syringes) can facilitate appropriate dosing and adherence.

14. **What resources are available for patients who require insulin but are not able to safely self-administer it?**
In many cases, caregivers, such as spouses or other family members, might administer insulin and monitor blood glucose levels for patients who cannot safely self-administer insulin because of cognitive or functional impairments. If this is not feasible, home health services may accommodate insulin administration and/or blood glucose checks. In other cases, patients may require placement in long-term care facilities for additional assistance with medication management and other care.

15. **What is deprescribing?**
Deprescribing is the practice of deintensifying a treatment regimen by dose reduction or discontinuation when the risks of a particular medication outweigh the benefits or when a medication is no longer necessary and medication burden and cost can be minimized. Complex treatment regimens can lead to a higher likelihood of medication errors, and deprescribing can help simplify diabetes regimens. In older adults with diabetes, deprescribing should be considered when A1C control improves to the point where the patient may be at risk of hypoglycemia or is simply taking unnecessary medications.

16. **How can complex insulin regimens be simplified?**
Older adults with type 2 diabetes on basal/bolus insulin regimens may be able to simplify their regimen by switching from mealtime insulin to a noninsulin agent, such as a GLP-1 receptor agonist. Patients taking 10 units or less per dose of mealtime insulin can often discontinue the mealtime insulin when starting a noninsulin agent. In patients taking more than 10 units of mealtime insulin per dose, reducing the mealtime insulin dose by 50% may be reasonable when adding a noninsulin agent, and the mealtime insulin doses can then be further reduced as appropriate.

17. **What is an appropriate blood pressure target in older adults with diabetes?**
Blood pressure targets vary slightly by organizational guidelines. The 2017 American College of Cardiology/American Heart Association (ACC/AHA) Hypertension Guidelines recommend a blood pressure target of <130/80 mm Hg in patients with diabetes and in ambulatory, community-dwelling adults age 65 and older. However, for older adults with multiple comorbidities and limited life expectancy, clinical judgment and shared decision making are recommended to determine blood pressure targets.
The ADA recommends a similar blood pressure target of <130/80 mm Hg in patients with ASCVD or with 10-year ASCVD risk of ≥15%. However, in lower-risk patients not meeting these criteria, the ADA recommends a blood pressure target of <140/90 mm Hg, regardless of age. In older adults, adverse effects from antihypertensive therapy may be more common, and gradual medication titration with monitoring for orthostatic hypotension is recommended. Antihypertensive medications that are more likely to cause orthostatic hypotension, such as alpha blockers and clonidine, should also be avoided in older adults when possible.

18. **Are statins recommended in older adults with diabetes?**
Statins are recommended for the primary prevention of ASCVD in patients with diabetes aged 40 to 75 years and for secondary prevention of ASCVD in adults of all ages, including those older than 75 years of age. The benefits of statin therapy for primary prevention in adults over 75 years of age with diabetes are less clear (Table 18.2).

Table 18.2 Statin Therapy Recommendations for Patients With Diabetes

INDICATION	AGE	RECOMMENDATION
Primary prevention of ASCVD	40–75 years	Statin therapy recommended
Primary prevention of ASCVD	>75 years	If already on statin therapy, it is reasonable to continue. It may be reasonable to start statin therapy after discussion of potential benefits and risks.
Secondary prevention of ASCVD	All ages	Statin therapy recommended.

Modified from Grundy SM, Stone NJ, Bailey AL, et al. 2018 AHA/ACC/AACVPR/AAPA/ABC/ACPM/ADA/AGS/APhA/ASPC/NLA/PCNA guideline on the management of blood cholesterol: a report of the American College of Cardiology/American Heart Association Task Force on Clinical Practice Guidelines [published correction appears in *Circulation.* 2019 Jun 18;139[25]:e1182–e1186]. *Circulation.* 2019;139[25]:e1082–e1143.
ASCVD, atherosclerotic cardiovascular disease.

19. **What is the role of aspirin in older adults with diabetes?**

Aspirin is recommended for the secondary prevention of ASCVD in patients with diabetes, regardless of age. For primary prevention, aspirin should be avoided in most older adults. Although aspirin may be considered for primary prevention in adults with diabetes and increased cardiovascular risk after discussion of benefits versus bleeding risk, recent evidence has shown a lack of benefit and an increased risk of bleeding with aspirin in adults over age 70 who do not have ASCVD. The 2019 ACC/AHA Guideline on the Primary Prevention of Cardiovascular Disease recommends against aspirin use for primary prevention in adults over 70 years of age.

20. **How should diabetes be managed in patients at the end of life?**

Measures should be taken to maximize comfort and quality of life. This should include avoiding both hypoglycemia and symptomatic hyperglycemia. Blood glucose monitoring should be reserved for cases when it is necessary to ensure the achievement of these goals, and injection frequency should be minimized when insulin therapy is still warranted. Many chronic oral medications, including statins, can be withdrawn to improve comfort by minimizing the medication burden.

KEY POINTS

1. Glycemic targets should be individualized in older adults to minimize the risk of hypoglycemia while still preventing microvascular complications of diabetes.
2. Age-related changes can complicate the management of diabetes in older adults and should be considered when selecting appropriate medication regimens.
3. Deprescribing diabetes medications in appropriate patients can simplify treatment regimens and reduce the risk of hypoglycemia.
4. Blood pressure targets for most older adults are similar to those recommended in younger patients, although antihypertensives should be titrated cautiously to avoid hypotension.
5. Statins and aspirin are recommended for the secondary prevention of ASCVD in older adults. The benefits of statin therapy for primary prevention in older adults with diabetes are less clear, and aspirin should not routinely be used for primary prevention in older adults.

BIBLIOGRAPHY

1. The 2019 American Geriatrics Society Beers Criteria® Update Expert Panel. American Geriatrics Society 2019 updated AGS Beers Criteria® for potentially inappropriate medication use in older adults. *J Am Geriatr Soc.* 2019;67(4):674–694.
2. American Diabetes Association. 12. Older adults: Standards of Medical Care in Diabetes-2020. *Diabetes Care.* 2021;44(Suppl 1): S168–S179.
3. Arnett DK, Blumenthal RS, Albert MA, et al. 2019 ACC/AHA guideline on the primary prevention of cardiovascular disease: a report of the American College of Cardiology/American Heart Association Task Force on Clinical Practice Guidelines [published correction appears in Circulation. 2019 Sep 10;140(11):e649–e650] [published correction appears in Circulation. 2020 Jan 28;141(4):e60] [published correction appears in Circulation. 2020 Apr 21;141(16):e774]. *Circulation.* 2019;140(11):e596–e646.
4. Carmeli E, Patish H, Coleman R. The aging hand. *J Gerontol A Biol Sci Med Sci.* 2003;58(2):146–152.
5. Choi HJ, Park C, Lee YK, Ha YC, Jang S, Shin CS. Risk of fractures and diabetes medications: a nationwide cohort study. *Osteoporos Int.* 2016;27(9):2709–2715.
6. Farrell B, Black C, Thompson W, et al. Deprescribing antihyperglycemic agents in older persons: evidence-based clinical practice guideline. *Can Fam Physician.* 2017;63(11):832–843.
7. Grundy SM, Stone NJ, Bailey AL, et al. 2018 AHA/ACC/AACVPR/AAPA/ABC/ACPM/ADA/AGS/APhA/ASPC/NLA/PCNA guideline on the management of blood cholesterol: a report of the American College of Cardiology/American Heart Association Task Force on Clinical Practice Guidelines [published correction appears in Circulation. 2019 Jun 18;139(25):e1182–e1186]. *Circulation.* 2019;139(25):e1082–e1143.
8. Leroith D, Biessels GJ, Braithwaite SS, et al. Treatment of diabetes in older adults: an Endocrine Society* Clinical Practice Guideline. *J Clin Endocrinol Metab.* 2019;104(5):1520–1574.
9. Watts NB, Bilezikian JP, Usiskin K, et al. Effects of canagliflozin on fracture risk in patients with type 2 diabetes mellitus. *J Clin Endocrinol Metab.* 2016;101(1):157–166.
10. Whelton PK, Carey RM, Aronow WS, et al. 2017 ACC/AHA/AAPA/ABC/ACPM/AGS/APhA/ASH/ASPC/NMA/PCNA guideline for the prevention, detection, evaluation, and management of high blood pressure in adults: a report of the American College of Cardiology/American Heart Association Task Force on Clinical Practice Guidelines. *Circulation.* 2018;138(17):e484–e594.

CHAPTER 19

DIABETES MANAGEMENT DURING EXERCISE, SPORTS, AND COMPETITION

Michael T. McDermott, MD

1. **Describe normal energy metabolism during exercise**

   After an overnight fast, approximately 4 to 5 g of glucose circulates in the bloodstream, 400 g is stored as glycogen in muscle, and 100 g is stored as glycogen in the liver. Muscle glycogen is the initial energy source during exercise but is depleted after about 30 to 60 minutes. Thereafter, blood glucose (BG) is maintained by a balance between hepatic glucose production (glycogenolysis and gluconeogenesis) and muscle glucose uptake. Non–insulin-mediated glucose uptake in muscle increases as much as 50-fold during exercise. Hormonal changes during exercise include suppression of insulin and a rise in counterregulatory hormone (epinephrine, cortisol, and growth hormone) secretion; epinephrine exhibits the most pronounced increment. After exercise, insulin levels increase, and counterregulatory hormone levels return to baseline.

2. **What are the main types of exercise?**

   Aerobic exercise involves the repetitive use of large muscle groups at relatively low intensity for prolonged periods of time; examples include distance running, cycling, swimming, and walking. Anaerobic (resistance) exercise involves using smaller groups of muscles against a resistive force; examples include weightlifting and work with resistance bands. High-intensity exercise involves short spurts of high-intensity, predominantly anaerobic, muscle work. Intermittent high-intensity exercise involves alternating spurts of high-intensity exercise with recovery periods of low to moderate exercise.

3. **Is there a difference in the effects of aerobic and anaerobic exercise on glucose levels?**

   BG levels generally decrease during aerobic exercise. Anaerobic (resistance) exercise causes less initial BG decline, along with smoother and more prolonged BG reductions after exercise. BG actually increases during anaerobic exercise in some individuals. BG levels often increase significantly during high-intensity exercise and competition.

4. **Does it make any difference in which order aerobic and anaerobic exercises are performed?**

   Anaerobic exercise performed prior to aerobic exercise reduces the BG decline that occurs during the subsequent aerobic exercise period. Furthermore, anaerobic exercise performed before or intermittently during aerobic exercise improves BG stability throughout both exercise periods and reduces the severity of postexercise BG fluctuations.

5. **What is the effect of short, high-intensity exercise on BG levels?**

   BG levels increase significantly during a 10-second sprint. This coincides with and appears to be attributable to an increase in circulating counterregulatory hormones (epinephrine, cortisol, and growth hormone); most significant among these is an abrupt increase in plasma epinephrine levels.

6. **How does intermittent high-intensity exercise affect BG levels?**

   Intermittent high-intensity exercise, consisting of 4-second sprints every 2 minutes during 30 minutes of moderate exercise, has been shown to reduce BG levels significantly less than moderate consistent exercise. This also appears to result from an increase in counterregulatory hormones, again most prominently epinephrine, during the high-intensity exercise periods. Sports competition, which often involves a mixture of aerobic activity and high-intensity activity, can affect BG in either direction, depending on the relative proportion of aerobic and high-intensity work and the level of competition.

7. **Does the time of day exercise is done affect glucose levels?**

   In people with type 1 diabetes, BG levels have been reported to increase during anaerobic exercise done in the morning before eating but to decrease during anaerobic exercise done in the afternoon. Postexercise BG levels were also higher after morning anaerobic exercise, and glucose variability was greater.

8. **What is the impact of the initial BG level on the glucose response to aerobic exercise?**

   When initial BG levels are <200 mg/dL, BG tends to decrease with aerobic exercise. However, when BG levels are >300 mg/dL, indicating low baseline insulin levels, BG usually remains the same or increases during aerobic exercise.

9. How many grams of carbohydrate are used during various types of exercise?
   See Table 19.1.

10. What are the primary drivers of hypoglycemia during exercise?
    See Table 19.2.

11. How do BG levels affect performance during exercise and sports?
    See Table 19.3.

12. What factors affect BG levels during exercise?
    See Table 19.4.

Table 19.1 Carbohydrate Utilization According to Exercise Intensity and Duration

EXERCISE INTENSITY	DURATION	CARBOHYDRATE USED (G/KG BODY WEIGHT)
Light	1 hour	3–5 g/kg
Moderate	1 hour	5–7 g/kg
Moderate–high	1–3 hours	7–10 g/kg
Moderate–high	4–5 hours	10–12 g/kg

Table 19.2 Primary Drivers of Hypoglycemia During Exercise

Non–insulin-mediated glucose uptake by muscle
Inability to reduce insulin levels during exercise
More rapid insulin absorption from subcutaneous sites
Inadequate carbohydrate intake during exercise
Variable insulin sensitivity during and after exercise

Table 19.3 The Effects of Blood Glucose Levels on Exercise and Sports Performance

BLOOD GLUCOSE	PERFORMANCE/SYMPTOMS
<100 mg/dL	Impaired performance/fatigue
100–200 mg/dL	Optimal performance
>200 mg/dL	Impaired performance
>250 mg/dL	Impaired performance/fatigue

Table 19.4 Factors Affecting Blood Glucose During Exercise

Type of exercise
Intensity of exercise
Duration of exercise
Level of training (fitness)
Time of day exercise is done
Nutritional state (fasting or fed)
Insulin on board during exercise
Blood glucose level before exercise
Blood glucose trend before exercise
Situation (training or competition)

13. **What are the key elements of diabetes management during exercise and sports?**
    See Table 19.5.

14. **How often should BG levels be tested during exercise and sports?**
    This depends significantly on the exercise and/or sport, but the general guidelines in Table 19.6 apply in most situations.

15. **How should a person respond to BG values prior to exercise?**
    See Table 19.7.

16. **What are general recommendations for nutritional intake during and after exercise?**
    See Table 19.8.

17. **Do nutritional recommendations vary with exercise intensity and duration?**
    Table 19.9 provides additional recommendations regarding carbohydrate intake based on exercise intensity and duration.

18. **How should bolus insulin doses be adjusted during aerobic exercise?**
    One published recommendation for bolus insulin adjustments is shown in Table 19.10. Dose reductions should focus on the insulin component that will be most active during the exercise. Insulin adjustments can also be combined with increased carbohydrate intake (Table 19.11). Again, dose reductions should focus on the insulin component that will be most active during the exercise.

19. **Does continuous glucose monitoring reduce the hypoglycemia risk during exercise?**
    Continuous glucose monitoring plus a carbohydrate-intake algorithm that makes recommendations based on current BG levels and trend arrows have been shown to significantly improve exercise glucose control in adolescents with type 1 diabetes. See Table 19.12.

Table 19.5 Key Elements of Diabetes Management During Exercise

Frequent blood glucose testing
Adequate nutritional intake
Appropriate insulin adjustments
Anticipation of exercise effects
Adequate hydration

Table 19.6 Recommended Blood Glucose Testing During Exercise

Blood Glucose Testing
Before exercise
Every hour during exercise
Every hour for 4 hours after exercise
At bedtime

Table 19.7 Recommended Responses to Preexercise Blood Glucose Testing

PREEXERCISE BLOOD GLUCOSE	RECOMMENDED ACTION
<90 mg/dL	Consume 10–20 g glucose. Delay exercise until BG > 90 mg/dL.
90–124 mg/dL	Consume 10 g glucose before aerobic work. Start exercise.
125–180 mg/dL	Start exercise. BG may rise with anaerobic/interval/high-intensity work.
181–270 mg/dL	Start exercise. BG may rise with anaerobic/interval/high- intensity work.
>270 mg/dL	Check ketones. Identify the cause of hyperglycemia and ketonemia. If blood ketones are low or urine ketones are less than 2+, moderate exercise can be initiated; BG levels should be monitored. If ketones are mildly elevated, light-intensity exercise for less than 30 minutes can be done. If ketones are moderately elevated or more, exercise should be delayed; BG and ketonemia should be managed as recommended by the healthcare provider.

Table 19.8 Recommended Carbohydrate Consumption During and After Exercise

TIME	CONSUME
During exercise	30–60 g of carbohydrate per hour
After exercise	30–60 g of carbohydrate every 2 hours for 4–6 hours

Notes:
Chocolate milk works well for many athletes after exercise.
Reducing insulin doses is an alternative when weight loss is one of the goals of exercise.

Table 19.9 Recommended Carbohydrate Intake During Exercise

EXERCISE INTENSITY	CARBOHYDRATE INTAKE (G/KG BODY WEIGHT/HOUR)
Mild aerobic exercise	0.25 g/kg/hour
Moderate aerobic exercise	0.50 g/kg/hour
Vigorous aerobic exercise	1.00 g/kg/hour

Table 19.10 Recommended Bolus Insulin Adjustments During Aerobic Exercise

EXERCISE INTENSITY	INSULIN ADJUSTMENT	
(VO$_2$ MAX)	30 MINUTES	60 MINUTES
25%	↓ 25%	↓ 50%
50%	↓ 50%	↓ 75%
75%	↓ 75%	↓ 100%

Table 19.11 Recommended Carbohydrate Intake and Insulin Adjustments According to Aerobic Exercise Intensity and Duration

EXERCISE INTENSITY (% MAX HEART RATE)	CARBOHYDRATE INTAKE AND BOLUS INSULIN ADJUSTMENT		
	<20 MINUTES	20–60 MINUTES	60 MINUTES
<60%	0	15 g	30 g/hour
60–75%	15 g	30 g	75 g/hour + ↓ insulin 20%
>75%	30 g	75 g/hour + ↓ insulin 0%–20%	100 g/hour + ↓ insulin 30%

Table 19.12 Recommended Carbohydrate Intake During Exercise When Wearing a Continuous Glucose Monitor With Trend-Arrow Data

BLOOD GLUCOSE	ARROWS	ACTION
109–124 mg/dL	↓ or ↓↓	8 g carbohydrate
90–108 mg/dL	↓	16 g carbohydrate
	↓↓	20 g carbohydrate
<90 mg/dL	—	16 g carbohydrate
	↓ or ↓↓	20 g carbohydrate

20. **Does insulin pump therapy improve glucose outcomes with exercise?**

Insulin pump therapy has been shown to limit postexercise hyperglycemia without increasing the risk for postexercise late-onset hypoglycemia compared with multiple daily insulin injections. Basal rate reductions of 25% to 50% usually work well for moderate exercise of $\geq$60 minutes in duration or strenuous exercise of $\geq$30 minutes in duration. The basal rate reduction should start 60 to 90 minutes before the exercise and continue for 60 to 90 minutes after the exercise is complete.

KEY POINTS

1. Aerobic exercise lowers BG levels during and after exercise in most people with diabetes. Resistance exercise causes less initial BG decline but smoother and more prolonged reductions in postexercise BG. Intermittent high-intensity exercise reduces BG less than moderate consistent exercise, and BG levels often rise during competition.

2. The primary drivers of hypoglycemia during exercise are noninsulin-mediated glucose uptake by muscle, inability to reduce insulin levels during exercise, more rapid insulin absorption from subcutaneous sites, inadequate carbohydrate intake during exercise, and variable insulin sensitivity during and after exercise.

3. BG levels during exercise are significantly affected by the type, intensity, and duration of exercise; level of training (fitness); time of day exercise is done; nutritional state (fasting or fed); insulin on board during exercise; BG level before exercise; BG trend before exercise; and situation (training or competition).

4. The key elements of diabetes management during exercise are frequent BG testing, adequate nutritional intake, appropriate insulin adjustments, anticipation of exercise effects, and adequate hydration.

5. Continuous glucose monitoring plus an algorithm that makes carbohydrate intake recommendations based on current BG levels and trend arrows has been reported to significantly improve exercise glucose control in adolescents with type 1 diabetes.

6. Insulin pump therapy limits postexercise hyperglycemia without increasing the risk for hypoglycemia compared with multiple daily insulin injections. Basal rate reductions starting 60 to 90 minutes before exercise and continuing for 60 to 90 minutes after exercise usually work well for moderate exercise of $\geq$60 minutes or strenuous exercise of $\geq$30 minutes.

BIBLIOGRAPHY

1. Aronson R, Brown RE, Li A, Riddell MC. Optimal insulin correction factor in post-high-intensity exercise hyperglycemia in adults with type 1 diabetes: the fit study. *Diabetes Care.* 2019 Jan;42(1):10–16.
2. Bally L, Thabit H. Closing the loop on exercise in type 1 diabetes. *Curr Diabetes Rev.* 2018;14(3):257–265.
3. Berger M, Berchtold P, Cüppers HJ, et al. Metabolic and hormonal effects of muscular exercise in juvenile type diabetics. *Diabetologia.* 1977 Aug;13(4):355–365.
4. Chu L, Hamilton J, Riddell MC. Clinical management of the physically active patient with type 1 diabetes. *Phys Sports Med.* 2011 May;39(2):64–77.
5. Diabetes Canada Clinical Practice Guidelines Expert Committee Sigal RJ, Armstrong MJ, Bacon SL, et al. Physical activity and diabetes. *Can J Diabetes.* 2018 Apr;42(Suppl 1):S54–S63.
6. Fahey AJ, Paramalingam N, Davey RJ, et al. The effect of a short sprint on post-exercise whole-body glucose production and utilization rates in individuals with type 1 diabetes mellitus. *J Clin Endocrinol Metab.* 2012 Nov;97(11):4193–4200.
7. Gallen IW, Hume C, Lumb A. Fueling the athlete with type 1 diabetes. *Diabetes Obes Metab.* 2011 Feb;13(2):130–136.
8. Grimm JJ, Ybarra J, Berné C, Muchnick S, Golay A. A new table for prevention of hypoglycaemia during physical activity in type 1 diabetic patients. *Diabetes Metab.* 2004 Nov;30(5):465–470.
9. Guelfi KJ, Jones TW, Fournier PA. The decline in blood glucose levels is less with intermittent high-intensity compared with moderate exercise in individuals with type 1 diabetes. *Diabetes Care.* 2005 Jun;28(6):1289–1294.
10. Guelfi KJ, Jones TW, Fournier PA. Intermittent high-intensity exercise does not increase the risk of early post-exercise hypoglycemia in individuals with type 1 diabetes. *Diabetes Care.* 2005 Feb;28(2):416–418.
11. Iscoe KE, Riddell MC. Continuous moderate-intensity exercise with or without intermittent high-intensity work: effects on acute and late glycaemia in athletes with Type 1 diabetes mellitus. *Diabet Med.* 2011 Jul;28(7):824–832.
12. Li A, Riddell MC, Potashner D, Brown RE, Aronson R. Time lag and accuracy of continuous glucose monitoring during high intensity interval training in adults with type 1 diabetes. *Diabetes Technol Ther.* 2019 May;21(5):286–294.
13. Manohar C, Levine JA, Nandy DK, et al. The effect of walking on postprandial glycemic excursion in patients with type 1 diabetes and healthy people. *Diabetes Care.* 2012 Dec;35(12):2493–2499.
14. Pasieka AM, Riddell MC. Advances in exercise, physical activity, and diabetes mellitus. *Diabetes Technol Ther.* 2017 Feb;19(S1):S94–S104.
15. Potashner D, Brown RE, Li A, Riddell MC, Aronson R. Paradoxical rise in hypoglycemia symptoms with development of hyperglycemia during high-intensity interval training in type 1 diabetes. *Diabetes Care.* 2019 Oct;42(10):2011–2014.
16. Rabasa-Lhoret R, Bourque J, Ducros F, Chiasson JL. Guidelines for premeal insulin dose reduction for postprandial exercise of different intensities and durations in type 1 diabetic subjects treated intensively with a basal-bolus insulin regimen (ultralente-lispro). *Diabetes Care.* 2001 Apr;24(4):625–630.
17. Riddell MC, Gallen IW, Smart CE, et al. Exercise management in type 1 diabetes: a consensus statement. *Lancet Diabetes Endocrinol.* 2017 May;5(5):377–390.
18. Riddell MC, Milliken J. Preventing exercise-induced hypoglycemia in type 1 diabetes using real-time continuous glucose monitoring and a new carbohydrate intake algorithm: an observational field study. *Diabetes Technol Ther.* 2011 Aug;13(8):819–825.
19. Tansey MJ, Tsalikian E, Beck RW, et al. The effects of aerobic exercise on glucose and counterregulatory hormone concentrations in children with type 1 diabetes. *Diabetes Care.* 2006 Jan;29(1):20–25.
20. Teich T, Zaharieva DP, Riddell MC. Advances in exercise, physical activity, and diabetes mellitus. *Diabetes Technol Ther.* 2019 Feb;21(S1):S112–S122.
21. Toghi-Eshghi SR, Yardley JE. Morning (fasting) vs afternoon resistance exercise in individuals with type 1 diabetes: a randomized crossover study. *J Clin Endocrinol Metab.* 2019;104:5217–5224.
22. Yardley JE, Iscoe KE, Sigal RJ, et al. Insulin pump therapy is associated with less post-exercise hyperglycemia than multiple daily injections: an observational study of physically active type 1 diabetes patients. *Diabetes Technol Ther.* 2013 Jan;15(1):84–88.

23. Yardley JE, Kenny GP, Perkins BA, et al. Resistance versus aerobic exercise: acute effects on glycemia in type 1 diabetes. *Diabetes Care*. 2013 Mar;36(3):537–542.
24. Yardley JE, Sigal RJ, Kenny GP, Riddell MC, Lovblom LE, Perkins BA. Point accuracy of interstitial continuous glucose monitoring during exercise in type 1 diabetes. *Diabetes Technol Ther*. 2013 Jan;15(1):46–49.
25. Yardley JE, Kenny GP, Perkins BA, et al. Effects of performing resistance exercise before versus after aerobic exercise on glycemia in type 1 diabetes. *Diabetes Care*. 2012 Apr;35(4):669–675.
26. Yardley JE, Hay J, Abou-Setta AM, Marks SD, McGavock J. A systematic review and meta-analysis of exercise interventions in adults with type 1 diabetes. *Diabetes Res Clin Pract*. 2014 Dec;106(3):393–400.
27. Yardley JE, Sigal RJ, Perkins BA, Riddell MC, Kenny GP. Resistance exercise in type 1 diabetes. *Can J Diabetes*. 2013 Dec;37(6):420–426.
28. Yardley JE, Iscoe KE, Sigal RJ, Kenny GP, Perkins BA, Riddell MC. Insulin pump therapy is associated with less post-exercise hyperglycemia than multiple daily injections: an observational study of physically active type 1 diabetes patients. *Diabetes Technol Ther*. 2013 Jan;15(1):84–88.
29. Zaharieva D, Yavelberg L, Jamnik V, Cinar A, Turksoy K, Riddell MC. The effects of basal insulin suspension at the start of exercise on blood glucose levels during continuous versus circuit-based exercise in individuals with type 1 diabetes on continuous subcutaneous insulin infusion. *Diabetes Technol Ther*. 2017 Jun;19(6):370–378.
30. Zaharieva DP, Cinar A, Yavelberg L, Jamnik V, Riddell MC. No disadvantage to insulin pump off vs pump on during intermittent high-intensity exercise in adults with type 1 diabetes. *Can J Diabetes*. 2020 Mar;44(2):162–168.
31. Zaharieva DP, Riddell MC. Insulin management strategies for exercise in diabetes. *Can J Diabetes*. 2017 Oct;41(5):507–516.
32. Zaharieva DP, Turksoy K, McGaugh SM, Pooni R, Vienneau T, Ly T, Riddell MC. Lag time remains with newer real-time continuous glucose monitoring technology during aerobic exercise in adults living with type 1 diabetes. *Diabetes Technol Ther*. 2019 Jun;21(6):313–321.
33. Zaharieva DP, McGaugh S, Pooni R, Vienneau T, Ly T, Riddell MC. Improved open-loop glucose control with basal insulin reduction 90 minutes before aerobic exercise in patients with type 1 diabetes on continuous subcutaneous insulin infusion. *Diabetes Care*. 2019 May;42(5):824–831.
34. Zaharieva DP, Riddell MC, Henske J. The accuracy of continuous glucose monitoring and flash glucose monitoring during aerobic exercise in type 1 diabetes. *J Diabetes Sci Technol*. 2019 Jan;13(1):140–141.
35. Zaharieva DP, McGaugh S, Davis EA, Riddell MC, et al. Advances in exercise, physical activity, and diabetes. *Diabetes Technol Ther*. 2020 Feb;22(S1):S109–S118.
36. Zisser H, Gong P, Kelley CM, Seidman JS, Riddell MC. Exercise and diabetes. *Int J Clin Pract (Suppl.)*. 2011 Feb;170:71–75.

CHAPTER 20

DIABETES MANAGEMENT IN HOSPITALIZED PATIENTS

Stacey A. Seggelke and R. Matthew Hawkins

1. **How common is diabetes and/or hyperglycemia in the inpatient setting?**
   Diabetes is a growing epidemic, with an estimated 1 out of every 10 people in the United States having a diagnosis of diabetes. The rate of prediabetes is even higher, at 1 out of every 3 American adults. Observation studies have reported a prevalence of diabetes and/or hyperglycemia ranging from 20% to 40% in hospitalized patients.

2. **What is considered hyperglycemia in the inpatient setting, and why is it a concern?**
   The American Diabetes Association (ADA) defines hyperglycemia in hospitalized patients as a blood glucose (BG) level of >140 mg/dL. Hyperglycemia in patients with or without diabetes is correlated with increased rates of infection, longer hospital lengths of stay, and higher morbidity and mortality rates. One study of general surgical patients reported an estimated increased risk of infection of 30% for every 40 mg/dL rise in BG above 110 mg/dL.

3. **What are the glycemic targets for the critically ill and noncritically ill inpatient population?**
   The ADA recommends a glycemic goal of 140 to 180 mg/dL for most critically ill and noncritically ill hospitalized patients. The glycemic goal can be further lowered to 110 to 140 mg/dL in select patients if that can be attained without hypoglycemia. Many people who have tight glycemic control in the outpatient setting prefer lower BG targets while hospitalized.

4. **What are the inpatient glycemic targets for pregnant patients?**
   BG goals for pregnancy are lower than those for the general population. Hyperglycemia during pregnancy is associated with many adverse outcomes, including macrosomia, congenital anomalies, fetal hyperinsulinemia, and fetal mortality. For people with gestational diabetes, type 1 diabetes, and type 2 diabetes, the recommendations are a fasting BG < 95 mg/dL, 1-hour postmeal BG ≤ 140 mg/dL, and 2-hour postmeal BG ≤ 120 mg/dL (Table 20.1). (Chapter 16 discusses the treatment of diabetes during pregnancy.)

5. **When should point-of-care (POC) BG testing be performed in the hospital setting?**
   Most hospitalized patients with diabetes should have POC BG testing before meals, at bedtime, and after any change in clinical status. Premeal testing should be completed as close to the meal as possible but ideally no more than 30 minutes before meals. For patients taking nothing by mouth (NPO) or receiving medical nutritional therapy, POC BG testing is recommended every 4 to 6 hours. Patients experiencing hypoglycemia, hyperglycemia, or other special circumstances may need POC BG testing more frequently.

6. **Should a hemoglobin A1c level be checked in hospitalized patients?**
   In all people with diabetes, a hemoglobin A1c should be checked on hospital admission unless they have had a value within the past 3 months. The A1c result can help evaluate home glycemic control and aid in discharge planning. For patients without known diabetes but who have a BG level of >140 mg/dL, an A1c should also be checked. If the A1c is ≥6.5%, it is likely that diabetes was present but undiagnosed prior to the hospital stay. If the A1c is <6.5%, this does not exclude a diagnosis of diabetes, and further testing with an oral glucose tolerance test should be completed in the outpatient setting. It is noteworthy that common inpatient comorbidities, such as anemia or sickle cell trait, and treatments such as hemodialysis, recent blood transfusions, or erythropoietin therapy can alter A1c results.

7. **What causes hyperglycemia in hospitalized patients with diabetes?**
   There are numerous factors that contribute to hyperglycemia in hospitalized patients with a preexisting diagnosis of diabetes. These situations include glucocorticoid therapy, enteral or parenteral nutrition, immunosuppressive agents, some chemotherapy agents, and/or metabolic changes caused by increased circulating counterregulatory hormones and proinflammatory cytokines (stress hyperglycemia). If hyperglycemia occurs (BG ≥ 180 mg/dL), appropriate treatment should be initiated, with glycemic goals of 140 to 180 mg/dL.

8. **What causes stress hyperglycemia?**
   Stress hyperglycemia is a common complication in hospitalized patients with or without underlying diabetes and is especially concerning for those with preexisting diabetes. Stress hyperglycemia results from increased circulating

Table 20.1 Target Glucose Levels for Hospitalized Patients

Critically ill: 140–180 mg/dL[a]

Noncritically ill: 140–180 mg/dL[a]

Pregnant: fasting < 95 mg/dL, 1 hr postprandial ≤ 140 mg/dL; 2 hr postprandial ≤ 120 mg/dL

[a]Glycemic goal can be lowered to 110–140 mg/dL in select patients if that can be attained without hypoglycemia.

Table 20.2 Inpatient Treatment of Hyperglycemia

Insulin is the most appropriate treatment agent for hyperglycemia in the hospital

Intravenous insulin infusion is the best therapy for critically ill patients

Basal/Bolus (prandial and correction) insulin is the best therapy for noncritically ill patients

Blood glucose levels should be evaluated daily and insulin adjusted as needed

proinflammatory cytokines and counterregulatory hormones (cortisol, catecholamines, growth hormone, and glucagon), leading to increased gluconeogenesis and glycogenolysis and decreased peripheral tissue glucose uptake. Additionally, a diminished incretin effect resulting in decreased insulin production has been described in critically ill patients.

9. **What is the best way to manage diabetes in hospitalized patients?**
   Insulin therapy, given as an intravenous (IV) infusion or as subcutaneous (SQ) injections, is the safest and most effective way to treat hyperglycemia in the hospital setting. The ADA recommends the initiation of insulin therapy for the treatment of hyperglycemia at a glucose threshold of ≥180 mg/dL. Insulin therapy should then be titrated to maintain BG levels between 140 and 180 mg/dL. Insulin dosing can be rapidly adjusted to adapt to changes in glucose levels or food intake. It is recommended that standardized insulin protocols be used whenever available.

10. **Does evidence support intensive management of BG in the hospital setting?**
    It is well established that hyperglycemia contributes to increased morbidity, mortality, and length of hospital stay. Improvement in inpatient glycemic control clearly facilitates better patient outcomes and shorter lengths of stay. However, there is controversy over what degree of glycemic control is most appropriate. The landmark study by Van den Berghe et al. demonstrated a 40% reduction in mortality in surgical intensive care patients treated to a BG goal of 80 to 110 mg/dL compared with those with a goal of 180 to 215 mg/dL. This initial study called for tight glycemic control, especially in the critical care setting. These glycemic goals were later modified by the Normoglycemia in Intensive Care Evaluation and Survival Using Glucose Algorithm Regulation (NICE-SUGAR) study. The NICE-SUGAR study was a large randomized controlled trial (RCT) that reported an increased risk of mortality in patients with tight glycemic control (BG target 81–108 mg/dL) compared with those with standard glycemic control (BG target 144–180 mg/dL). The increased mortality was considered to be due partially to the high hypoglycemia (≤40 mg/dL) rate that occurred in the intensively treated group. Although this study corroborated previous evidence that glycemic control is important, it did underscore the risks of hypoglycemia and led to a relaxing of glycemic targets. Thus, recommended inpatient BG targets were modified to 140 to 180 mg/dL to reduce the risk of hypoglycemia (Table 20.2).

11. **What is an IV insulin infusion, and why is it used in critically ill patients?**
    An IV insulin infusion or insulin drip (gtt) is composed of 1 unit of regular human insulin per 1 mL of 0.9% NaCl (normal saline). When given IV, regular insulin has a rapid onset and short half-life, allowing for quick adjustment of insulin doses to achieve appropriate glycemic control.

12. **How should the IV insulin infusion rate be started and adjusted?**
    An insulin infusion is usually initiated at 0.1 unit/hour/kg body weight. Insulin infusions should be adjusted hourly based on the current BG level and the rate of change from the previous BG level. If BG levels do not change by 30 to 50 mg/dL within an hour, the insulin infusion rate should be increased. Conversely, if BG levels drop more than 30 to 50 mg/dL in an hour, the insulin drip rate should be reduced. We strongly recommend that written insulin infusion protocols or computer-generated algorithms be used. These should include the key elements noted in Table 20.3.

13. **How do I transition a patient off an insulin infusion?**
    Because of the short duration of action of IV regular insulin, it is ideal to give SQ basal insulin, a long-acting or intermediate-acting form, 2 to 4 hours before or rapid-acting insulin 1 to 2 hours before discontinuation of the insulin infusion. An appropriate transition from IV insulin to scheduled SQ insulin is important to decrease the risk

Table 20.3 Key Elements of an Intravenous Insulin Infusion Protocol
• Identify appropriate BG targets
• Nurse-driven, easy to use insulin titration protocols
• Frequent POC BG checks and insulin adjustments
• Titration based on direction of BG change (decrease, no change, increase)
• Titration based on velocity of BG change (decrease rate faster if larger drop in BG values)
• Included guidelines for treatment of hypoglycemia and subsequent adjustment of insulin rate

BG, Blood glucose; *POC*, point of care.

of rebound hyperglycemia. This is imperative in people with type 1 diabetes, in whom just a few hours without insulin can result in diabetic ketoacidosis (DKA). Three different methods we use to transition patients from IV insulin infusions to SQ insulin injections are as follows:

1. **Preferred method:** Estimate the basal SQ insulin dose based on the total amount of IV insulin given in the last 6 hours. Calculate the total amount of insulin given during the last 6 hours of the IV insulin infusion and multiply by 4 for an estimate of the 24-hour insulin requirement; then reduce that amount by 20% for an initial SQ basal insulin dose. This calculation assumes the patient was NPO while on the insulin infusion.
2. Calculate a weight-based SQ basal insulin dose and order rapid-acting bolus insulin according to oral intake (see following discussion).
3. Resume home SQ basal dosing and order bolus insulin according to oral intake (see following discussion).

14. **How should you select a basal insulin dose if a patient is not on an insulin infusion?**
Basal insulin coverage can be achieved using (preferably) long-acting insulin (glargine, detemir) dosed once or twice daily or intermediate-acting insulin (neutral protamine Hagedorn [NPH]) dosed twice daily. Long-acting insulins generally provide more consistent coverage with minimal insulin peaks, whereas NPH insulin is more likely to cause hypoglycemia as a result of variable insulin action and peaks. Degludec insulin has been shown to reduce hypoglycemia in the outpatient setting, but its long duration of action makes titration difficult, and it is not recommended for inpatient use. Regardless of insulin type, basal insulin usually accounts for approximately 50% of the total daily dose (TDD) of insulin.

The initial basal insulin dose is based on the diabetes type and the patient's nutritional status. For those with type 1 diabetes, a starting basal dose of 0.1 to 0.2 units/kg is appropriate; *these patients require basal insulin at all times*, including when they are NPO. For patients with type 2 diabetes who are NPO or have poor PO intake, a starting basal dose of 0.2 to 0.3 units/kg is best. A recommended starting basal dose for patients with type 2 diabetes with adequate oral intake is 0.4 to 0.5 units/kg.

Before continuing a home basal insulin dose, assessment of the current A1c, reported home BG profiles, and hypoglycemia frequency should be conducted. Outpatient basal insulin doses are often excessive to cover basal requirements, along with a mistaken attempt to cover some postprandial BG rises (overbasalization). If a patient reports hypoglycemia at home, especially nocturnal, a decrease in the basal dose of 20% to 50% may be warranted.

> **Important**
> Impaired renal function increases the risk of hypoglycemia through decreased insulin clearance and metabolism and decreased renal contribution to gluconeogenesis, so doses may need to be decreased accordingly.

15. **How should you select a prandial dose for patients on insulin?**
Prandial insulin should include both nutritional (meal coverage) and correctional (treatment of hyperglycemia) components. Rapid-acting insulin analogs (lispro, aspart, glulisine) should be given 0 to 15 minutes prior to meals, whereas short-acting insulin (regular) should be given 30 minutes prior to meals. Rapid-acting analogs provide increased flexibility in dosing and have a shorter duration of action, making them the preferred method of treatment. In general, the total bolus insulin doses each day should be about 50% of the TDD of insulin delivery. However, in the hospital setting, a reduced prandial dose may be needed because of decreased appetite or variance in PO intake. Correction insulin dosing can be calculated based on the patient's insulin sensitivity. This insulin is either added to the nutritional dose or given alone if the patient is not receiving calories. For patients with type 1 diabetes or who are insulin sensitive, a good starting point for correction dosing is 1 unit of insulin for every 50 mg/dL above a goal of 100 mg/dL. For patients with type 2 diabetes or insulin resistance, 1 unit of insulin for every 25 mg/dL above 100 to 150 mg/dL is recommended. (See Table 20.4 for example). To prevent hypoglycemia resulting from the "stacking" of insulin, correction insulin doses should not be given more often than every 4 hours (Fig. 20.1).

Table 20.4 Example of Nutritional and Correctional Insulin Dosing Chart

BLOOD GLUCOSE (MG/DL)	INSULIN-SENSITIVE TYPE 1 DM STRESS HYPERGLYCEMIA NORMAL BODY WEIGHT		INSULIN-RESISTANT TYPE 2 DM STEROIDS OVERWEIGHT/OBESE		EXTRA-INSULIN-RESISTANT BLOOD GLUCOSE UNCONTROLLED BY "RESISTANT TO INSULIN" RECOMMENDATIONS		CUSTOMIZED INDIVIDUALIZED	
≤70	IMPLEMENT HYPOGLYCEMIA ORDERS		IMPLEMENT HYPOGLYCEMIA ORDERS		IMPLEMENT HYPOGLYCEMIA ORDERS		IMPLEMENT HYPOGLYCEMIA ORDERS	
	RECEIVING CALORIES	NO CALORIES	RECEIVING CALORIES	NO CALORIES	RECEIVING CALORIES	NO CALORIES	RECEIVING CALORIES	NO CALORIES
71–124	3 units	No insulin	6 units	No insulin	10 units	No insulin	___ units	___ units
125–149	3 units	No insulin	7 units	1 unit	12 units	1 unit	___ units	___ units
150–199	4 units	1 unit	8 units	2 units	14 units	3 units	___ units	___ units
200–249	5 units	2 units	10 units	4 units	16 units	5 units	___ units	___ units
250–299	6 units	3 units	12 units	6 units	18 units	7 units	___ units	___ units
300–349	7 units	4 units	14 units	8 units	20 units	9 units	___ units	___ units
350–399	8 units	5 units	16 units	10 units	22 units	11 units	___ units	___ units
≥400	Call MD		Call MD		Call MD		Call MD	

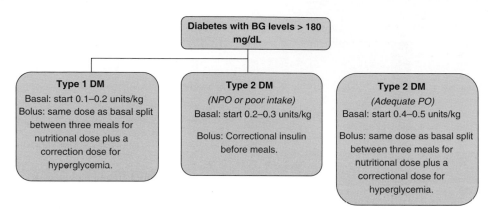

Fig. 20.1 Treatment of inpatient hyperglycemia.

16. **How should you adjust insulin dosages?**

BG profiles should be evaluated daily. Basal insulin doses are assessed mainly by reviewing fasting morning BG levels compared with bedtime BG levels the night before. With ideal basal insulin dosing, BG levels should remain relatively stable through the night. A significant rise or drop in BG during the night necessitates a change in basal insulin dosing. Prandial insulin is assessed by prelunch, predinner, and bedtime BG values. If BG levels rise during the day and oral intake is stable, the bolus insulin doses should be increased. Similarly, if oral intake is stable and BG levels decrease during the day, a bolus insulin decrease is recommended. For more precise prandial insulin dosing, a 2-hour postprandial BG check can be performed. It is expected that this postprandial BG value will be about 30 to 50 mg/dL higher than the preprandial BG reading.

17. **Is "sliding-scale" insulin still used?**

Sliding-scale insulin is not an effective treatment for hyperglycemia and therefore should not be used. A sliding scale was a set amount of bolus insulin, usually regular insulin, which was given to treat high BG levels, generally above 200 mg/dL. The insulin was given without thought as to mealtimes, previous dosages, carbohydrate content of meals, or the patient's insulin sensitivity. This often resulted in a wide fluctuation of BG levels because hyperglycemia was not treated preemptively but instead was treated after the fact.

18. **What is hypoglycemia, and what contributes to it?**

Hypoglycemia is defined as a BG < 70 mg/dL, which is considered the initial threshold for counterregulatory hormone release. The ADA further classifies hypoglycemia into three levels:

Level 1: BG < 70 mg/dL and ≥ 54 mg/dL

Level 2: BG < 54 mg/dL

Level 3: Severe hypoglycemic event where the patient has altered mental or physical status and requires assistance for the treatment of hypoglycemia

Patients at high risk for hypoglycemia include those with renal or liver failure, altered nutrition, older age, sepsis, and a history of severe hypoglycemia.

19. **How should hypoglycemia be treated?**

Treatment of hypoglycemia is based on the situation. For a patient who can take oral treatment, 15 to 30 g of quick-acting carbohydrates, such as juice, regular soda, or glucose tablets, is the preferred treatment. If unconscious or unable to take oral treatment, the patient can be given 50 g (1 ampule) of Dextrose 50% IV or glucagon 1 mg intramuscularly (IM). This is also the preferred treatment for patients with level 2 hypoglycemia in the hospital setting. BG levels should be rechecked within 15 to 20 minutes of treatment to assess hypoglycemia resolution. If the BG is still <70 mg/dL, treatment should be repeated.

20. **Are oral agents or noninsulin injectables appropriate to use in hospitalized patients?**

Limited data are available on the safety and efficacy of using oral agents or noninsulin injectables (glucagon-like peptide-1 [GLP-1] analogs or pramlintide) in hospital settings. In most cases of hospital hyperglycemia, noninsulin treatment options are not effective in lowering BG to goal levels, especially in acute illness. Recent studies have demonstrated the efficacy and safety of using dipeptidyl peptidase-4 (DPP-4) inhibitors (linagliptin and sitagliptin) in the hospital setting. When used alone or in combination with basal insulin or correctional bolus insulin, DPP-4 inhibitors proved to be an effective treatment. Caution is recommended with the use of saxagliptin and alogliptin in patients with established heart or kidney disease because of a potential increased risk of heart failure, according to a U.S. Food and Drug Administration (FDA) safety communication. Safety concerns for other oral agents include a risk of lactic acidosis with metformin, delayed onset of action and fluid retention with thiazolidinediones, increased risk of urinary and genital tract infections and dehydration with sodium–glucose cotransporter 2 (SGLT-2) inhibitors, and sustained hypoglycemia with sulfonylureas. Oral agents may be initiated or resumed in clinically stable patients in anticipation of discharge. Inpatient use of GLP-1 agonist therapies for the management of hyperglycemia is generally not recommended because of the known gastrointestinal side effects. One study compared exenatide 5 μg administered twice daily both with and without basal insulin with a standard basal-bolus insulin regimen in general medicine and surgery patients with diabetes. Glycemic control was similar in the two groups, but patients receiving exenatide experienced higher rates of nausea.

21. **What is the best treatment for steroid-induced hyperglycemia?**
Steroids cause both insulin resistance and diminished insulin secretion, manifested largely by excessive post-prandial BG excursions. The extent of BG elevation is dependent on the type, amount, and duration of steroid therapy. Individuals who are on low steroid doses and who are insulin naive may be treated with bolus insulin at mealtimes. If a patient is receiving higher steroid doses (prednisone 20 mg daily or an equivalent dose of another steroid) or has a history of insulin-treated diabetes, a good treatment option is intermediate basal insulin. NPH insulin can be dosed at the same time as administration of the steroid. The NPH dosage can be based on the patient's weight and the steroid dose ordered. One recommended regimen is 0.1 unit/kg of NPH for each 10 mg of prednisone equivalent to a maximum of 0.4 units/kg for doses ≥40 mg of prednisone equivalent.
   For patients on steroids with a long duration of action (dexamethasone) or multiple daily doses of shorter-acting steroids, long-acting basal insulin may be used. Insulin needs should be assessed and adjusted as steroid therapy is later tapered or discontinued. If BG levels remain uncontrolled with SQ insulin therapy, an IV insulin fusion may be needed.

22. **What is the best treatment for hyperglycemia with parenteral nutrition (PN)?**
For PN, the addition of regular insulin to the PN bag is the safest approach to glycemic control. The initial dosing recommendation is 1 unit for every 10 to 12 g of dextrose in the PN solution. A rapid-acting insulin correction scale every 4 to 6 hours is also recommended for hyperglycemia if the initial dose of regular insulin in the PN is not adequate. The TDD of correctional insulin needed to maintain euglycemia can then be added to the total regular insulin dose in the PN the next day. Another approach to treatment is the use of an SQ basal/bolus regimen. The latter poses an increased risk of hypoglycemia if PN is unexpectedly discontinued or the PN dextrose concentration is changed without adjustment of insulin dosing. When using SQ insulin regimens, it is important to include orders that a dextrose-containing IV solution, such as D10W, be initiated at the same rate of PN if nutritional therapy is unexpectedly interrupted. Reducing or holding the next dose of long-acting or intermediate-acting insulin may also be necessary. Additionally, patients receiving PN are in a consistent postprandial state, and BG goals should be adjusted accordingly.

23. **What is the best treatment for hyperglycemia with enteral nutrition (EN)?**
There are many approaches to treatment for hyperglycemia associated with EN. Depending on whether EN is continuous or cyclic, basal or intermediate-acting insulin can be administered once or twice daily in combination with a rapid-acting insulin correction scale every 4 to 6 hours. Alternatively, intermediate-acting 70/30 human insulin given every 8 hours with a correctional rapid-acting insulin scale every 4 hours is an approach that the authors use. Hypoglycemia is a concern in these patients because feeding can be interrupted unexpectedly with dislodging of the feeding tube or discontinuation of EN because of nausea or diagnostic testing. It is important that all EN insulin orders recommend that a dextrose-containing IV solution, such as D10W, be initiated at the same rate as EN if nutritional therapy is unexpectedly interrupted and that the next dose of long-acting or intermediate-acting insulin be reduced or withheld. Importantly, these patients are in a consistent postprandial state, and BG goals should be adjusted accordingly.

24. **Can concentrated insulins be used in the hospital?**
The use of concentrated insulin in the outpatient setting has become more commonplace; however, there are numerous concerns about continuing these insulins in the inpatient setting. U-500 regular insulin is a concentrated insulin that delivers the same unit amount in one-fifth the volume as U-100 insulin and is used either as SQ injections or in insulin pumps. Because of its concentration, there is potential for adverse events related to insulin dosing calculations. It is recommended that pharmacy staff confirm the dosing and deliver predrawn syringes to the wards for patients. However, most people who use U-500 at home do not need to continue use in the hospital. One study found that patients required significantly lower insulin doses while hospitalized and that glucose could be managed with conventional insulin formulations.
   Other concentrated insulins on the market, such as insulin glargine 300 U/mL, insulin degludec 200 U/mL, and insulin lispro 200 U/mL, come in pen devices that adjust the volume of insulin given to avoid calculation errors. The efficacy and safety of these insulins in the hospital setting have not been determined.

25. **Can a continuous subcutaneous insulin infusion be used in the inpatient setting?**
    Continuous subcutaneous insulin infusion (CSII), also known as an *insulin pump*, can be safely used in the inpatient setting. Most patients who are well controlled on their insulin pump as outpatients will become frustrated if the insulin pump is removed during their inpatient stay. However, it is imperative that patients be mentally and physically able to operate their own insulin pumps. It is also recommended that ward personnel with CSII experience help manage these patients. For patient and staff safety, an insulin pump agreement should be completed that outlines expectations that the patient will collaborate with the hospital team and report symptoms of hypoglycemia, BG levels not performed by hospital staff, and all boluses given for nutritional or correctional coverage. Current pump settings, including basal rates, bolus settings, and bolus dosages, should be manually reviewed and documented on hospital admission and daily thereafter by the treating hospital team. Insulin pump companies recommend that patients disconnect or remove the pump for many tests where there is a risk of exposure to radiation or strong magnetic fields, such as used with magnetic resonance imaging (MRI). Patients who use a continuous glucose monitor (CGM) in combination with an insulin pump should be allowed to continue the use of this device in the hospital; however, all insulin dosing decisions should be made based on fingerstick BG testing. Closed-loop insulin delivery systems, where the pump and CGM are linked to control BG levels, may be continued in the inpatient setting if the hospital team feels it is appropriate (Table 20.5).

26. **Can a CGM be used in the inpatient setting?**
    Through continuous testing of interstitial glucose levels, a CGM provides current glucose values in addition to directional glucose trend arrows. Alarms, which are built into most CGM devices, can alert patients to projected and current hypo- or hyperglycemia. Most studies using either real-time or intermittently scanned CGM in the hospital setting reported reductions in hypoglycemia events but did not demonstrate overall improvement in glycemia. The use of a real-time or intermittently scanned CGM can be continued in the hospital; however, at present, all insulin dosing decisions should be made based on fingerstick BG testing.

27. **How do you adjust diabetes medications prior to surgery?**
    Hypoglycemia is a considerable risk for patients undergoing surgery because of their NPO status and inability to sense hypoglycemic symptoms while under the influence of anesthesia. Oral agents should be held the morning of the procedure. SGLT2-inhibitors should be held for 48 to 72 hours prior to surgery because of the increased risk of ketoacidosis when NPO. For patients on long-acting insulin (glargine/detemir/degludec), it is recommended that they take about 80% of their usual dose the night before or morning of surgery. Patients on intermediate-acting insulin (NPH) should take 50% of their typical dose the morning of the procedure. Correctional doses of rapid-acting insulin analogs can be given in the perioperative period every 4 hours to maintain BG levels of <180 mg/dL. If a procedure is prolonged or if prolonged NPO status is expected, the use of an insulin infusion is recommended.

28. **How do I decide what home regimen to order at discharge?**
    Patients who had good glycemic control as outpatients, which can be determined by an A1c drawn at admission, can be sent home on the regimen they were on prior to admission. For those with a new diagnosis of diabetes or those requiring a change in their previous therapy because of poor antecedent glycemic control, recommendations should be based on the patients' preference/ability and the cost of and contraindications to new medications. It is also recommended that medication administration instructions, especially for insulin, be given in both oral and written formats. Details of discharge medications and instructions should be communicated promptly and clearly to the patients' outpatient diabetes providers. In addition, patients' diabetes self-management knowledge should be assessed prior to discharge to determine their understanding of their diabetes diagnosis, the technique and goals of BG self-monitoring, treatment of hypoglycemia, sick-day management, and how/when to take glucose-lowering medications.

29. **What is unique about treating patients with diabetes with COVID-19?**
    COVID-19 has provided a unique challenge in inpatient diabetes management. It has been well established that patients with uncontrolled diabetes who contract COVID-19 have more severe disease progression and increased

Table 20.5 Contraindications to Insulin Pump Use in the Hospital

Altered mental status
Suicidal ideation
Diabetic ketoacidosis
Concern for insulin pump malfunction
Lack of appropriate insulin pump supplies
Patient/family inability to participate in pump self-management

mortality. Many of these patients have demonstrated severe insulin resistance, requiring 300 to 500 units of insulin per day to maintain euglycemia while in the intensive care unit (ICU) setting. These extreme insulin needs are thought to be secondary to the acute inflammatory and metabolic effects of COVID-19 and the need for medical nutrition and steroid therapy. Significant reductions in insulin requirements are generally seen with clinical improvement. Vigilant monitoring of BG levels is imperative.

KEY POINTS

1. Insulin is the most appropriate treatment agent for hyperglycemia in the hospital.
2. BG levels should be evaluated daily because changes in clinical status can directly affect insulin needs.
3. In all patients with diabetes, a hemoglobin A1c should be checked on admission unless patients have a value within the past 3 months.
4. Insulin pumps can be continued in the inpatient setting if patients are mentally and physically able to operate their own insulin pumps.

WEBSITES

1. American Diabetes Association Standards of Diabetes Care 2020 – Diabetes Care in the Hospital
   https://care.diabetesjournals.org/content/43/Supplement_1/S193
2. American Association of Clinical Endocrinologist Inpatient Glycemic Control Resource Center
   http://resources.aace.com
3. Society of Hospital Medicine Glycemic Control Resource Room:
   http://www.hospitalmedicine.org/ResourceRoomRedesign/RR_LandingPage.cfm
4. Center for Disease Control and Prevention Diabetes Home Page
   https://www.cdc.gov/diabetes/index.html

BIBLIOGRAPHY

1. American Diabetes Association. Standards of medical care in diabetes 2020. *Diabetes Care*. 2020;43:S193–S202.
2. Davis GM, Galindo RJ, Migdal AL. Diabetes technology the inpatient setting for management of hyperglycemia. *Endocrinology & Metabolism Clinics*. 2020;49(1):79–93.
3. Lorenzo-Gonzalez C, Atienza-Sanchez E, Reyes-Umpierrez D. Safety and efficacy of DDP-4 inhibitors for the management of hospitalized general medicine and surgical patients with type 2 diabetes. *Endocrine Practice*. 2020;26(7):722–729.
4. Umpierrez GE, Smiley D, et al. Randomized study of basal-bolus insulin therapy in the inpatient management of patients with type 2 diabetes (RABBIT 2 trial). *Diabetes Care*. 2018;30(9):2181–2186.
5. Umpierrez Smiley D, et al. Randomized study of basal-bolus insulin therapy in the inpatient management of patients with type 2 diabetes undergoing surgery. *Diabetes Care*. 2011;34:256–261.
6. Umpierrez GE, Pasquel FJ. Management of inpatient hyperglycemia and diabetes in older adults. *Diabetes Care*. 2017;40(4):509–517.
7. Umpierrez GE, Pasquel FJ. Management of inpatient hyperglycemia and diabetes in older adults. *Diabsetes Care*. 2017;10(4):509–517.
8. Van den Berghe G, Wilmer A, et al. Intensive insulin therapy in the medical ICU. *N Engl J Med*. 2006;354:449–446.

CHAPTER 21

CONTINUOUS GLUCOSE MONITORING

Michael T. McDermott, MD

1. **What is the perfect glucose sensor?**

   Pancreatic islet cells are the perfect glucose sensors. Through cell-membrane glucose transporters that bring glucose into the intracellular compartment, these cells assess ambient blood glucose (BG) concentrations continually. Beta cells respond instantaneously to this information by producing the appropriate amounts of insulin, and alpha cells respond by producing the necessary amounts of glucagon.

2. **Is there a correlation between the number of fingerstick BG tests done per day and glucose control?**
   Yes. Published studies have demonstrated unequivocally that BG control improves in direct proportion to the number of fingerstick BG tests done per day.

3. **What is a continuous glucose monitor (CGM)?**
   A CGM is a device that consists of a sensor, a transmitter, and a receiver. The sensor is inserted under the skin and measures interstitial glucose levels almost continuously (every 1–5 minutes). The sensor is connected to a transmitter that wirelessly transmits the glucose values to a receiver, which can be a monitor, cellphone, watch, or an insulin pump. The receiver displays the glucose values in real time or intermittently and shows trend arrows that inform the user about the direction and magnitude of glucose-level changes.

4. **What is a professional CGM?**
   Professional CGM devices are owned by providers and are loaned to users for periods of 1 to 2 weeks, during which glucose values and patterns are blindly recorded and/or displayed in real time. The devices are then returned to the office, where CGM data are downloaded and analyzed. The user is instructed to keep careful records of insulin dosing, meals, snacks, and physical activity to enable the provider and/or certified diabetes education specialist (CDES) to relate the glucose patterns to these events. The user's carbohydrate-counting skills and proper use of correction insulin doses can also be evaluated. Currently available professional CGM systems are the Abbott FreeStyle Libre Pro, the Dexcom G6 Pro, and the Medtronic iPro2.

5. **What is a personal CGM?**
   Personal CGM devices are prescribed by providers and owned by users. They are worn daily or intermittently, but the best results occur when they are worn continuously or frequently. The devices display real-time or intermittent glucose values along with trend arrows to help people make day-to-day decisions regarding accurate insulin dosing for meals, high-BG corrections, and physical activity. The devices also have audible or vibratory alarms to alert the user when glucose values are high or low; some also have alarms for predictive low and predictive high glucose trends. Currently available personal CGM devices are the Abbott FreeStyle Libre and Libre 2, Dexcom G5 and G6, Guardian Connect 3, and Senseonics Eversense.

6. **How accurate are CGM devices?**
   CGM devices measure interstitial fluid glucose and not BG. When BG levels are stable, interstitial glucose values are usually very close to BG levels. However, when BG levels are changing, interstitial glucose values lag by 15 to 30 minutes and thus will give lower glucose readings when BG levels are rising and higher glucose readings when BG values are falling. Current CGM devices have a mean absolute relative difference (MARD) of ≤10%, which means that over a range of glucose values, the sensors report glucose levels that are within 10% of a gold-standard lab BG measurement.

7. **What are the features of the various personal CGM devices, and how do they differ?**
   Table 21.1 lists the currently available personal CGM devices with their MARDs, wear-time durations, need for calibration, audible alerts, and current integration with or U.S. Food and Drug Administration (FDA) approval for future integration with insulin pumps.

8. **What information do people receive from a personal CGM?**
   Without the need for fingerstick BG testing (Abbott FreeStyle Libre and Libre 2, Dexcom G5 and G6) or only twice-a-day BG testing for instrument calibration (Guardian Connect/Sensor 3, Senseonics Eversense), a personal CGM provides people with real-time or intermittent interstitial glucose values, trend arrows showing the direction and

Table 21.1 Personal Continuous Glucose Monitors

CGM	MARD	WEAR TIME	NEED TO CALIBRATE	AUDIBLE ALERTS	PUMP INTEGRATION
Abbott FreeStyle Libre 2	9.3%	14 days	No	Yes	Approved
Dexcom G5, G6	9.0%	10 days	No	Yes	Tandem T-Slim X2
Guardian Connect 3	8.7%–10.6%	7 days 2×/day	Yes	Yes	Medtronic 670/770 G
Senseonics Eversense	8.5%	90 days 2×/day	Yes	No	No

CGM, Continuous glucose monitor; *MARD*, mean absolute relative difference (compared with gold-standard lab values).

Table 21.2 Continuous Glucose Monitoring Time in Range (TIR) Targets in Nonpregnant Adults (2021)

GLUCOSE	TYPE 1 + TYPE 2 TARGET TIR	OLDER/HIGH-RISK TYPE 1 + TYPE 2 TARGET TIR
>250 mg/dL	<5%	<10%
>180 mg/dL	<25%	<50%
70–180 mg/dL	>70%	>50%
<70 mg/dL	<4%	<1%
<54 mg/dL	<1%	0%

magnitude of glucose changes, and alarms that alert for hypoglycemia and hyperglycemia; some also alert for predicted hypoglycemia and hyperglycemia so that preventive action can be taken.

9. **What information do providers get from a professional or personal CGM?**
Data recorded by CGM devices can be downloaded directly or virtually to display an ambulatory glucose profile (AGP), mean glucose levels throughout the day, postmeal glucose excursions, glucose variability, and user wear time.

10. **What is the AGP?**
The AGP is generated from the CGM download (usually for a 2-week period). It consists of a glucose management indicator (GMI), which is an estimate of the equivalent A1c for that 2-week period; the overall average glucose value; the percent of time in range (TIR) at various levels; glucose variability (coefficient of variation and/or standard deviation); and active CGM wear time. A suggested system for recording the AGP in a person's chart is as follows:
Glucose Management Indicator (GMI): ___%
Average BG: ___ mg/dL
TIR:
TIR > 250 mg/dL: ___%
TIR > 180 mg/dL: ___%
TIR 70 to 180 mg/dL: ___%
TIR < 70 mg/dL: ___%
TIR < 54 mg/dL: ___%
Coefficient of variation: ___% Standard deviation: ___ mg/dL
Time (%) CGM active: ___%

11. **What are the TIR targets for people using personal CGM devices?**
See Table 21.2.

Table 21.3 Continuous Glucose Monitoring Interpretation Worksheet

Continuous Glucose Monitor (CGM) Glucose Pattern Interpretation

Fasting glucose: _____

Postprandial glucose: _____

Bedtime glucose: _____

Overnight glucose: _____

High glucose: _____

Low glucose: _____

Glucose variability: _____

Overall: _____

Recommendations: _____

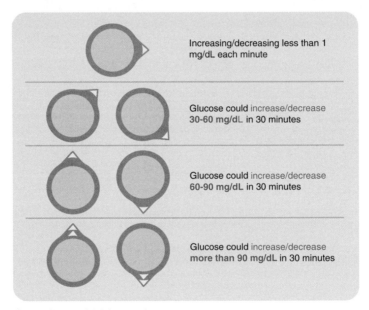

Fig. 21.1 Dexcom G6 arrow figures and their interpretation.

12. **Is there a standardized approach for interpreting CGM downloads?**
Standardized approaches to CGM interpretation, such as those used for electrocardiograms (ECGs), have not been formalized; however, in addition to analyzing the AGP, we recommend using a systematic method for evaluating CGM data. We use the following approach: first, the AGP is analyzed for overall glucose control and time spent in various glucose ranges; next, the fasting glucose values, postprandial glucose values after each meal, bedtime glucose values, and the glucose changes overnight are serially analyzed. We then summarize when glucose is most often high, most often low, and most variable. We finish with an overall impression and recommendations for management.
It is often helpful to use a standardized form. We use the worksheet shown in Table 21.3.

13. **How are CGM trend arrows used to help with optimal insulin dosing decisions?**
Trend arrows show the direction and magnitude of glucose changes. The changes are depicted differently by the different CGM devices. Figs. 21.1 and 21.2 show the arrow figures as they appear on the Dexcom G6 and Freestyle Libre, respectively. Trend-arrow interpretation is shown in Table 21.4 for the Dexcom G6 and in Table 21.5 for the Freestyle Libre. Recent publications have recommended how to use trend arrows to adjust bolus doses.

FreeStyle Libre System Trend Arrows		
Reader	Glucose Direction	Change in Glucose
↑	Rising quickly	**Glucose is rising quickly** Increasing >2 mg/dL/min or >60 mg/dL in 30 minutes
↗	Rising	**Glucose is rising** Increasing 1–2 mg/dL/min or 30–60 mg/dL in 30 minutes
→	Changing slowly	**Glucose is changing slowly** Not increasing/decreasing >1 mg/dL/min
↘	Falling	**Glucose is falling** Decreasing 1–2 mg/dL/min or 30–60 mg/dL in 30 minutes
↓	Falling quickly	**Glucose is falling quickly** Decreasing >2 mg/dL/min or >60 mg/dL in 30 minutes
No arrow present indicates that the system cannot calculate the velocity and direction of the glucose change.		

Fig. 21.2 Freestyle Libre arrow figures and their interpretation.

Table 21.4 Dexcom G6 Trend Arrows: Interpretation and Recommended Insulin Changes

ARROWS	GLUCOSE CHANGE	BOLUS DOSE CHANGE
Two 90° arrows up	Rising >3 mg/dL/min	Add 3 units
One 90° arrow up	Rising 2 to 3 mg/dL/min	Add 2 to 3 units
One 45° arrow up	Rising 1 to 2 mg/dL/min	Add 1 to 2 units
Horizontal arrow	Changing <1 mg/dL/min	Take usual bolus dose
One 45° arrow down	Falling 1 to 2 mg/dL/min	Subtract 1 to 2 units
One 90° arrow down	Falling 2 to 3 mg/dL/min	Subtract 2 to 3 units or omit
Two 90° arrows down	Falling >3 mg/dL/min	Don't take a bolus

Table 21.5 Freestyle Libre 2 Trend Arrows: Interpretation and Recommended Insulin Changes

ARROWS	GLUCOSE CHANGE	BOLUS DOSE CHANGE
One 90° arrow up	Rising >2 mg/dL/min	Add 2–3 units
One 45° arrow up	Rising 1 to 2 mg/dL/min	Add 1–2 units
Horizontal arrow	Changing <1 mg/dL/min	Take usual bolus dose
One 45° arrow down	Falling 1 to 2 mg/dL/min	Subtract 1–2 units
One 90° arrow down	Falling >2 mg/dL/min	Subtract 2–3 units or omit

A simple approach works best, in our experience, for real-life situations. Tables 21.4 and 21.5 also show (right columns) what bolus dose changes we recommend in response to trend arrows on these two systems. Whatever method is used, it is important to individualize the plan for each person and make sure these adjustments can be made during a person's day-to-day life.

14. How do CGM devices integrate with insulin pumps?
The current integrated technology is referred to as a *hybrid closed-loop system*. It is termed a *hybrid* rather than a fully closed-loop because these systems use CGM data to adjust basal insulin delivery rates and correction doses

but do not provide automatic meal boluses; therefore people must still count carbohydrates accurately and manually to determine the bolus to cover meals adequately. This topic is covered more fully in Chapter 23.

15. **Is there evidence that CGM improves glycemic control in people with type 1 diabetes?**

    Multiple studies in people with type 1 diabetes, treated with multiple daily insulin injections or insulin pumps, have demonstrated that CGM use reduces A1c, increases glucose time in target range, reduces time in hypoglycemia, improves hypoglycemia awareness in those who have hypoglycemia unawareness, and improves quality of life.

16. **Does CGM improve glycemic control in people with type 2 diabetes?**

    Personal CGM in people with type 2 diabetes who are taking multiple daily insulin injections has been reported to significantly reduce A1c levels but not hypoglycemia. Professional CGM done intermittently (3-month intervals) in people with type 2 diabetes in general practices has been shown to reduce A1c and improve glucose time in target range.

17. **Can CGM be used in hospitalized patients, including those in intensive care?**

    CGM devices have not yet (as of the date of this writing) been FDA approved for inpatient use. Although there are previously published and currently ongoing studies addressing this issue, there is still insufficient evidence that interstitial glucose values obtained in the inpatient setting, especially in intensive care, are accurate enough to inform insulin dosing decisions. However, consensus guidelines have been published supporting CGM use in hospitalized individuals.

18. **Let's practice some CGM interpretations**

    Practice exercises in CGM interpretation are presented in the next chapter.

KEY POINTS

1. A CGM has three components: (1) a sensor that is inserted under the skin and measures interstitial glucose levels almost continuously (every 1–5 minutes), (2) a transmitter that wirelessly transmits the glucose values, and (3) a receiver that displays the glucose values in real time or intermittently and shows trend arrows to inform the user about the direction and magnitude of glucose changes.
2. Professional CGM devices are owned by providers and are loaned to users for 1 to 2 weeks at a time, either recording blinded glucose patterns or displaying real-time glucose values that can later be downloaded by providers for analysis.
3. Personal CGM devices are prescribed by the provider and are owned by the user to be worn every day or intermittently. Without the need for fingerstick glucose testing or with only twice-a-day testing, personal CGM provides people with real-time or intermittent interstitial glucose values; trend arrows showing the direction and magnitude of glucose changes; and alarms that alert for hypoglycemia, predicted hypoglycemia, hyperglycemia, and predicted hyperglycemia.
4. The AGP is generated from the CGM download and consists of the GMI, an estimate of the equivalent A1c for the preceding 2-week period; the overall average glucose value; the percentage of TIR at various levels; glucose variability; and active CGM wear time.
5. CGM devices measure interstitial fluid glucose and not BG. When BG values are stable, interstitial glucose values are usually very close to BG values. However, when BG levels are changing, interstitial glucose values lag by 15 to 30 minutes and thus will give lower glucose readings when BG values are rising and higher glucose readings when BG values are falling.
6. Multiple studies in people with type 1 diabetes, treated with multiple daily insulin injections or insulin pumps, have demonstrated that CGM use reduces A1c, increases glucose time in target range, reduces time in hypoglycemia, improves hypoglycemia awareness in people with hypoglycemia unawareness, and improves quality of life.

BIBLIOGRAPHY

Ahmadi SS, Westman K, Pivodic A, et al. The association between HbA1c and time in hypoglycemia during CGM and self-monitoring of blood glucose in people with type 1 diabetes and multiple daily injections: a randomized clinical trial (GOLD-4). *Diabetes Care.* 2020;43:2017–2024.

Aleppo G, Laffel LM, Ahmann AJ, et al. A practical approach to using trend arrows on the Dexcom G5 CGM System for the management of adults with diabetes. *J Endocr Soc.* 2017 Nov 20;1(12):1445–1460.

American Diabetes Association. Clinical Practice Recommendations 2020. *Diabetes Care.* 2020 Jan;43(Suppl 1):S1–S123.

Bailey TS, Grunberger G, Bode BW, et al. American Association of Clinical Endocrinologists and American College of Endocrinology 2016 Outpatient Glucose Monitoring Consensus Statement. *Endocr Pract.* 2016 Feb;22(2):231–261.

Battelino T. Effect of continuous glucose monitoring on hypoglycemia in type 1 diabetes. *Diabetes Care.* 2011;34:795–800.

Battelino T. The use and efficacy of continuous glucose monitoring in type 1 diabetes treated with insulin pump therapy: a randomized controlled trial. *Diabetologia.* 2012;55:3155–3162.

Battelino T, Danne T, Bergenstal RM, et al. Clinical targets for continuous glucose monitoring data interpretation: recommendations from the international consensus on time in range. *Diabetes Care.* 2019 Aug;42(8):1593–1603.

Beck RW, Riddlesworth T, Ruedy K, et al. Effect of continuous glucose monitoring on glycemic control in adults with type 1 diabetes using insulin injections: the DIAMOND randomized clinical trial. *JAMA.* 2017 Jan 24;317(4):371–378.

Beck RW, Riddlesworth TD, Ruedy K, et al. Continuous glucose monitoring versus usual care in patients with type 2 diabetes receiving multiple daily insulin injections: a randomized trial. *Ann Intern Med.* 2017 Sep 19;167(6):365–374.

Carlson AL, Mullen DM, Bergenstal RM. Clinical use of continuous glucose monitoring in adults with type 2 diabetes. *Diabetes Technol Ther.* 2017 May;19(S2):S4–S11.

Chamberlain JJ, Doyle-Delgado K, Peterson L, Skolnik N. Diabetes technology: review of the 2019 American Diabetes Association standards of medical care in diabetes. *Ann Intern Med.* 2019;171:415–420.

Deshmukh H, Wilmot EG, Gregory R, et al. Effect of flash glucose monitoring on glycemic control, hypoglycemia, diabetes-related distress, and resource utilization in the Association of British Clinical Diabetologists (ABCD) nationwide audit. *Diabetes Care*. 2020;43:2153–2160.

Engler R, Routh TL, Lucisano JY. Adoption barriers for continuous glucose monitoring and their potential reduction with a fully implanted system: results from patient preference surveys. *Clin Diabetes*. 2018 Jan;36(1):50–58.

Feig DS, Donovan LE, Corcoy R, et al. Continuous glucose monitoring in pregnant women with type 1 diabetes (CONCEPTT): a multicentre international randomised controlled trial. *Lancet*. 2017 Nov 25;390(10110):2347–2359.

Fonseca VA, Grunberger G, Anhalt H, et al. Continuous glucose monitoring: a consensus conference of the American Association of Clinical Endocrinologists and American College of Endocrinology. *Endocr Pract*. 2016 Aug;22(8):1008–1021.

Furler J, O'Neal D, Speight J, et al. Use of professional-mode flash glucose monitoring, at 3-month intervals in adults with type 2 diabetes in general practice (GP-OSMOTIC): a pragmatic, open-label, 12-month, randomised, controlled trial. *Lancet Diabetes Endocrinol*. 2020;8:17–26.

Galindo RJ, Umpierrez GE, Rushakoff RJ, et al. Continuous glucose monitors and automated insulin dosing systems in the hospital consensus guideline. *J Diab Sci Technol*. 2020, Sep 28:1–30.

Garg K. Use of continuous glucose monitoring in subjects with type 1 diabetes on multiple daily injections versus continuous subcutaneous insulin infusion therapy. *Diabetes Care*. 2011;34:574–579.

Grunberger G, Handelsman Y, Bloomgarden ZT, et al. American Association of Clinical Endocrinologists and American College of Endocrinology 2018 position statement on integration of insulin pumps and continuous glucose monitoring in patients with diabetes mellitus. *Endocr Pract*. 2018 Mar;24(3):302–308.

Klonoff DC. Continuous glucose monitoring: an Endocrine Society clinical practice guideline. *J Clin Endocrinol Metab*. 2011;96:2968–2979.

Kudva YC, Ahmann AJ, Bergenstal RM, et al. Approach to using trend arrows in the FreeStyle Libre Flash glucose monitoring systems in adults. *J Endocr Soc*. 2018 Nov 14;2(12):1320–1337.

Laffel LM, Aleppo G, Buckingham BA, et al. A practical approach to using trend arrows on the Dexcom G5 CGM System to manage children and adolescents with diabetes. *J Endocr Soc*. 2017 Nov 20;1(12):1461–1476.

Leelarathna L, English SW, Thabit H, et al. Accuracy of subcutaneous continuous glucose monitoring in critically ill adults: improved sensor performance with enhanced calibrations. *Diabetes Technol Ther*. 2014 Feb;16(2):97–101.

Lin YK, Groat D, Chan O, et al. Alarm settings of continuous glucose monitoring systems and associations to glucose outcomes in type 1 diabetes. *J Endocr Soc*. 2019 Nov 19;4(1):bvz005 http://doi.org/10.1210/jendso/bvz005. eCollection 2020 Jan 1.

Lind M, Polonsky W, Hirsch IB, et al. Continuous glucose monitoring vs conventional therapy for glycemic control in adults with type 1 diabetes treated with multiple daily insulin injections: the GOLD randomized clinical trial. *JAMA*. 2017 Jan 24;317(4):379–387.

Pease A, Lo C, Earnest A, et al. Time in range for multiple technologies in type 1 diabetes: a systematic review and network meta-analysis. *Diabetes Care*. 2020;43:1967–1975.

Rickels MR, Peleckis AJ, Dalton-Bakes C, et al. Continuous glucose monitoring for hypoglycemia avoidance and glucose counter-regulation in long-standing type 1 diabetes. *J Clin Endocrinol Metab*. 2018 Jan 1;103(1):105–114.

Shah V, DuBose SN, Li Z, et al. Continuous glucose monitoring profiles in healthy nondiabetic participants: a multicentre prospective study. *J Clin Endocrinol Metab*. 2019;104:4356–4364.

Spanakis EK, Levitt DL, Siddiqui T, et al. The effect of continuous glucose monitoring in preventing inpatient hypoglycemia in general wards: the glucose telemetry system. *J Diabetes Sci Technol*. 2018 Jan;12(1):20–25.

Umpierrez GE, Klonoff DC. Diabetes technology update: use of insulin pumps and continuous glucose monitoring in the hospital. *Diabetes Care*. 2018 Aug;41(8):1579–1589.

van Beers CA, DeVries JH, Kleijer SJ, et al. Continuous glucose monitoring for patients with type 1 diabetes and impaired awareness of hypoglycaemia (IN CONTROL): a randomised, open-label, crossover trial. *Lancet Diabetes Endocrinol*. 2016 Nov;4(11):893–902.

van Beers CAJ, de Wit M, Kleijer SJ, et al. Continuous glucose monitoring in patients with type 1 diabetes and impaired awareness of hypoglycemia: also effective in patients with psychological distress? *Diabetes Technol Ther*. 2017 Oct;19(10):595–599.

Wallia A, Umpierrez GE, Rushakoff RJ, et al. Consensus statement on inpatient use of continuous glucose monitoring. *J Diabetes Sci Technol*. 2017 Sep;11(5):1036–1044.

WEBSITES

DANAtech. www.danatech.org
DiabetesWise. www.diabeteswise.org

CHAPTER 22

CONTINUOUS GLUCOSE MONITORING INTERPRETATION: PRACTICE CASES

Michael T. McDermott, MD

CONTINUOUS GLUCOSE MONITOR INTERPRETATION CASES

In the following cases, CGM = continuous glucose monitor; GMI = glucose management indicator.

CASE 1

The patient is a 72-year-old man who has had type 1 diabetes mellitus for 67 years. He has developed diabetic retinopathy, peripheral neuropathy, and coronary artery disease. He manages his glucose with a hybrid closed-loop insulin pump and CGM. A1C = 6.6%. GMI = 6.5%. CGM data are shown.

What is your interpretation?
What are your recommendations?

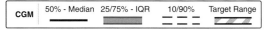

Glucose Statistics	Avg Glucose mg/dL	Very Low < 54 mg/dL	Low < 70 mg/dL	In Target Range 70 - 180 mg/dL	High > 180 mg/dL	Very High > 250 mg/dL	Coefficient of Variation	SD mg/dL	% Time CGM Active
	134	**1.6%**	**8.2%**	**73.4%**	**18.4%**	**1.0%**	**35.1%**	**47**	**96.9%**
	Glucose Exposure			Glucose Ranges			Glucose Variability		Data Sufficiency

CGM	50% - Median	25/75% - IQR	10/90%	Target Range

Curves/plots represent glucose frequency distibutions by time regarless of date.

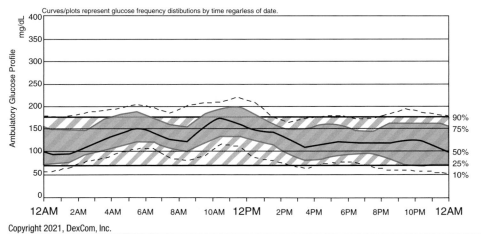

Copyright 2021, DexCom, Inc.

CASE 2

The patient is a 68-year-old woman who has had type 1 diabetes mellitus for 12 years. She has developed background diabetic retinopathy. She manages her glucose with an insulin pump and a CGM. A1c = 7.5%. GMI = 7.6%. CGM data are shown.

What is your interpretation?
What are your recommendations?

Avg Glucose mg/dL	Very Low	Low	In Target Range	High	Very High	Coefficient of Variation	SD mg/dL	% Time CGM Active
	< 54 mg/dL	< 70 mg/dL	70 - 180 mg/dL	> 180 mg/dL	> 250 mg/dL			
172	**0.7%**	**5.3%**	**53.5%**	**41.2%**	**15.6%**	**43.7%**	**75**	**87.1%**
Glucose Exposure			Glucose Ranges			Glucose Variability		Data Sufficiency

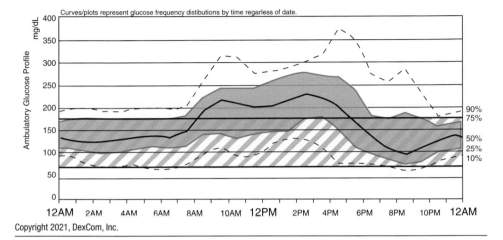

Curves/plots represent glucose frequency distibutions by time regarless of date.

Copyright 2021, DexCom, Inc.

CASE 3

The patient is a 76-year-old woman who has had type 2 diabetes mellitus for 14 years. She has developed microalbuminuria, background diabetic retinopathy, and peripheral neuropathy. Diabetes medications are metformin and basal-bolus insulin therapy. She uses a CGM. A1c = 7.9%. GMI = 7.6%. CGM data are shown.

What is your interpretation?

What are your recommendations?

Avg Glucose mg/dL	Very Low	Low	In Target Range	High	Very High	Coefficient of Variation	SD mg/dL	% Time CGM Active
	< 54 mg/dL	< 70 mg/dL	70 - 180 mg/dL	> 180 mg/dL	> 250 mg/dL			
183	**0.0%**	**0.0%**	**57.6%**	**42.4%**	**14.5%**	**35.2%**	**64**	**98.3%**
Glucose Exposure			Glucose Ranges			Glucose Variability		Data Sufficiency

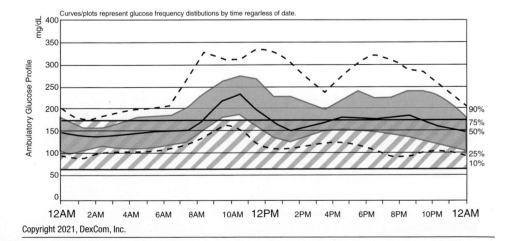

Curves/plots represent glucose frequency distibutions by time regarless of date.

Copyright 2021, DexCom, Inc.

CASE 4

The patient is a 48-year-old woman who has had type 1 diabetes mellitus for 34 years and has no chronic complications. She manages her glucose with an insulin pump and a CGM. A1c = 7.0%. GMI = 6.9%. CGM data are shown.

What is your interpretation?

What are your recommendations?

Glucose Statistics									
Avg Glucose mg/dL	**Very Low**	**Low**	**In Target Range**	**High**	**Very High**		**Coefficient of Variation**	**SD mg/dL**	**% Time CGM Active**
	< 54 mg/dL	< 70 mg/dL	70 - 180 mg/dL	> 180 mg/dL	> 250 mg/dL				
159	**0.6%**	**2.7%**	**68.8%**	**25.5%**	**9.7%**		**40.9%**	**65**	**96.6%**
Glucose Exposure			Glucose Ranges				Glucose Variability		Data Sufficiency

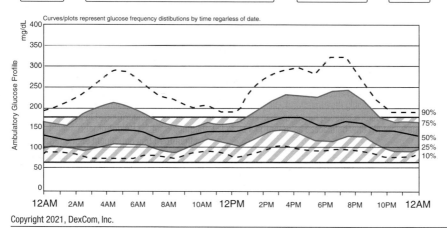

Copyright 2021, DexCom, Inc.

CASE 5

The patient is a 57-year-old woman who has had type 1 diabetes mellitus for 28 years and has no chronic complications. She manages her glucose with a hybrid closed-loop insulin pump and CGM. A1c = 6.5%. GMI = 6.4%. CGM data are shown.

What is your interpretation?

What are your recommendations?

Glucose Statistics									
Avg Glucose mg/dL	**Very Low**	**Low**	**In Target Range**	**High**	**Very High**		**Coefficient of Variation**	**SD mg/dL**	**% Time CGN Active**
	< 54 mg/dL	< 70 mg/dL	70 - 180 mg/dL	> 180 mg/dL	> 250 mg/dL				
136	**3.3%**	**11.1%**	**68.8%**	**20.1%**	**6.3%**		**44.1%**	**60**	**64.8%**
Glucose Exposure			Glucose Ranges				Glucose Variability		Data Sufficiency

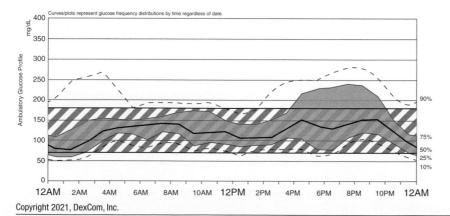

Copyright 2021, DexCom, Inc.

CASE 6

The patient is a 61-year-old man who has had type 1 diabetes mellitus for 48 years. He has developed diabetic nephropathy, retinopathy, peripheral neuropathy, and coronary artery disease. He manages his glucose with an insulin pump and a CGM. A1c = 7.6%. GMI = 7.4%. CGM data are shown.

What is your interpretation?

What are your recommendations?

Glucose Statistics	Avg Glucose mg/dL	Very Low	Low	In Target Range	High	Very High	Coefficient of Variation	SD mg/dL	% Time CGN Active
		< 54 mg/dL	< 70 mg/dL	70 - 180 mg/dL	> 180 mg/dL	> 250 mg/dL			
	197	**2.1%**	**5.6%**	**39.8%**	**54.6%**	**24.5%**	**43.8%**	**86**	**81.4%**
	Glucose Exposure			Glucose Ranges			Glucose Variability		Data Sufficiency

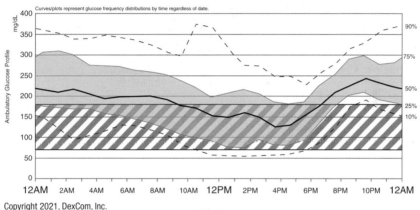

Curves/plots represent glucose frequency distributions by time regardless of date.

Copyright 2021, DexCom, Inc.

CASE 7

The patient is a 29-year-old woman who has had type 1 diabetes mellitus for 2 years and has no chronic complications. She manages her glucose with a hybrid closed-loop insulin pump and CGM. A1c = 7.2%. GMI = 6.8%. CGM data are shown.

What is your interpretation?

What are your recommendations?

Glucose Statistics	Avg Glucose mg/dL	Very Low	Low	In Target Range	High	Very High	Coefficient of Variation	SD mg/dL	% Time CGM Active
		< 54 mg/dL	< 70 mg/dL	70 - 180 mg/dL	> 180 mg/dL	> 250 mg/dL			
	165	**0.0%**	**0.3%**	**68.8%**	**30.9%**	**10.1%**	**33.8%**	**56**	**99.0%**
	Glucose Exposure			Glucose Ranges			Glucose Variability		Data Sufficiency

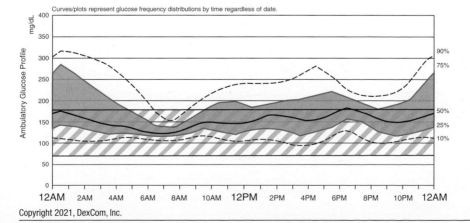

Curves/plots represent glucose frequency distributions by time regardless of date.

Copyright 2021, DexCom, Inc.

CASE 8

The patient is a 41-year-old man who has had type 1 diabetes mellitus for 11 years and has no chronic complications. He manages his glucose with a hybrid closed-loop insulin pump and CGM. A1C = 7.0%. GMI = 6.7%. CGM data are shown.

What is your interpretation?

What are your recommendations?

Avg Glucose mg/dL	Very Low < 54 mg/dL	Low < 70 mg/dL	In Target Range 70 - 180 mg/dL	High > 180 mg/dL	Very High > 250 mg/dL	Coefficient of Variation	SD mg/dL	% Time CGM Active
158	**0.5%**	**4.4%**	**63.8%**	**31.8%**	**11.5%**	**44.2%**	**70**	**93.6%**
Glucose Exposure			Glucose Ranges			Glucose Variability		Data Sufficiency

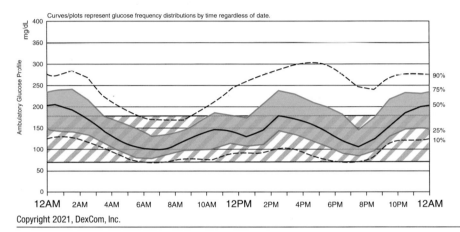

Curves/plots represent glucose frequency distributions by time regardless of date.

Copyright 2021, DexCom, Inc.

CASE 9

The patient is a 56-year-old woman who has had type 1 diabetes mellitus for 45 years. She has developed mild diabetic nephropathy and diabetic retinopathy. She manages her glucose with a hybrid closed-loop insulin pump and CGM. A1c = 8.0%. GMI = 8.1%. CGM data are shown.

What is your interpretation?

What are your recommendations?

Avg Glucose mg/dL	Very Low < 54 mg/dL	Low < 70 mg/dL	In Target Range 70 – 180 mg/dL	High > 180 mg/dL	Very High > 250 mg/dL	Coefficient of Variation	SD mg/dL	% Time CGM Active
168	**0.0%**	**0.2%**	**58.8%**	**41.0%**	**5.5%**	**29.2%**	**49**	**98.5%**
Glucose Exposure			Glucose Ranges			Glucose Variability		Data Sufficiency

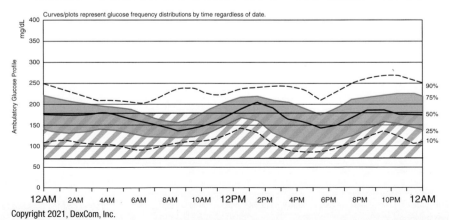

Curves/plots represent glucose frequency distributions by time regardless of date.

Copyright 2021, DexCom, Inc.

CASE 10

The patient is a 90-year-old woman who has had type 2 diabetes mellitus for 34 years. She has developed background diabetic retinopathy and peripheral neuropathy. Diabetes medications include basal-bolus insulin therapy. She uses a CGM. A1c = 8.0%. GMI = 8.0%. CGM data are shown.
What is your interpretation?
What are your recommendations?

Glucose Statistics									
Avg Glucose mg/dL	**Very Low**	**Low**	**In Target Range**	**High**	**Very High**		**Coefficient of Variation**	**SD mg/dL**	**% Time CGM Active**
	< 54 mg/dL	< 70 mg/dL	70 - 180 mg/dL	> 180 mg/dL	> 250 mg/dL				
188	0.0%	0.0%	51.4%	48.6%	8.3%		21.8%	41	100.0%
Glucose Exposure			Glucose Ranges				Glucose Variability		Data Sufficiency

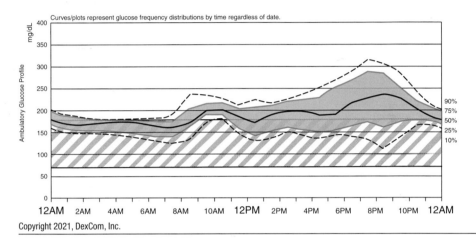

Curves/plots represent glucose frequency distributions by time regardless of date.

Copyright 2021, DexCom, Inc.

CASE 11

The patient is a 50-year-old man who has had type 1 diabetes mellitus for 19 years. He has developed diabetic retinopathy and peripheral neuropathy. He manages his glucose with a hybrid closed-loop insulin pump and CGM. A1c = 8.0%. GMI = 7.8%. CGM data are shown.
What is your interpretation?
What are your recommendations?

Glucose Statistics									
Avg Glucose mg/dL	**Very Low**	**Low**	**In Target Range**	**High**	**Very High**		**Coefficient of Variation**	**SD mg/dL**	**% Time CGN Active**
	< 54 mg/dL	< 70 mg/dL	70 - 180 mg/dL	> 180 mg/dL	> 250 mg/dL				
197	0.0%	0.3%	45.1%	54.6%	18.5%		32.5%	64	96.0%
Glucose Exposure			Glucose Ranges				Glucose Variability		Data Sufficiency

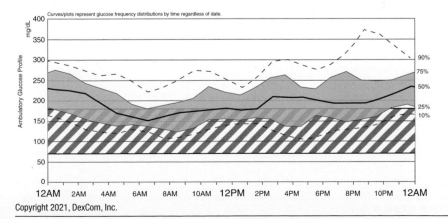

Curves/plots represent glucose frequency distributions by time regardless of date.

Copyright 2021, DexCom, Inc.

CASE 12

The patient is a 43-year-old woman who has had type 1 diabetes mellitus for 13 years. She has developed diabetic peripheral neuropathy. She manages her glucose with an insulin pump and a CGM. A1 = 10.3%. GMI = 10.1%. CGM data are shown (blousing after meals and missing boluses).
What is your interpretation?
What are your recommendations?

	Avg Glucose mg/dL	Very Low < 54 mg/dL	Low < 70 mg/dL	In Target Range 70 - 180 mg/dL	High > 180 mg/dL	Very High > 250 mg/dL	Coefficient of Variation	SD mg/dL	% Time CGN Active
Glucose Statistics	**226**	**0.0%**	**0.6%**	**29.0%**	**70.4%**	**45.5%**	**33.7%**	**76**	**99.3%**
	Glucose Exposure			Glucose Ranges				Glucose Variability	Data Sufficiency

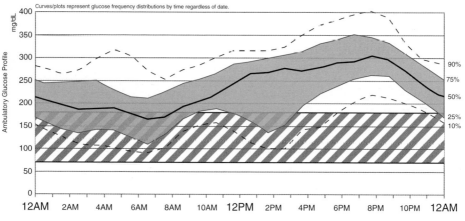

Curves/plots represent glucose frequency distributions by time regardless of date.

Copyright 2021, DexCom, Inc.

CONTINUOUS GLUCOSE MONITOR INTERPRETATION CASES—MY BEST ANSWERS

Following are my best interpretations and recommendations for the 12 continuous glucose monitoring cases in this chapter. My answers are not necessarily better than yours. Feel free to agree or disagree.

For all of the case answers, we will use the following abbreviations: BG = blood glucose, FBG = fasting blood glucose, PPBG = postprandial blood glucose, HS BG = bedtime BG.

CASE 1

Patient: 72-year-old man with type 1 diabetes mellitus for 67 years

Ambulatory Glucose Profile (AGP) Interpretation
Excess time in the hypoglycemic ranges.

Blood Glucose (BG) Pattern Interpretation
FBG: Mostly in or near target range.
PPBG: Glucose excursions after breakfast are often excessive, but excursions after lunch and dinner are appropriate.
HS BG: Mostly in target range or below.
BG Overnight: Decreases overnight with hypoglycemia occurring most often during this time.
BG Highs: Most often 4 AM to 6 AM following an overnight low glucose and after breakfast.
BG Lows: Mostly overnight from 10 PM to 1 AM.
BG Variability: After breakfast, after dinner, and overnight.
Overall: Excessive hypoglycemia mostly during the night, with some rebound hyperglycemia in the early morning and hyperglycemia after breakfast.

Recommendations
Reduce basal rate from 9 PM to 1 AM and/or weaken bedtime correction factor. Strengthen carbohydrate-to-insulin ratio at breakfast modestly. Troubleshoot lifestyle causes of variability.

CASE 2

Patient: 68-year-old woman with type 1 diabetes mellitus for 12 years

AGP Interpretation

Slightly excessive time in hypoglycemic ranges and excessive time in hyperglycemic ranges.

BG Pattern Interpretation

FBG: Mostly in or near target range.

PPBG: Glucose excursions after breakfast are excessive. Glucose remains high all morning and after lunch, returning to the target range after late-afternoon correction insulin doses. Some low glucose values after dinner.

HS BG: Mostly in target range.

BG Overnight: Stable overnight without significant change.

BG Highs: After breakfast and after lunch.

BG Lows: After dinner.

BG Variability: After all meals

Overall: BG excursions are excessive after breakfast and remain high prelunch. Postlunch BG levels remain high until late afternoon, then decrease into the target range. BG levels after dinner are sometimes low.

Recommendations

Strengthen carbohydrate-to-insulin ratio at breakfast. Strengthen carbohydrate-to-insulin ratio and/or correction factor at lunch. Reduce late-afternoon basal rates. Improve carbohydrate-counting skills. Troubleshoot lifestyle causes of variability.

CASE 3

Patient: 76 year old woman with type 2 diabetes mellitus for 14 years

AGP Interpretation

No significant hypoglycemia. Excess time in the hyperglycemic ranges.

BG Pattern Interpretation

FBG: Most often in or near target range.

PPBG: Glucose excursions after breakfast are excessive. Glucose excursions after lunch and dinner are mostly appropriate.

HS BG: Most often in target range.

BG Overnight: Generally stable without significant drift.

BG Highs: After breakfast.

BG Lows: None.

BG Variability: High after breakfast and after dinner.

Overall: Excessive glucose excursions after breakfast, resulting in overall high glucose levels throughout the remainder of the day. Significant variability after breakfast and after dinner.

Recommendations

Strengthen carbohydrate-to-insulin ratio or increase fixed insulin dose at breakfast and evaluate breakfast correction factor. Improve carbohydrate-counting skills. Troubleshoot lifestyle causes of variability.

CASE 4

Patient: 48-year-old woman with type 1 diabetes mellitus for 34 years

AGP Interpretation

Infrequent hypoglycemia. Time spent in hyperglycemic ranges moderately excessive.

BG Pattern Interpretation

FBG: Most often in or near target range.

PPBG: Glucose excursions after lunch are excessive. Glucose levels remain elevated throughout the afternoon, eventually coming down after dinner.

HS BG: Mostly in or near target range

BG Overnight: Stable without a significant slope.

BG Highs: Most common after lunch, during the afternoon, and after dinner.

BG Lows: Uncommon but occasionally occur in the early mornings.

BG Variability: Highest after lunch and dinner and in the early-morning hours.

Overall: Excessive glucose excursions after lunch, with hyperglycemia persisting through the afternoon, with significant postlunch and afternoon variability. Moderate variability overnight with few hypoglycemic episodes.

Recommendations

Strengthen carbohydrate-to-insulin ratio at lunch and evaluate lunchtime correction factor. Improve carbohydrate-counting skills. Troubleshoot lifestyle causes of variability.

CASE 5

Patient: 57-year-old woman with type 1 diabetes mellitus for 28 years

AGP Interpretation

Excessive time in the hypoglycemic ranges and slightly excessive time in hyperglycemic ranges.

BG Pattern Interpretation

> FBG: Usually in or near the target range.
> PPBG: Glucose rises in the late afternoon, usually in response to snacking prior to dinner, and remains high for a while after dinner.
> HS BG: Often in target range but also frequently low.
> BG Overnight: Drops significantly starting at about 9 PM, with nadirs from 12 AM to 2 AM.
> BG Highs: After afternoon snacks and after dinner.
> BG Lows: Most often from 12 AM to 2 AM.
> BG Variability: After dinner and in the first few hours after midnight.
> Overall: Excessive glucose excursions in the afternoon in response to late-afternoon snacks followed by dinner. BG drops significantly between 9 PM and 2 PM, sometimes into the hypoglycemic range between midnight and 2 PM.

Recommendations

Encourage her to bolus for late-afternoon snacks. Evaluate carbohydrate-to-insulin ratio at dinner once predinner glucose is better controlled. Reduce basal rate from 9 PM to 2 AM. Correction factor in the late evening and at bedtime should be reduced.

CASE 6

Patient: 61-year-old man with type 1 diabetes mellitus for 48 years

AGP Interpretation

Excessive time spent in both the hypoglycemic and hyperglycemic ranges.

BG Pattern Interpretation

> FBG: Elevated most often.
> PPBG: Glucose excursions after breakfast and lunch are minimal, but glucose excursions after dinner are excessive.
> HS BG: Consistently elevated.
> BG Overnight: Moderate glucose drop overnight, toward but not into the target range by morning.
> BG Highs: After dinner and throughout the night.
> BG Lows: Between 12 noon and 5 PM.
> BG Variability: All times of the day.
> Overall: Excessive glucose excursions after dinner with a gradual drop overnight, but glucose remains above target levels by morning. Glucose excursions after breakfast and lunch are mostly appropriate, but hypoglycemia occurs most frequently after lunch. There is significant variability throughout the day.

Recommendations

Strengthen carbohydrate-to-insulin ratio at dinner. Overnight basal rates may need to be decreased if glucose values at bedtime become consistently in the target range. Troubleshoot lifestyle causes of high variability. Improve carbohydrate-counting skills.

CASE 7

Patient: 29-year-old woman with type 1 diabetes mellitus for 2 years

AGP Interpretation

Appropriately low amount of time in hypoglycemic ranges. Moderately excessive time in hyperglycemic ranges.

BG Pattern Interpretation

> FBG: Most often in or near target range.
> PPBG: Mildly excessive glucose excursions after breakfast. Glucose rises in the late afternoon because of snacking. Significant glucose rises after 10 PM because of late-night snacks that are not covered with bolus insulin doses.
> HS BG: Usually above target.
> BG Overnight: Moderate glucose drop overnight as a result of either correction doses or basal insulin rates.

BG Highs: Most often between 10 PM and 2 AM.
BG Lows: Rare but most often in the late afternoon.
BG Variability: Highest during the afternoon and at bedtime.
Overall: Excessive glucose excursions after afternoon snacks and especially after late-evening snacks.

Recommendations

Take boluses for afternoon snacks and late-evening snacks and evaluate carbohydrate-to-insulin ratio at those times. Overnight basal rate may need to be decreased if glucose levels at bedtime are improved to prevent overnight hypoglycemia. This may occur automatically with her hybrid closed-loop system.

CASE 8

Patient: 41-year-old man with type 1 diabetes mellitus for 11 years

AGP Interpretation

Appropriately low time spent in hypoglycemic ranges. Moderately excessive time in hyperglycemic ranges.

BG Pattern Interpretation

FBG: Most often in or near target range but occasionally low.
PPBG: Moderate glucose excursions after breakfast. Excessive glucose excursions after lunch and dinner.
HS BG: Generally above target range.
BG Overnight: Significant drop in glucose values overnight as a result of either correction bolus doses at bedtime or overnight basal rates.
BG Highs: After lunch, after dinner, and from 12 midnight to 2 AM.
BG Lows: Morning hours from 5 AM to 7 AM.
BG Variability: After lunch, after dinner, and overnight.
Overall: Excessive glucose excursions after lunch and dinner, resulting in high bedtime glucose values and a significant glucose drop overnight.

Recommendations

Strengthen carbohydrate-to-insulin ratio at lunch and dinner. Reduce overnight basal rate to prevent low blood glucose values during the night and early-morning hours once bedtime blood glucose levels are in or near target range from better mealtime coverage. This may occur automatically with his hybrid closed-loop system. Improve carbohydrate-counting skills. Troubleshoot lifestyle causes of high variability.

CASE 9

Patient: 56-year-old woman with type 1 diabetes mellitus for 45 years

AGP Interpretation

Appropriately low time in the hypoglycemic ranges. Excessive time in the moderately hyperglycemic range.

BG Pattern Interpretation

FBG: Most often in or near target range.
PPBG: Glucose excursions after lunch and dinner are moderately excessive.
HS BG: Usually above target range as a result of excessive glucose rise after dinner.
BG Overnight: Moderate downward trend overnight, driven by the basal rate.
BG Highs: Mostly after lunch and after dinner.
BG Lows: Most often in late afternoon from 4 PM to 6 PM.
BG Variability: Mostly after dinner and overnight.
Overall: Excessive glucose rise after lunch and dinner, requiring a higher-than-optimal basal rate to lower glucose to target range by morning.

Recommendations

Strengthen carbohydrate-to-insulin ratio at lunch and dinner. Reduce overnight basal rate modestly to prevent hypoglycemia once bedtime blood glucose values are within target range. Troubleshoot lifestyle causes for high variability. Improve carbohydrate-counting skills.

CASE 10

Patient: 90-year-old woman with type 2 diabetes mellitus for 34 years

AGP Interpretation

No time spent in hypoglycemic ranges. Moderately excessive time spent in hyperglycemic ranges, although her A1c and glucose management index are appropriate for her age.

BG Pattern Interpretation

> FBG: Most often in or near target range.
>
> PPBG: Glucose excursions after breakfast are moderately excessive. Glucose excursions after dinner are frequently excessive and variable.
>
> HS BG: Slightly above target range but not excessive, considering her age.
>
> BG Overnight: Mild downward drift of glucose values overnight without hypoglycemia.
>
> BG Highs: After breakfast and after dinner.
>
> BG Lows: No significant hypoglycemia.
>
> BG Variability: After dinner.
>
> Overall: Moderately excessive glucose excursions after breakfast and frequently high but variable excursions after dinner, with overall good control.

Recommendations

Increase breakfast bolus dose slightly. Increase dinner insulin dose slightly. Troubleshoot causes of variability after dinner.

CASE 11

Patient: 50-year-old man with type I diabetes mellitus for 19 years

AGP Interpretation

Appropriately low amount of time spent in hypoglycemic ranges. Moderately excessive time spent in hyperglycemic ranges.

BG Pattern Interpretation

> FBG: Most often in or near target range.
>
> PPBG: Moderately excessive glucose excursions after breakfast, lunch, and dinner.
>
> HS BG: Usually well above target range following excessive glucose excursions after dinner.
>
> BG Overnight: Significant decline overnight following elevated bedtime glucose values.
>
> BG Highs: After breakfast, throughout the afternoon, especially in the evenings, and during the night from 12 midnight to 3 AM.
>
> BG Lows: Occur infrequently.
>
> BG Variability: After breakfast, lunch, and dinner.
>
> Overall: BG excursions after all three meals are excessive and result in progressive increases in glucose values throughout the day and especially high values at bedtime, with subsequent declines overnight into the target range as a result of either bedtime correction doses or, more likely, his basal rates.

Recommendations

Strengthen carbohydrate-to-insulin ratio at all three meals. Reduce overnight basal rate to reduce the risk of hypoglycemia once his bedtime glucose values are in or near target range. Troubleshoot causes of variability after dinner. Improve carbohydrate-counting skills.

CASE 12

Patient: 43-year-old woman with type 1 diabetes mellitus for 13 years

AGP Interpretation

Appropriately low amount of time in hypoglycemic ranges but also low amount of time in the target range. Excessive amount of time in the hyperglycemic ranges.

BG Pattern Interpretation

> FBG: Fairly consistently above target range.
>
> PPBG: Significant glucose excursions after breakfast, lunch, and dinner.
>
> HS BG: Usually above target range.
>
> BG Overnight: Glucose begins to decline at about 8 PM following correction doses and continues to decline overnight, driven by her basal rates.
>
> BG Highs: All day, especially after meals, with progressive increases throughout the day.
>
> BG Lows: None.
>
> BG Variability: High all day long, especially after lunch and after dinner.
>
> Overall: High glucose values throughout the day with significant postmeal glucose excursions and high degrees of variability. This is suggestive of poor adherence to her regimen, with frequent missed bolus doses.

Recommendations

Query the patient regarding missed bolus doses. (She admitted that she misses at least half of her mealtime bolus doses upon questioning.) Encourage her to avoid missed bolus doses. Once boluses are taken on a regular basis, reevaluate carbohydrate-to-insulin ratios. The evening correction factor and overnight basal rate will then need to be reevaluated to avoid hypoglycemia during the night once bedtime glucose values are in or near target range.

INSULIN PUMPS AND INTEGRATED SYSTEMS

Michael T. McDermott, MD

CHAPTER 23

1. What is an insulin pump?

An insulin pump is a mechanical device that delivers insulin continuously through a subcutaneous site. Insulin pumps consist of an insulin reservoir, a pumping mechanism, and an infusion set. The reservoir typically holds a 3-day insulin supply and is filled with insulin drawn from a vial into a syringe. The infusion set consists either of tubing that terminates in a plastic cannula or a plastic cannula that extends directly from the pump without tubing; a small needle inside the cannula is used to insert the cannula through the skin and is then withdrawn to leave the hollow cannula under the skin.

2. How does an insulin pump deliver insulin?

There are two basic components of insulin delivery by an insulin pump: basal insulin and bolus insulin. Basal insulin is a continuous 24-hour infusion of insulin that maintains a background serum insulin level that controls hepatic glucose production overnight and between meals. Bolus insulin is an acute dose of insulin that is given to cover a meal, to correct a high blood glucose (BG) level, or both. Bolus insulin, therefore, has two discrete components: a nutritional dose and a correction dose. The nutritional dose is the amount of insulin required to cover a meal a person is preparing to eat. The correction dose is the amount of additional insulin a person adds to the nutritional dose if the premeal BG is elevated; correction boluses may also be taken alone between meals to correct high BG values.

3. What type of insulin is used in insulin pumps?

Insulin pumps should only be filled with rapid-acting insulin analogs such as lispro, aspart, and glulisine. Occasionally, regular insulin is used, and people with very high insulin requirements (>200 units daily) may use U500 regular insulin in their pumps. However, regular insulin and U500 regular insulin provide less effective coverage of the rapid glucose rise that occurs after meals.

4. What are the benefits of using insulin pump therapy?

The basal insulin infusion rate can be varied throughout the day to match a person's activities and individual glucose patterns, something that cannot be adequately done with injected basal insulin. Pumps also have bolus calculators that accurately compute exact bolus insulin doses based on the carbohydrate content of the meal to be consumed, the current glucose level, and the carbohydrate-to-insulin (C:I) ratios and correction factors (CFs) that are preprogrammed into the pump; this avoids math errors and leaves only carbohydrate counting as user input. Some pumps can also integrate with continuous glucose monitors (CGMs). Finally, insulin pumps eliminate the need for multiple daily insulin injections.

5. How do you determine initial basal rates and bolus dosing when starting insulin pump therapy?

Most people who are starting insulin pump therapy are already taking multiple daily insulin injections with both basal and bolus components. The current dose of injected basal (long-acting) insulin can be used to calculate the initial insulin pump basal rates. If the A1c is ≤8.0%, the current injected basal dose should be reduced by 10% to 20%, and this value is then divided by 24 to determine the initial hourly basal infusion rate. If the A1c is >8% and the person is not having frequent hypoglycemia, the current full injected basal dose can be used and similarly be divided by 24 to determine the initial hourly basal infusion rate. Most people who transition to insulin pump therapy are already using a C:I ratio and a CF for their injections; if these ratios are working properly, the same ratios can be used with the insulin pump.

If a person does not already have an established C:I ratio and CF, the initial C:I ratio can be calculated by the following equation: C:I ratio = 500/TDD (TDD = current total daily dose of insulin). Similarly, the CF can be calculated by the following equation: CF = 1650/TDD. Some providers recommend other equations for these initial calculations, but we find these to be very accurate in our clinic population. However, these are only initial estimates; both the basal rates and bolus doses must be modified by analyzing the subsequent glucose profiles.

6. Let's look at an example of calculating initial basal rates, the C:I ratio, and the CF

A 22-year-old woman who has had type 1 diabetes mellitus for 3 years has decided to transition to insulin pump therapy. Her current A1c is 8.9%, and she has hypoglycemia approximately once a month. Her current dose of injected basal insulin is 20 units daily. Her bolus insulin consists of 6 units for breakfast, 7 units for lunch, 7 units for dinner, and a CF of 50:1 with a target of 100 mg/dL. You have her attend carbohydrate-counting classes, and she does well.

    Her initial insulin pump settings could be calculated as follows:

        Basal rates: 20 units/24 hours = 0.8 units/hour

        Bolus doses: C:I ratio (500/40) = 13:1; CF (1650/40) = 40:1

7. **How are basal insulin infusion rates evaluated and adjusted in standard insulin pumps?**
Basal insulin infusion rates should be set and adjusted to maintain BG at a stable level, with changes of no more than 30 mg/dL overnight and during intervals in which no food or bolus doses are taken. Generally, if bedtime (HS) BG is in the range of 110 to 150 mg/dL and no HS snacks or bolus doses are taken, the next morning fasting BG (FBG) should be in the range of 80 to 130 mg/dL. Basal rates are adjusted by assessing HS BG levels, overnight BG patterns, morning FBG levels, and BG trends $\geq$4 hours after meals.

    Formal nighttime basal rate assessment can be done by testing serial BG values overnight with a CGM or with fingerstick BG values every 2 to 3 hours on a night when the HS BG is 110 to 180 mg/dL so that no HS snacks or correction doses are needed. Daytime basal rate testing is done by skipping select meals to verify that the basal rates between meals appropriately stabilize BG trends in the absence of food.

8. **How are the bolus insulin doses evaluated and adjusted in standard insulin pumps?**
When the C:I ratio is correct and carbohydrate counting is accurate, BG excursions from premeal to 2 hours post-meal should be about 30 to 50 mg/dL. C:I ratio accuracy is best tested by eating a meal of known carbohydrate content and with <20 gm of fat, taking the calculated amount of premeal insulin based on the C:I ratio, and then rechecking the BG level 2 hours after the meal; this test is valid only if the premeal BG is at a level that does not require a correction dose. If premeal to 2-hour postmeal BG excursions are not in the range of 30 to 50 mg/dL, the C:I ratio should be adjusted and testing repeated, with further adjustments made as needed. The accuracy of the CF can be tested by rechecking a BG level 4 hours after a nonmeal correction dose to determine whether the BG has decreased into the target range.

9. **What input, knowledge, and skills are required for using a standard insulin pump?**
Insulin pump therapy does not improve glucose control without significant user input, skill, and knowledge. Most insurance companies will cover the cost of a pump and supplies only for people who are taking four or more insulin injections per day and are doing self-monitoring of blood glucose (SMBG) at least four times a day or are using a CGM. Once approved, the following skills are critical for optimal benefit from pump therapy: motivation to continue SMBG $\geq$ 4 times per day or use a CGM, development of accurate carbohydrate-counting skills, adequate numeracy skills, knowledge of the various pump functions, manual dexterity sufficient to insert the infusion sets and manipulate the pump settings, and problem-solving ability to troubleshoot high and low BG values when they occur.

10. **What are the potential causes of a sudden deterioration in glucose control in a person on insulin pump therapy?**
When a person who usually has good BG control with pump therapy suddenly develops unexplained hyperglycemia, the problem may be in one or several areas. The following should be considered and evaluated: infection, stress, medication changes, diet changes, physical activity changes, nonadherence, insertion-site problems (scar tissue), infusion-set issues (occlusion, kinking), and insulin problems (bad insulin). Affected individuals should also check for ketones, ensure adequate oral hydration, and correct whatever problems are identified.

11. **A woman with type 1 diabetes, well controlled on insulin pump therapy, calls you from her beach vacation to inform you that her insulin pump fell into the ocean and no longer works; she called the help-line, and a new pump will be mailed to her within 48 hours. You learn that her total basal insulin dose is 21.2 units per day, her C:I ratio is 15:1, and her CF is 50:1 to a target of 120 mg/dL. What actions should be taken now?**
You should call in prescriptions to her local pharmacy for injectable basal and rapid-acting insulins and advise her to inject 16 units daily of basal insulin (75% of her usual total basal requirement; 80% or 17 units would also be fine) and to inject rapid-acting insulin before each meal using her current C:I ratio and CF estimates. Once her new pump arrives, you can help her program it over the phone using the settings on her previous pump or have her visit your office soon after she returns home from her vacation.

12. **What insulin pumps are currently available in the United States?**
There are four major brands of insulin pumps available in the United States (as of the date of this writing). Medtronic (MiniMed 530 G, 630 G, 670 G, and 770 G), Tandem (t:slim X2), Insulet (Omnipod), and V-Go. The Medtronic, Tandem, and Omnipod are all computer-controlled mechanical pumps; V-Go is a purely mechanical

pump. The Medtronic and Tandem pumps use hollow tubing to connect the pump to a subcutaneous insertion site. The Omnipod and V-Go connect directly to the insertion site from the underside of the pump, which is attached with adhesive to the skin. The Medtronic (670 G and 770 G) and Tandem (t:slim X2) can integrate with CGM to make hybrid closed-loop systems. Omnipod has not yet developed that capability, but work is in progress. Table 23.1 lists the available pumps and their features.

13. **What is a hybrid closed-loop system?**
A hybrid closed loop is an integrated system in which CGM data are transmitted directly to an insulin pump, which responds through an algorithm that adjusts the basal rates and/or correction doses to maintain glucose levels within a prespecified target range. The most commonly used hybrid closed-loop systems currently are the MiniMed 670 G and 770 G/Guardian 3 and the Tandem t:slim X2/Dexcom G6 Control IQ. These are called *hybrid closed-loop systems* because the CGM responsive algorithms drive the basal rates and can give correction doses but do not deliver mealtime boluses. People using these systems must therefore still count carbohydrates accurately and have an appropriate C:I ratio. A fully closed-loop system (true artificial pancreas) that controls basal and bolus insulin delivery without user input is not yet available.

14. **Describe the Medtronic MiniMed 670 G and 770 G hybrid closed-loop systems**
The Medtronic MiniMed 670 G and 770 G systems integrate with the Guardian-3 CGM, which has a 7-day wear time and requires two fingerstick glucose calibrations per day. The 670 G and 770 G pumps respond to CGM data by adjusting basal insulin delivery in response to rising or falling glucose levels. The target glucose level is 120 mg/dL; a temporary target of 150 mg/dL can be used under circumstances where hypoglycemia may be more likely, such as exercise. Correction boluses are estimated by a system learning algorithm. Nutritional boluses are calculated according to the preprogrammed C:I ratio and the meal carbohydrate content that must be determined by the user.

15. **What features are available on the Tandem t:slim X2 hybrid closed-loop systems?**
The Tandem t:slim X2 Basal IQ system integrates with the Dexcom G6 CGM, which has a 10-day wear time and requires no fingerstick glucose calibrations. The pump responds to CGM data by decreasing basal insulin delivery in response to falling glucose levels or frank hypoglycemia. The Basal IQ system is designed specifically to prevent hypoglycemia.

      The Tandem t:slim X2 Control IQ system, designed to prevent both hyperglycemia and hypoglycemia, uses Dexcom G6 CGM data to predict glucose values 30 minutes ahead, enabling the system to adjust basal insulin in response to rising or falling glucose values or frank hypoglycemia; the target glucose range is 70 to 180 mg/dL. If glucose values exceed or are predicted to exceed 180 mg/dL, the system can also give an automatic correction bolus, which is 60% of the dose needed to reduce the glucose to 110 mg/dL, and can repeat the correction bolus up to once an hour if needed. Additional settings can be used for sleep and exercise. Nutritional boluses are calculated from the preprogrammed C:I ratio and the meal carbohydrate content estimated by the user. The system also has smartphone data integration.

16. **What automated insulin delivery systems that are in development are anticipated to be available soon?**
The Medtronic MiniMed 780 G will integrate with the Guardian-3 CGM, which has a 7-day wear time and requires two fingerstick glucose calibrations per day. The 780 G pump responds to CGM data by adjusting basal insulin delivery in response to rising or falling glucose levels. The target glucose level is adjustable down to 100 mg/dL. Correction boluses are estimated by a system learning algorithm and are given automatically. Nutritional boluses are calculated according to the preprogrammed C:I ratio and the user-estimated meal carbohydrate content. The system will also have smartphone data integration.

Table 23.1 Insulin Pumps Available in the United States (2021)

INSULIN PUMP	TUBING	CGM INTEGRATION
Medtronic MiniMed 530 G, 630 G, 670 G, 770 G	Yes	Yes (670 G or 770 G/Guardian 3)
Tandem t:slim X2	Yes	Yes (t:slim X2/Dexcom G6)
Insulet Omnipod	No	No
V-Go	No	No

CGM, Continuous glucose monitor.

The Insulet Omnipod Horizon will integrate with the Dexcom G6 CGM, which has a 10-day wear time and requires no fingerstick glucose calibrations. The target glucose level is adjustable down to 100 mg/dL. Correction boluses are estimated by a system learning algorithm and are given automatically. Nutritional boluses are given according to the preprogrammed C:I ratio and the user-estimated meal carbohydrate content. Smartphone integration will be available for pump control functions.

17. What other types of automated insulin delivery systems are in development?
Beta Biologics iLet: This pump will integrate with the Dexcom G6 or Senseonics CGM. It will have the capacity to infuse insulin alone or insulin plus glucagon. Nutritional boluses will be automatic, without the need for carbohydrate counting by the user. It will only require users to enter their body weight for the system to initialize therapy. In December 2019, the U.S. Food and Drug Administration (FDA) granted the Breakthrough Device designation for the development and approval of this system.

Bigfoot Biomedical Unlty: This pump will integrate with the Libre Freestyle CGM. Smartphone integration for control of function will also be a feature.

Lilly pump: This pump will integrate with the Dexcom G6 and will have several pump options, including a patch pump and a detached pump with a short infusion set or a long infusion set.

18. What is a bihormonal pump?
Currently available insulin pumps are uni-hormonal; they only deliver insulin. Although the hybrid closed-loop systems decrease basal insulin delivery when glucose levels are dropping and stop delivery when glucose levels are low, correction of hypoglycemia may still be delayed because insulin that has already been delivered remains under the skin and will still be absorbed. A bihormonal pump not only delivers insulin to prevent hyperglycemia and shuts it off during hypoglycemia, but this device also gives glucagon boluses in response to hypoglycemia. Glucagon, by stimulating hepatic glycogenolysis, raises glucose values more rapidly than can occur by simply turning off the insulin infusion. Bihormonal systems are in development but are not yet FDA approved (as of the date of this writing).

19. What is Tidepool Loop?
The Tidepool Loop pump will integrate with the Dexcom G6 or Senseonics CGM. It will have the capacity to infuse insulin alone or insulin plus glucagon. Correction boluses will be estimated by the system based on a learning algorithm and will be given automatically. Nutritional boluses will also be automatic, without the need for carbohydrate counting by the user. The insulin-only pumps will reduce or stop insulin for predicted or existing hypoglycemia, whereas the insulin-plus-glucagon pump will stop the insulin infusion and give a glucagon bolus in response to hypoglycemia.

20. What is looping?
Looping is a process of hacking into and reprogramming older insulin pumps (without safeguards against hacking) so that they respond to glucose values and trends provided by a CGM. Similar in principle to available hybrid closed-loop insulin pumps, these systems are not FDA approved and are currently considered off-label uses. The FDA released a warning about these do-it-yourself (DIY) systems that was reported in the *Washington Post* (December 13, 2019): "a worldwide community of engineers, software developers and designers who do not want to wait for the big medical device corporations to release another mediocre diabetes product," so they take "a do-it-yourself approach to diabetes management." The #WeAreNotWaiting movement members, who "have diabetes, or have family members with the ailment," are not "afraid to tweak the technology to meet their needs." Still, people should "consider the inherent risks of DIY devices and services, which have not been approved by the Food and Drug Administration."

Information on how to set up a looping system is available on the Internet and must be done by each individual user. The next chapter gives significantly more detail regarding looping. Note again that this is an off-label use and is provided only for the reader's education.

KEY POINTS
1. Insulin pumps consist of an insulin reservoir, a pumping mechanism, and an infusion set through which insulin is delivered continuously into a subcutaneous site. Rapid-acting insulin analogs are the most common type of insulin used in pumps.
2. The two basic components of insulin delivery by an insulin pump are basal insulin and bolus insulin. Basal insulin is a continuous infusion that maintains a background serum insulin level to control hepatic glucose production overnight and between meals. Bolus insulin consists of the acute doses of insulin that are given to cover meals, to correct high BG levels, or both.
3. Basal insulin infusion rates can be varied throughout the day to match a person's activities and individual glucose patterns.
4. Bolus insulin has two discrete components: a nutritional dose and a correction dose. The nutritional dose is given to cover the meal a person is preparing to eat. The correction dose is the amount of additional insulin that is added to the nutritional dose if the premeal BG is elevated; correction boluses may also be taken alone between meals for high BG values.
5. Insulin pumps have bolus calculators that accurately compute the exact bolus insulin doses needed based on the user-estimated carbohydrate content of a meal, the current glucose level, and the C:I ratios and CFs that are preprogrammed into the pump to avoid math errors.

6. Hyperglycemia developing suddenly in someone who usually has good BG control with pump therapy requires careful evaluation. Potential causes that should be considered include infection; stress; changes in medications, diet, or physical activity; nonadherence; insertion-site problems (scar tissue); infusion-set issues (occlusion, kinking); and bad insulin.

7. A hybrid closed loop is an integrated system in which CGM data are transmitted directly to an insulin pump, which uses an embedded algorithm to adjust the basal insulin infusion rate and/or give correction boluses to maintain glucose levels within a prespecified target range. These are called *hybrid closed-loop systems* because the CGM responsive algorithms can drive basal rates and correction doses, but do not yet have the capability to deliver accurate mealtime boluses.

BIBLIOGRAPHY

American Diabetes Association. Clinical practice recommendations 2020. *Diabetes Care*. 2020 Jan; 43;Suppl 1:S1–S204.

Bally L, Thabit H, Hartnell S, et al. Closed-loop insulin delivery for glycemic control in noncritical care. *N Engl J Med*. 2018 Aug 9;379(6):547–556.

Bally L, Thabit H, Kojzar H, et al. Day-and-night glycaemic control with closed-loop insulin delivery versus conventional insulin pump therapy in free-living adults with well controlled type 1 diabetes: an open-label, randomised, crossover study. *Lancet Diabetes Endocrinol*. 2017 Apr;5(4):261–270.

Bally L, Thabit H, Ruan Y, et al. Bolusing frequency and amount impacts glucose control during hybrid closed-loop. *Diabet Med*. 2018 Mar;35(3):347–351.

Bergenstal RM, Garg S, Weinzimer SA, et al. Safety of a hybrid closed-loop insulin delivery system in patients with type 1 diabetes. *JAMA*. 2016 Oct 4;316(13):1407–1408.

Bergenstal RM, Klonoff DC, Garg SK, et al. Threshold-based insulin-pump interruption for reduction of hypoglycemia. *N Engl J Med*. 2013 Jul 18;369(3):224–232.

Breton MD, Cherñavvsky DR, Forlenza GP, et al. Closed-loop control during intense prolonged outdoor exercise in adolescents with type 1 diabetes: the artificial pancreas ski study. *Diabetes Care*. 2017 Dec;40(12):1644–1650.

Brown SA, Beck RW, Raghinaru D, et al. Glycemic outcomes of use of CLC versus PLGS in type 1 diabetes: a randomized controlled trial. *Diabetes Care*. 2020;43:1822–1828.

Brown SA, Breton MD, Anderson SM, et al. Overnight closed-loop control improves glycemic control in a multicenter study of adults with type 1 diabetes. *J Clin Endocrinol Metab*. 2017 Oct 1;102(10):3674–3682.

Brown SA, Kovatchev BP, Raghinaru D, et al. Six-month randomized, multicenter trial of closed-loop control in type 1 diabetes. *N Engl J Med*. 2019 Oct 31;381(18):1707–1717.

Chamberlain JJ, Doyle-Delgado K, Peterson L, Skolnik N. Diabetes technology: review of the 2019 American Diabetes Association standards of medical care in diabetes. *Ann Intern Med*. 2019;171:415–420.

Grunberger G, Handelsman Y, Bloomgarden ZT, et al. American Association of Clinical Endocrinologists and American College of Endocrinology 2018 position statement on integration of insulin pumps and continuous glucose monitoring in patients with diabetes mellitus. *Endocr Pract*. 2018 Mar;24(3):302–308.

Haidar A, Legault L, Dallaire M, et al. Glucose-responsive insulin and glucagon delivery (dual-hormone artificial pancreas) in adults with type 1 diabetes: a randomized crossover controlled trial. *CMAJ*. 2013 Mar 5;185(4):297–305.

Karges B, Schwandt A, Heidtmann B, et al. Association of insulin pump therapy vs insulin injection therapy with severe hypoglycemia, ketoacidosis, and glycemic control among children, adolescents, and young adults with type 1 diabetes. *JAMA*. 2017 Oct 10;318(14):1358–1366.

Kovatchev B, Cheng P, Anderson SM, et al. Feasibility of long-term closed-loop control: a multicenter 6-month trial of 24/7 automated insulin delivery. *Diabetes Technol Ther*. 2017 Jan;19(1):18–24.

Lal RA, Basina M, Maahs DM, et al. One-year clinical experience of the first commercial hybrid closed-loop system. *Diabetes Care*. 2019;42:2190–2196.

Lal RA, Ekhlaspour L, Hood K, Buckingham B. Realizing a closed-loop (artificial pancreas) system for the treatment of type 1 diabetes. *Endocrine Reviews*. 2019;40(6):1521–1546.

Muller L, Habif S, Leas S, Aranoff-Spencer E. Reducing hypoglycemia in the real world: a retrospective analysis of predictive low-glucose suspend technology in an ambulatory insulin-dependent cohort. *Diabetes Technol Ther*. 2019;21(9):478–484.

Pickup JC. Insulin pumps. *Diabetes Technol Ther*. 2017 Feb;19(S1):S19–S26.

Pickup JC, Reznik Y, Sutton AJ. Glycemic control during continuous subcutaneous insulin infusion versus multiple daily insulin injections in type 2 diabetes: individual patient data meta-analysis and meta-regression of randomized controlled trials. *Diabetes Care*. 2017 May;40(5):715–722.

Ruan Y, Bally L, Thabit H, et al. Hypoglycaemia incidence and recovery during home use of hybrid closed-loop insulin delivery in adults with type 1 diabetes. *Diabetes Obes Metab*. 2018 Aug;20(8):2004–2008.

Russell SJ, El-Khatib FH, Sinha M, et al. Outpatient glycemic control with a bionic pancreas in type 1 diabetes. *N Engl J Med*. 2014 Jul 24;371(4):313–325.

Spaic T, Driscoll M, Raghinaru D, et al. Predictive hyperglycemia and hypoglycemia minimization: in-home evaluation of safety, feasibility, and efficacy in overnight glucose control in type 1 diabetes. *Diabetes Care*. 2017 Mar;40(3):359–366.

Stewart ZA, Wilinska ME, Hartnell S, et al. Closed-loop insulin delivery during pregnancy in women with type 1 diabetes. *N Engl J Med*. 2016 Aug 18;375(7):644–654.

Tauschmann M, Thabit H, Bally L, et al. Closed-loop insulin delivery in suboptimally controlled type 1 diabetes: a multicentre, 12-week randomised trial. *Lancet*. 2018 Oct 13;392(10155):1321–1329.

Thabit H, Hartnell S, Allen JM, et al. Closed-loop insulin delivery in inpatients with type 2 diabetes: a randomised, parallel-group trial. *Lancet Diabetes Endocrinol*. 2017 Feb;5(2):117–124.

Thabit H, Tauschmann M, Allen JM, et al. Home use of an artificial beta cell in type 1 diabetes. *N Engl J Med*. 2015 Nov 26;373(22): 2129–2140.

Umpierrez GE, Klonoff DC. Diabetes technology update: use of insulin pumps and continuous glucose monitoring in the hospital. *Diabetes Care*. 2018 Aug;41(8):1579–1589.

Weisman A, Bai JW, Cardinez M, Kramer CK, Perkins BA. Effect of artificial pancreas systems on glycaemic control in patients with type 1 diabetes: a systematic review and meta-analysis of outpatient randomised controlled trials. *Lancet Diabetes Endocrinol*. 2017 Jul;5(7):501–512.

WEBSITES

DANAtech. www.danatech.org

DiabetesWise. www.diabeteswise.org

American Diabetes Association, 2015. How Do Insulin Pumps Work? http://www.diabetes.org/living-with-diabetes/treatment-and-care/medication/insulin/how-do-insulin-pumps-work.html

American Association of Diabetes Educators, 2018. Continuous Subcutaneous Insulin Infusion (CSII) Without and With Sensor Integration. http://main.diabetes.org/dforg/pdfs/2017/2017-cg-insulin-pumps.pdf

Manderfeld, A, 2018, May 28. Everything You Need to Know About Insulin Pumps. Thediabetescouncil.com

CHAPTER 24

LOOPING

Gregory Schleis, MD

INTRODUCTION

This chapter is designed to answer basic questions about do-it-yourself artificial pancreas systems (DIY APSs). Many users have discovered these systems on their own and may bring questions about them to their diabetes team. This chapter is not an endorsement or condemnation but an educational tool intended for readers to better understand and collaborate with patients on their diabetes care. In this rapidly evolving field, the goal of this chapter is to explain our current (at the time of publication) understanding of the field.

1. **What is "looping"?**
   Although there is an official definition, "looping" is the process of using continuous glucose monitor (CGM) data to automate insulin delivery. Looping relies on computerized algorithms to adjust insulin delivery in response to various inputs by the user, including CGM data, exercise, carbohydrate intake, and previous insulin pump settings. These inputs are used to predict future glucose levels to enable the algorithms to make insulin dosing adjustments to maintain glucose levels in the desired range. None of the DIY APSs have been approved by the U.S. Food and Drug Administration (FDA).

   The systems can operate either as an open loop that makes recommendations for the user to implement or as a closed loop that automatically implements the recommendations.

2. **What is the difference between Loop, AndroidAPS, and OpenAPS?**
   Looping is a generalized term that describes the process of automated insulin delivery, whereas the different vehicles for this process are Loop, AndroidAPS, and OpenAPS. Loop uses an Apple device with iOS. AndroidAPS uses an Android-based device. OpenAPS uses a small computer (e.g., a Raspberry Pi). All these options allow for different algorithms to be used, but all require that the user build the applications themselves. They cannot be downloaded like conventional applications through the app store on iOS or Google Play store on Android. Tidepool is a group that is working on creating an FDA-approved looping application that could possibly be downloaded in the future.

3. **How does looping work?**
   Looping works by using various algorithms that determine the best manner to achieve target blood glucose (BG) levels. Users can choose from the various algorithms depending on their preferences and understanding of the system. For example, if the person is hyperglycemic, the algorithm may decide to increase the basal rate for a preset amount of time. The algorithm will readjust every 30 minutes in order to prevent overcorrection. If the deviation is too great for the algorithm, the default settings will take over as a safety measure.

   There are four main components of a DIY APS: (1) a Bluetooth radio that can communicate with both an insulin pump and a computer/phone; (2) a CGM; (3) an insulin pump (not all types of insulin pumps can do this); (4) a computer stick/phone that is able to run the algorithm. There are insulin pumps not currently available in the United States that are able to use Bluetooth and do not require the communicative radio.

   Many of the systems that people currently use are based on the OpenAPS reference design protocol. There are embedded safety principles that were originally designed in 2015. The idea behind the safety features is that if there is any error or unexpected value during the process, the system defaults back to the standard therapy that is programmed into the insulin pump.

4. **How does the algorithm know what to do?**
   Disclaimer: This section is not essential for the average user to comprehend completely. As users become more advanced, this may be useful for optimizing their settings.

   OpenAPS was initially designed for safety. To safely dose insulin, the algorithm from OpenAPS does not rely conclusively on a single glucose measurement. OpenAPS continuously recalculates insulin dosing requirements to bring BG levels into the target range. If there is a variance between the expected BG level and the actual BG level, the algorithm for OpenAPS will withhold any insulin dosing changes and revert to the original preprogrammed insulin pump settings. Erroneous data may occur because CGMs are not 100% accurate for many reasons; these include faulty or dying sensors, compression events, and temperature changes. The algorithm relies on accurate data from the CGM and multiple user variables, including carbohydrates consumed, physical activity, carbohydrate-to-insulin ratio, insulin sensitivity factor, and duration of insulin action. As the CGM continues to measure interstitial glucose every 5 minutes, the algorithm makes adjustments based on the incoming data by either canceling or creating new temporary basal rates.

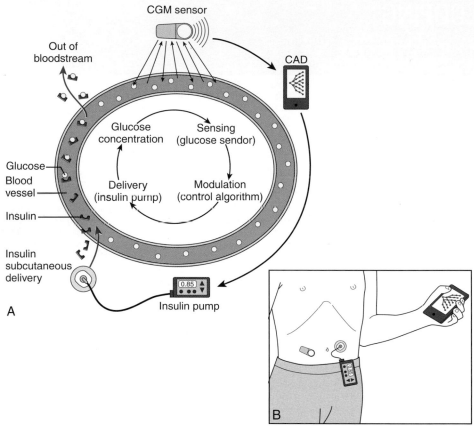

Fig. 24.1 Looping system. (From Boughton CK, Hovorka R. Advances in artificial pancreas systems. *Science Translational Medicine.* 2019;11[484].)

If the user becomes hypoglycemic (typically 30 mg/dL below the target range), OpenAPS will revert to the traditional "low-glucose suspend" behavior until the glucose level is rising fast enough to return to the desired range.

The original algorithm was based on the concept of a temporary basal rate algorithm known as *open reference design zero* (oref0). One of the safety constraints is that oref0 cannot issue insulin boluses but can only change temporary basal rates. The second design constraint is a maximum allowable temporary basal rate. Users can program into their settings a maximum basal rate, but OpenAPS will choose the minimum of three options: programmed maximum temporary basal, 3× the maximum daily scheduled basal rate, and 4× the current scheduled basal rate. Although the temporary basal rates are designed to act without the person actively changing the basal rates, users must still choose their own bolusing patterns for meals or corrections.

OpenAPS uses the insulin pump's bolus and temporary basal history, along with settings that are programmed by the user, such as the duration of insulin action and the published insulin-on-board curves, to calculate the net insulin on board (insulin that is active in the body can include both boluses and basal rates, whereas insulin pump insulin on board only uses the bolus history). More advanced versions use the rate of BG change (increasing or decreasing) and subsequently use the difference between the observed BG change and the predicted BG change to allow for a continued duration of higher temporary basal rates than previously allowed by the algorithm.

Also included in the system is the concept of "bolus snooze." This activity allows for the system to avoid issuing the lower temporary basal rates when the user has bolused or prebolused for a meal but the BG has not yet started to rise from the meal. The system only takes action when the BG drops below the low-glucose suspend threshold, increases more than expected, stays persistently elevated after a mealtime rise, or decreases faster than expected. The process works in advanced OpenAPS by comparing bolus insulin on board separately from net insulin on board and re-adding the BG impact of the bolus insulin on board when deciding whether to set a lower temporary basal rate. This decreases the variation that can occur in the postprandial setting on the system and will take over to ensure that the person's BG reaches the target range. In the postprandial setting, immediately after a bolus, the target BG range is widened but then narrowed over the next couple of hours until it is back to the preprogrammed range.

As the systems began to evolve, the people with diabetes who work on these algorithms have also developed algorithms such as "advanced meal assist" (AMA). This algorithm still requires users to enter carbohydrate counts when eating meals, but it also addresses meal variations in absorption, digestion, and meal composition in order to prevent postprandial BG spikes while avoiding hypoglycemia in the setting where carbohydrate absorption is delayed.

A further development stemming from oref0 is oref1, which is based on the use of small super-microboluses of insulin at mealtimes to more quickly administer the required insulin. In the postprandial setting, this technique sets the temporary basal rate at 0 units/h for the duration to make sure the BG returns to a safe range even in the setting of variable absorption, inaccurate carbohydrate counting, or a missed meal.

The oref1 algorithm continues to recalculate insulin requirements every 5 minutes and continues to issue new super-microboluses depending on the insulin requirements. If the BG starts decreasing, there is already a temporary basal rate set at 0 units/h, so the insulin on board will be quickly reduced as the super-microboluses are reduced. In order to ensure safety, the system ensures that the insulin pump is not currently delivering insulin before ordering another insulin dose. The system also checks the pump reservoir and the bolus history before calculating the next dose after calculating the current dose to ensure there has not been any other delivery of insulin via the insulin pump. All super-microboluses are limited to one-third of the insulin known to be required based on the current information.

If communication is disrupted or there is a lack of BG readings, oref1 reverts to oref0 with AMA and sets an appropriately high temporary basal rate. oref1's super-microbolus features are only active when carbohydrates are still present. The system returns to oref0 overnight or when the user is not interacting with the system.

The development of fully closed-loop systems that do not require entering carbohydrates consumed has also begun. Many other advanced features are also currently in development. As the features go through alpha and beta phases, they can be incorporated into the long-term support (LTS) branches. In many of the system instruction documents, users are advised to use the LTS branches and not the development branches.

5. **What does a person need to begin looping?**
   To use Loop, the user will need an iOS-compatible phone with Bluetooth, an iOS developer account (approximately $100 a year), a Bluetooth radio corresponding to the insulin pump of choice, a "loopable" insulin pump (see the Loop website—the list can change), a MacBook with macOS, and a compatible CGM (see the Loop website—the list can change).

   To use AndroidAPS, the user will need application developer software such as Android Studio, a Windows- or Linux-based computer, an Android smartphone with Bluetooth, a Bluetooth radio corresponding to the insulin pump of choice, a "loopable" insulin pump (see the AndroidAPS website—the list can change), and a compatible CGM (see the AndroidAPS website—the list can change). The user may need to work through some of the system basics while answering questions to unlock more advanced features in the system.

   OpenAPS requires a computer to run the algorithm, as well as Bluetooth (e.g., a Raspberry Pi), app development software, a Bluetooth radio corresponding to the insulin pump of choice, a "loopable" insulin pump (see the OpenAPS website—the list can change), and a compatible CGM (see the OpenAPS website—the list can change).

6. **Which insulin pumps/CGMs/phones can be used?**
   There is a list of compatible insulin pumps that can be used, but many of them available within the United States are older models of Medtronic or OmniPod pumps. Outside the United States, there are available models of insulin pumps, such as the DanaRS, that do not require Bluetooth radio because they are Bluetooth enabled via smartphone. The older Medtronic insulin pumps require certain firmware that has not been upgraded and that allows for the ability to set temporary basal rates remotely.

   A true CGM, such as a Dexcom or the older Medtronic Enlite, is also needed; many people use a Dexcom G6. Freestyle Libre sensors can be used, but they require extra hardware, such as a Miao Miao or Bluecon, which helps convert glucose monitors to CGMs. These are not recommended by most within the community because of the lack of a true CGM.

   Many of the iPhones can be used for Loop. With AndroidAPS, the documents list the smartphones and smartwatches that can run the application and have been tested by the community.

   For older insulin pumps such as the Medtronic 722, a Bluetooth radio that communicates between the smartphone and the insulin pump is required. Each type of insulin pump requires a different type of radio because the communication with the insulin pump has a different frequency depending on the company that built it. The radio that communicates with the Medtronic pump will not communicate with an Omnipod pump.

   Many users purchase a Bluetooth radio that communicates with their insulin pump of choice. They can buy this device from a website called RileyLink and customize certain aspects (e.g., wireless charging) for various price points. Users can also build their own Bluetooth radio. Fig. 24.2 shows an example.

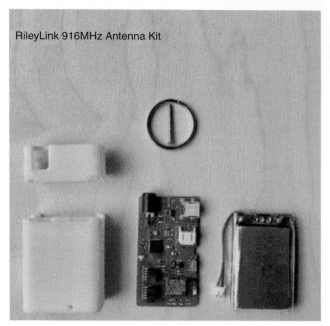

RileyLink 916MHz Antenna Kit

Fig. 24.2 RileyLink breakdown. (From Get RileyLink Order Site. https://getrileylink.org/; 2016.)

7. Where do people get these pumps if they do not have one?

Many people use older pumps they already own. If the user doesn't have one, they may buy one on the Internet from various sources, including Facebook. Those outside the United States can get pumps that are Bluetooth enabled; they will not require a RileyLink. Some may want to buy a backup pump because these pumps are currently out of warranty.

8. Where do people learn about this?

There are separate websites for Loop, AndroidAPS, and OpenAPS. For troubleshooting, different forums are available online through social media (e.g., Facebook) that allow users to post their questions and for others to offer guidance. Again, there is no downloadable application, so the application must be built by the user. Users should read the documentation online multiple times before attempting to install the system themselves. They should also continue to read the documentation online as the systems change. Multiple groups around the world regularly meet to troubleshoot issues and learn about the systems available. The documents online are cited in the Bibliography for their respective system.

9. I'm not a computer person; how do I do this?

Some people have minimal or no coding experience before setting up the applications. If they read the documents online and follow the instructions in a stepwise manner, they will be able to build the application as necessary. It is like a cookbook. It is recommended that users read the documents multiple times to be familiar with each step before attempting to build the application themselves. Various users post issues/questions on online forums such as Facebook.

10. If a person has new-onset type 1 diabetes mellitus, can they just be put on this immediately?

With new-onset type 1 diabetes, there are ongoing changes that occur in the individual's pathophysiology, such as improved insulin production after the glucotoxic period. The looping systems still rely on accurate carbohydrate counting, carbohydrate-to-insulin ratios, insulin sensitivity factors, duration of insulin action, and appropriate basal rates. In someone with a new diagnosis, these may not be known but can be deduced after some work with their provider. People can be overwhelmed with the initiation of DIY APSs, and this may exacerbate distress. Users must have a solid foundation of understanding their diabetes before the initiation of a DIY APS.

11. Can a person start looping with a new insulin pump?

No. Looping can only be done with certain insulin pumps as listed in the documents. It requires the capability of being controlled through Bluetooth, but many of the newer pumps have shut down this access. If users are outside the United States and have access to Bluetooth-enabled insulin pumps (e.g., the DanaRS), they will be able to loop with a new insulin pump. The list of usable insulin pumps for each system can be found in the online documents.

12. Why not use the FDA-approved hybrid closed-loop systems instead of looping?

Depending on insurance coverage, some people do not have the option of obtaining a Medtronic 670 G or Tandem t-slim X2 with Control-IQ with all the required equipment. The DIY APS programs allow people to use whatever products they can obtain. Some people also prefer different CGMs. In the setting of DIY APS, people can use a CGM from one company and an insulin pump from another. For example, a user can be looping with a Dexcom G6 CGM and a Medtronic insulin pump.

Many of the commercial systems were not available until recently and may not offer features that some people desire. The customization bed found in DIY APS attracts many people to these systems rather than to the commercial systems, which adhere to preset guidelines and rules as required by the FDA. The innovation in the DIY APS space also allows users to obtain new features as they become available, whereas some of the commercial products require upgrades that can only happen with newer hardware. Users can also incorporate remote monitoring, which is enticing for people who want to be monitored remotely by others.

13. When a person begins looping, has the diabetes team been replaced?

No. The diabetes team is even more essential because the user will need help with backups because systems or hardware can fail. The fundamentals of treating type 1 diabetes, such as accurate carbohydrate-counting skills, appropriate carbohydrate-to-insulin ratios and insulin sensitivity factors, screening for complications, and discussion of other comorbidities, won't be changed by looping. Users must continue to work with their diabetes team to discuss the other aspects of diabetes besides glucose control.

14. What are good recommendations providers can offer to people who want to loop?

Although diabetes providers cannot recommend DIY APSs currently and there are no formal guidelines, there is advice that can be offered to help users and prevent potential issues:

1. Users should always have backup long-acting insulin because insulin pumps that are currently being used in the United States for DIY APSs are out of warranty and can fail.
2. If users can afford to have backup RileyLink and other equipment, it is recommended because systems can fail, and they will need to wait for a replacement or may not even be able to get a replacement (e.g., an older Medtronic pump that is out of warranty).
3. Patience is necessary to see results. People should have tempered expectations, especially in the beginning of this process, because it is not perfected.
4. Looping is not FDA approved, and insurance may not cover things such as a RileyLink, developer accounts, and cell phones.
5. Because the systems rely on cell phones (except OpenAPS), people should have backup cell-phone batteries that can also charge both the cell phone and the RileyLink.
6. Diligent carbohydrate counting is essential to obtain the desired results. Although the system can make up for small errors, users still need to understand the concepts behind carbohydrate counting, mealtime insulin dosing, and correction insulin dosing.
7. The system will not know if the insulin pump is disconnected or if the insertion site is not absorbing insulin adequately. There are many links in the chain that can be broken in the system, and all of those must be considered when troubleshooting. For example, if the CGM sensor is dying, there can be inaccurate readings sent to the DIY APS, resulting in improper insulin dosing. There are safety measures set up within the algorithms, but none of these is perfect.

15. How safe is this? Can it be hacked?

None of the systems have been studied yet in true randomized controlled trials, and none of these systems have received FDA approval. The data are mostly self-reported and retrospective. There has been a prospective comparison of AndroidAPS to the older Medtronic low-glucose suspend insulin pump. In the retrospective studies, there has been self-reported improvement in hemoglobin A1c, increased time in range, decreased glucose variability, decreased episodes of hypoglycemia, less reliance on accuracy of carbohydrate counting, improved overnight control, and reduced mental burden. Highly motivated individuals have self-reported great success, but potential users must be aware of the risks of hypoglycemia.

16. How does someone troubleshoot?

People can troubleshoot using various online forums and Facebook groups. There are several groups on Facebook, and each of them has its own rules on how to publish questions and concerns. Much of the support is community and user driven; there is no central company that provides troubleshooting help. The documents that are published online, along with the online repositories such as GitHub, are openly available to all. Users can also use the Slack channels regarding topics or use the messaging application Gitter.

17. **Is this covered by insurance?**

    Some components of the systems, such as CGMs, insulin pumps, and pump supplies, can be covered by insurance, but other parts are not covered. The RileyLink costs about $150 but can be built cheaper if the user has the time and expertise. The developer account for Apple products is not typically covered by insurance but is required if the user wants to use the Loop app.

18. **How can people on DIY APS be remotely monitored?**

    People using DIY APSs can be remotely monitored by friends and family members using Nightscout. This is similar to Dexcom Share. Nightscout can also be used with the Medtronic 670 G system if desired. It displays real-time CGM data and can also create reports that users and providers can use for making adjustments. Some people also use Nightscout (http://www.nightscout.info/) to put their glucose data on different applications, such as smartphones, computers, or other devices.

19. **How can I see users' data when they come to the office?**

    People can share their data through Nightscout reports (as mentioned previously) or through Dexcom Clarity if they are using a Dexcom device. Some users upload their data to Tidepool, which can also be shared with the diabetes team.

20. **Where can I find more information?**

    This field is rapidly evolving as technology continues to change. This chapter is a basic introduction, but continued reading is necessary to stay up to date. The online community is a source of information and troubleshooting. There are various Facebook groups, such as Looped, AndroidAPS Users, and CGM in the Cloud, that are user forums where people can post questions along with recommendations for others. The documents for the various DIY APS branches that are located online are also great sources of information. They are listed in the recommended sources of reading. Some of the main contributors and creators within the community can also be found on respective social media sites such as Twitter. Dana Lewis, Kate Farnsworth, Milos Kozak, and Katie DiSimone are some examples. Dana Lewis also wrote a book; she was one of the original pioneers in the field. Her book is available as a free PDF online, but the book can also be purchased on various sites. The link for the book is listed in the Bibliography.

KEY POINTS

1. DIY APSs are not FDA approved, but people are using these systems to obtain the desired results for their diabetes.
2. The systems are built by the user and have various external equipment requirements in addition to the requirement for the use of older insulin pumps, which can be out of warranty.
3. The design of each system can be individualized by the user, but the systems still require user inputs that rely on a fundamental understanding of diabetes.
4. The diabetes care team has not been replaced by these systems because the user needs to have proper diabetes education and guidance on safety and other potential issues that may arise.
5. It is recommended that backup systems be in place because many of the insulin pumps are out of warranty, and there is no formal troubleshooting support.
6. As the systems progress, information can continue to be found online in forums or the documents that users follow to build the application for themselves.

BIBLIOGRAPHY

Boughton CK, Hovorka R. Advances in artificial pancreas systems. *Science Translational Medicine.* 2019;11(484). https://doi.org/10.1126/scitranslmed.aaw4949.

GetRileyLink Order Site. https://getrileylink.org/

Jennings P, Hussain S. Do-it-yourself artificial pancreas systems: a review of the emerging evidence and insights for healthcare professionals. *J Diabetes Sci Technol.* Published online December 17, 2019:1932296819894296. https://doi.org/10.1177/1932296819894296.

Kesavadev J, Srinivasan S, Saboo B, Krishna BM, Krishnan G. The Do-it-yourself artificial pancreas: a comprehensive review. *Diabetes Ther.* Published online April 30, 2020. https://doi.org/10.1007/s13300-020-00823z.

Lewis D. History and perspective on DIY closed looping. *J Diabetes Sci Technol.* 2018;13(4):790–793. https://doi.org/10.1177/1932296818808307.

Lewis DM. Do-it-yourself artificial pancreas system and the OpenAPS movement. *Endocrinology and Metabolism Clinics of North America.* 2020;49(1):203–213. https://doi.org/10.1016/j.ecl.2019.10.005.

LoopDocs. https://loopkit.github.io/loopdocs/

OpenAPS Reference Design – OpenAPS.org. https://openaps.org/reference-design/

Petruzelkova L, Soupal J, Plasova V, et al. Excellent glycemic control maintained by open-source hybrid closed-loop androidAPS during and after sustained physical activity. *Diabetes Technology & Therapeutics.* 2018;20(11):744–750. https://doi.org/10.1089/dia.2018.0214.

Racklyeft N. The history of Loop and LoopKit. *Medium.* Published October 3, 2016. https://medium.com/@loudnate/the-history-of-loop-and-loopkit-59b3caf13805

Welcome to OpenAPS's documentation! — OpenAPS 0.0.0 documentation. https://openaps.readthedocs.io/en/latest/index.html

Welcome to the AndroidAPS documentation — AndroidAPS 2.6.1 documentation. https://androidaps.readthedocs.io/en/latest/EN/index.html

Welcome to Nightscout. The Nightscout Project. Accessed August 9, 2020. http://www.nightscout.info/

CHAPTER 25

HYPOGLYCEMIA

Diana Isaacs, PharmD, BCPS, BCACP, BC-ADM, CDCES, FADCES, FCCP

1. **How is hypoglycemia defined?**

   Hypoglycemia is defined as a glucose level of less than 70 mg/dL. This is the point at which neuroendocrine symptoms develop in people without diabetes. Hypoglycemia is classified into three levels. Level 1 hypoglycemia is a glucose level from 54 to <70 mg/dL. Level 2 hypoglycemia is a glucose level below 54 mg/dL. Level 3 hypoglycemia is not defined by a specific number but rather as a severe event causing altered mental status or physical functioning that requires assistance from another person for recovery. Level 2 hypoglycemia can lead to level 3 hypoglycemia if not quickly treated. See Table 25.1 for the classification of hypoglycemia.

2. **What are the symptoms of hypoglycemia?**

   There are neurogenic and neuroglycopenic symptoms of hypoglycemia. Neurogenic symptoms include those that are catecholamine mediated and cholinergic mediated. Catecholamine-mediated symptoms are rapid heart rate, anxiety, and shakiness. Cholinergic-mediated symptoms include hunger, sweating, and paresthesia. During level 2 hypoglycemia, neuroglycopenic symptoms occur and can include changes in mental status, confusion, irritability, behavioral changes, seizures, loss of consciousness, coma, and even death. See Fig. 25.1.

3. **What are the health implications of hypoglycemia?**

   Hypoglycemia is potentially fatal and may be a contributor to up to 6% of deaths in people with diabetes younger than 40 years of age. There is an increased risk for cardiovascular and all-cause mortality in insulin-treated individuals with type 1 diabetes (T1D) and type 2 diabetes (T2D) who experience hypoglycemia. An association of severe hypoglycemia and mortality was found in the landmark ADVANCE trial, which assessed outcomes of intensive glucose management to an A1c of <6.5%.

   Cognitive changes from hypoglycemia are linked to higher rates of motor vehicle accidents in people with diabetes. Children experiencing recurrent episodes of hypoglycemia may develop permanent neurologic deficiencies and learning differences.

   Even level 1 hypoglycemia can cause fatigue and other symptoms that impair the ability to concentrate up to hours after the event. Hypoglycemia commonly leads to rebound hyperglycemia from overtreatment. Avoidance of hypoglycemia makes it more difficult to achieve glycemic targets, which can contribute to hyperglycemia and indirectly contribute to microvascular and macrovascular complications of diabetes.

4. **Does hypoglycemia affect quality of life?**

   Hypoglycemia is associated with reduced perceived quality of life and reduced health satisfaction. It has also been correlated to reduced school and work performance, absenteeism, reduced productivity, and disability. Another important aspect is the potential fear of hypoglycemia that some people with diabetes experience, which can be a deterrent to diabetes self-management and can negatively affect quality of life.

5. **What causes hypoglycemia?**

   The most common cause of hypoglycemia is treatment with insulin. The insulin secretagogues— sulfonylureas and meglitinides—cause the pancreas to release insulin and are also contributors to hypoglycemia. Other diabetes medication classes have a very low risk of hypoglycemia and are not expected to cause hypoglycemia based on their mechanism of action. However, when combined with insulin or a secretagogue, they can increase the incidence of hypoglycemia, especially if the insulin or secretagogue dose is not adjusted prior to combining. Treatment-associated hypoglycemia occurs most commonly from a missed meal, insufficient carbohydrate intake, inaccurate carbohydrate or insulin calculations, alcohol use, and inadequate carbohydrate replacement during activity or exercise.

   It has been estimated that 9.2% of emergency department (ED) visits are a result of insulin-related hypoglycemia. Precipitating factors leading to ED visits are most often related to issues with mealtime insulin dosing, such as taking the wrong dose, taking the insulin and not eating, or taking the wrong insulin. For example, people may accidentally take the fast-acting mealtime insulin instead of the long-acting insulin.

6. **Are there any nonmedication causes of hypoglycemia?**

   Other, less common causes of hypoglycemia include insulinoma, which is an insulin-secreting tumor; post–gastric bypass hypoglycemia; insulin autoimmune syndrome (antibody to insulin or insulin receptor); adrenal insufficiency; and critical illness.

Table 25.1 Classification of Hypoglycemia		
LEVEL	**GLYCEMIC CRITERIA**	**DESCRIPTION**
Level 1	Glucose ≤ 70 mg/dL (3.9 mmol/L) and glucose ≥ 54 mg/dL (3.0 mmol/L)	Hypoglycemia alert
Level 2	<54 mg/dL (3.0 mmol/L)	Clinically significant hypoglycemia
Level 3	No specific glucose threshold	A severe event characterized by altered mental status and/or physical status requiring assistance for treatment of hypoglycemic

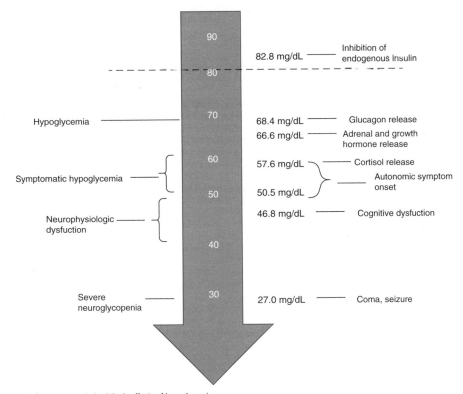

Fig. 25.1 Symptoms and physiologic effects of hypoglycemia.

7. **Who is most at risk of hypoglycemia?**
   Anyone who takes insulin or a secretagogue could be at risk of hypoglycemia. Older people are at greater risk because of some of the changes that happen with advanced age, such as reduced kidney function, changes in vision, changes in taste, cognitive impairment, and poor nutrition.
   Other people at risk are those who have erratic mealtimes, changes in physical activity, a long-standing history of diabetes, alcohol use, malnutrition, or psychiatric conditions and those with coexisting chronic conditions, including renal and hepatic impairment.
   Additional factors that have been associated with increased hypoglycemia include low socioeconomic status, high school education or less, unstable living situation, lack of insurance, and food insecurity.

8. **What is the physiologic mechanism that occurs during hypoglycemia?**
   For those who can produce insulin, the body decreases its own insulin production when glucose drops to try to prevent hypoglycemia. Counterregulatory hormones, including glucagon and epinephrine, are released when glucose is 65 to 70 mg/dL. Glucagon stimulates gluconeogenesis in the liver. Epinephrine stimulates hepatic glycogenolysis and hepatic and renal gluconeogenesis. However, glucagon secretion is partially or fully lost among

people with established T1D. The epinephrine response to falling glucose levels is typically reduced in T1D as well. For those with T2D, these counterregulatory hormone mechanisms are usually initially intact but can decrease over time. See Fig. 25.1.

9. How common is hypoglycemia?
   Hypoglycemia affects people with diabetes of all ages and diabetes types, although it is more common in people with T1D. The actual number of cases is higher among people with T2D simply because more people overall are diagnosed with T2D. The overall rates vary and are likely underreported. It is estimated that each year, 245,000 people with diabetes report to the ED for treatment-related hypoglycemia. Hypoglycemia events occur in more than 40% of long-term care residents with diabetes.

10. Can we eliminate hypoglycemia?
    Unfortunately, hypoglycemia is a common occurrence because it is challenging to perfectly pair carbohydrate intake with insulin doses. In fact, it is so common that an international consensus report advises that up to 4% of time spent in hypoglycemia is acceptable to achieve glycemic targets, acknowledging that it is challenging to limit hypoglycemia with the currently available antihyperglycemic agents. This equates to nearly 1 hour per day. Of note, the guideline does state that for those with more advanced age or complications, less than 1% of the time should be spent in hypoglycemia. This is still around 15 minutes per day.

11. Why is it so challenging to eliminate hypoglycemia?
    The main limiting factor to tight glycemic management is hypoglycemia. For this reason, the American Diabetes Association (ADA) recommends higher glycosylated hemoglobin (A1c) targets, of up to <8.5%, for older adults and those with more comorbidities at the greatest risk of hypoglycemia. Current insulin options do not perfectly mimic true physiologic insulin. For example, compared with physiologic insulin secretion after a meal, current bolus insulin options take longer to start working and stay in the body past the point when they are needed.

12. What is impaired awareness of hypoglycemia?
    Hypoglycemic unawareness is when a person may not feel any symptoms despite a glucose level that is below 70 mg/dL. Many people with diabetes have impaired counterregulatory responses to hypoglycemia or experience hypoglycemia unawareness. Some people with diabetes may lose all ability to sense hypoglycemia and must rely on other people to notice signs or symptoms or on technology (e.g., continuous glucose monitor [CGM]) to alert them.

13. Are there certain drugs that can mask the symptoms of hypoglycemia?
    People who take certain medications, such as beta blockers, may not experience the neurogenic symptoms of hypoglycemia because they are blocked by the drug. The cholinergic-mediated symptoms, such as sweating, are still expected to occur.

14. What should a person do if they think they are experiencing symptoms of hypoglycemia?
    If a person feels like they may be experiencing symptoms of hypoglycemia, the first thing to do is to check glucose. This is an important first step to confirm hypoglycemia because some of the symptoms could be confused with other conditions, such as hypotension or even hyperglycemia.

15. How is hypoglycemia treated?
    For individuals with confirmed hypoglycemia who are able to eat, 15 to 20 g of glucose is the preferred treatment. Examples include 4 to 6 oz of juice, three to four glucose tablets, or three to five hard candies (not chocolate). If glucose remains below 70 mg/dL after 15 minutes, then an additional 15 to 20 g should be ingested. This can be repeated up to three times as needed. Once the glucose reading or glucose pattern is trending up, the individual should consume a meal or snack to prevent the recurrence of hypoglycemia.

16. Why shouldn't chocolate be used to treat hypoglycemia?
    Chocolate contains fat, which can delay the absorption of the carbohydrate, and it will take longer for glucose to rise and to have a resolution of symptoms.

17. What is the role of glucagon?
    Glucagon is a counterregulatory hormone that is secreted by the pancreatic alpha cells to stimulate gluconeogenesis, which is the breakdown and release of glycogen in the liver. This leads to increased glucose concentrations. In glucose homeostasis, glucagon works with insulin to regulate and maintain normal glucose concentrations.

18. When should glucagon be prescribed?
    Glucagon is the preferred treatment option for severe hypoglycemia and should be prescribed for all people with diabetes who are at increased risk of level 2 hypoglycemia. This should generally include all people with T1D and

Table 25.2 Comparison of Glucagon Products

	INTRANASAL GLUCAGON (BAQSIMI)	LIQUID STABLE GLUCAGON (GVOKE)	LYOPHILIZED GLUCAGON POWDER INJECTION (GLUCAGON EMERGENCY KIT)	LYOPHILIZED GLUCAGON POWDER INJECTION (GLUCAGEN)
Available doses	3 mg	0.5 mg, 1 mg	0.5 mg, 1 mg	0.5 mg, 1 mg
FDA-approved ages	Over 4 years	Over 2 years	Any age	Any age
Route of administration	Nasal	SC	SC, IM, IV	SC, IM, IV
Location of administration	Nose	Lower abdomen, outer thigh, or outer upper arm	Upper arms, thighs, or buttocks	Upper arms, thighs, or buttocks
Dosage	3 mg	Over 12 years of age: 1 mg Under 12 years of age and <45 kg: 0.5 mg	Adults and pediatrics weighing >20 kg: 1 mg Pediatrics weighing <20 kg: 0.5 mg or dose equivalent to 20–30 mcg/kg	Adults and pediatrics weighing >25 kg or >6 years: 1 mg Pediatrics weighing <25 kg or <6 years: 0.5 mg
Requires reconstitution prior to use	No	No	Yes	Yes
Shelf-life stability	24 months	24 months	24 months If reconstituted, must use immediately	24 months If reconstituted, must use immediately

FDA, U.S. Food and Drug Administration; *IM*, intramuscular; *IV*, intravenous; *SC*, subcutaneous.

many insulin-treated people with T2D. Caregivers, school personnel, or family members of the person with diabetes should know where the person's glucagon is and how to administer it.

19. **What types of glucagon are available to treat hypoglycemia?**
Glucagon was originally only available in a dry powder, requiring reconstitution before administration because of its lack of stability when premixed. The original kit is still available and contains a vial of powdered glucagon, a syringe prefilled with diluent, and instructions for reconstitution and administration. There are two types of kits by two separate manufacturers.

Liquid stable glucagon is a native glucagon stabilized in dimethyl sulfoxide-based solvent. It is stable at room temperature. There are prefilled syringe and autoinjector pen options; both have two available dosing options of 0.5 mg or 1 mg. The autoinjector pen has no visible needle and auto-locks after use. Nasal glucagon is available as a 3-mg dose for ages 4 years and older. It is a white powder in an intranasal device with β-cyclodextrin (Betadex) and dodecylphosphocholine as excipients. They all should be stored at room temperature and are shelf stable for 2 years. See Table 25.2 for more information.

20. **Are there advantages of one glucagon formulation over another?**
Nasal and liquid stable glucagon are easier to administer compared with the traditional glucagon kit that requires reconstitution, although cost is lower with the traditional kit, and some insurance formularies prefer it. There are no direct comparisons from clinical trials between nasal and liquid stable glucagon. However, there are some differences that may entice a person to pick one product over another. For example, the autoinjector pen and prefilled syringe are approved for ages 2 years and older, whereas nasal glucagon is approved for ages 4 years and older. The autoinjector and prefilled syringe have two dosing options, which may be preferred for younger children or individuals with low body weight. Another important difference is comfort with using a needle. Some caregivers may be more comfortable with nasal glucagon or the autoinjector pen, where the needle is never seen by the patient or caregiver. However, if a person were having a seizure, the injection may be potentially easier to

administer than a nasal dose because there are more available sites for administration. Another consideration is the comfort from seeing the drug going into the person, which occurs with the traditional glucagon emergency kit and the glucagon prefilled syringe. Other considerations may include the perceived ease of administration and the size of the product to carry.

21. **What are the side effects of glucagon?**
The most commonly reported adverse events include nausea, vomiting, and headache. The injectables have the additional side effect of injection-site reactions, and the nasal spray can cause nasal discomfort and upper respiratory tract infection.

22. **Are there any warnings to using glucagon?**
All glucagon formulations are contraindicated in pheochromocytoma, insulinoma, and glucagon hypersensitivity. There are warnings about use in pheochromocytoma because it may stimulate the release of catecholamines from the tumor. It is not recommended to use in patients with insulinoma because it may actually worsen hypoglycemia. There is a warning about a lack of efficacy in patients with decreased hepatic glycogen, which can occur in states of starvation, adrenal insufficiency, and chronic hypoglycemia. Long periods of activity, such as marathon running or heavy alcohol use, may deplete glucagon stores. In these situations, glucagon will not be effective, and intravenous (IV) or oral glucose sources would be required to treat hypoglycemia.

23. **What are important educational points about hypoglycemia treatment?**
People with diabetes should be counseled that glucagon is an emergency medication. If a person is able to eat or drink, that should be the first-line treatment. Any time glucagon is used, the health team should be notified. Even if a patient becomes alert and oriented, emergency help may be needed because it is possible for the hypoglycemic episode to reoccur. It is also important to put a person onto their side after the glucagon is administered. It is common to experience nausea and vomiting. Turning to the side will ensure the airway stays open. Once a person becomes alert and is able to swallow, they should receive a rapidly absorbed source of carbohydrate, such as fruit juice, followed by a snack or meal containing both protein and carbohydrates, such as peanut butter crackers. This helps to restore liver glycogen and prevent secondary hypoglycemia. The injectable formulations should be discarded in a sharps container.

24. **What is the preferred treatment for hypoglycemia in the inpatient setting?**
Similar to the outpatient setting, 15 to 20 g of glucose is the preferred treatment. However, if level 3 hypoglycemia occurs, then IV dextrose is used to quickly raise glucose. Concentrated IV dextrose 50% (D50W) is most appropriate for severe hypoglycemia.

25. **What is the role of technology in preventing hypoglycemia?**
CGMs offer the ability to set alarms when hypoglycemia occurs. There are also options for predictive alerts. These alerts can be customized, and there are additional features, including fall rate, which provides an alert to let a person know that glucose is dropping rapidly. There are additional alerts to remind a person to recheck glucose after it was low. In addition to CGMs, there are now sensor-augmented insulin pumps. These insulin pumps can suspend insulin when glucose is predicted to go low to reduce the incidence of hypoglycemia. There are also hybrid closed-loop insulin pumps that can automatically adjust insulin rates to help reduce hypoglycemia. It is important to know that even with the current technology, most people will still experience some hypoglycemia.

26. **What is the role of diabetes self-management in hypoglycemia?**
According to the ADA standards of medical care, all individuals with diabetes should be educated on the signs and symptoms of hypoglycemia, along with prevention and treatment strategies. Those with T1D or insulin-treated T2D should be counseled on the frequency of self-monitoring of blood glucose concentrations in response to a hypoglycemic episode. People with diabetes should learn their glucose targets and learn how to problem-solve possible causes of and solutions to hypoglycemia.

KEY POINTS

1. Hypoglycemia is a common occurrence in diabetes management and often a barrier to achieving more intensive glycemic targets.
2. Hypoglycemia can be classified into three levels. Level 3 is the most severe and requires assistance from another person.
3. Consuming fast-acting carbohydrates is the treatment of choice if a person is able to eat or drink. When a person can't eat or drink, glucagon can be administered by another person, or IV dextrose can be given by the healthcare team.
4. New technologies can help reduce hypoglycemia through glucose alerts and automated insulin delivery based on glucose levels.

BIBLIOGRAPHY

LaManna J, Litchman ML, Dickinson JK, et al. Diabetes education impact on hypoglycemia outcomes: a systematic review of evidence and gaps in the literature. *Diabetes Educ.* 2019 Aug;45(4):349–369. https://doi.org/10.1177/0145721719855931. Epub 2019 Jun 18. PMID: 31210091.

American Diabetes Association. 6. Glycemic targets: standards of medical care in diabetes—2020. *Diabetes Care*. 2020;43(Suppl 1):S66–S76.

Freeman J. Management of hypoglycemia in older adults with type 2 diabetes. *Postgraduate Medicine*. 2019;131(4):241250. https://doi.org/10.1080/00325481.2019.1578590.

Lin YK, Fisher SJ, Pop-Busui R. Hypoglycemia unawareness and autonomic dysfunction in diabetes: lessons learned and roles of diabetes technologies. *J Diabetes Investig*. 2020 May 13 https://doi.org/10.1111/jdi.13290.

Mathew P, Thoppil D. *Hypoglycemia. 2020 Mar 16. StatPearls [Internet]*. Treasure Island, FL: StatPearls Publishing; 2020 Jan. PMID: 30521262.

Pratiwi C, Mokoagow MI, Made Kshanti IA, Soewondo P. The risk factors of inpatient hypoglycemia: a systematic review. *Heliyon*. 2020 May 11;6(5):e03913. https://doi.org/10.1016/j.heliyon.2020.e03913.

Evans Kreider K, Pereira K, Padilla BI. Practical approaches to diagnosing, treating and preventing hypoglycemia in diabetes. *Diabetes Ther*. 2017;8:1427–1435. https://doi.org/10.1007/s13300-017-0325-9.

Tourkmani AM, Alharbi TJ, Rsheed AMB, et al. A. Hypoglycemia in type 2 diabetes mellitus patients: a review article. *Diabetes Metab Syndr*. 2018 Sep;12(5):791–794. https://doi.org/10.1016/j.dsx.2018.04.004. Epub 2018 Apr 12. PMID: 29678605.

Battelino T, Danne T, Bergenstal RM, et al. Clinical targets for continuous glucose monitoring data interpretation: recommendations from the international consensus on time in range. *Diabetes Care*. 2019 Aug;42(8):1593–1603. https://doi.org/10.2337/dci19-0028. Epub 2019 Jun 8. PMID: 31177185; PMCID: PMC6973648.

CHAPTER 26

WEIGHT MANAGEMENT IN PATIENTS WITH TYPE 2 DIABETES

Christina Ramirez Cunningham, ANP-BC, CDCES, and David Saxon, MD

1. **Explain body mass index and how it is used to categorize overweight and obesity**
   The National Institutes of Health and the World Health Organization use body mass index (BMI) as a screening tool for overweight and obesity. BMI is calculated as a person's weight in kilograms (kg) divided by the square of their height in meters (m). BMI helps identify those individuals who are at higher risk of weight-related comorbidities. A BMI of 25 to 29.9 kg/m^2 (23–24.9 kg/m^2 in Asians) identifies someone as overweight, and BMI $\geq$ 30 kg/m^2 ($\geq$25 kg/m^2 in Asians) as having obesity. Several groups have further classified obesity by BMI cutoff points: 30 to 34.9 kg/m^2 (class I), 35 to 39.9 kg/m^2 (class II), $\geq$40 kg/m^2 (class III), $\geq$50 kg/m^2 (class IV), and $\geq$60 kg/m^2 (class V). BMI should be considered in the context of a person's gender, age, ethnicity, and muscularity.

2. **What is the prevalence of obesity and type 2 diabetes in the United States?**
   In 2017 to 2018, the age-adjusted prevalence of obesity among U.S. adults was 42.4%, and no significant differences existed between men and women. Severe obesity (class III–V obesity) had a prevalence of 9.2% and was more common in women than in men. Recent Centers for Disease Control and Prevention (CDC) estimates suggest that 34.2 million Americans have diabetes (10.5% of the U.S. population), and 88 million have prediabetes (34.5% of the adult U.S. population). Of those with type 2 diabetes (T2DM), 85% are obese.

3. **What impact does weight loss have on people with prediabetes?**
   There is substantial and consistent evidence that moderate weight loss (5%–10% of body weight) can delay the progression from prediabetes to T2DM. Weight loss in people with prediabetes decreases insulin resistance and preserves β-cell function. The greater the weight loss, the more substantial and clinically meaningful the benefits tend to be for dysglycemia, blood pressure, and lipids. In the Diabetes Prevention Program (DPP), lifestyle intervention for 2.8 years reduced the risk of converting from prediabetes to T2DM by 58%, compared with a 31% risk reduction in the group treated with metformin.

4. **How much weight loss is needed to modify outcomes in people with type 2 diabetes?**
   Proper diet, consistent physical activity, and behavioral therapy intended to achieve and maintain $\geq$5% weight loss for >1 year are recommended for individuals with T2DM who are overweight or obese. The Look AHEAD trial showed that a loss of 5% to 10% body weight in those with overweight/obesity and T2DM could improve cardiovascular disease (CVD) risk factors, reduce Hb A1c, improve fitness, and reduce medication use for T2DM, hypertension, and hyperlipidemia. The greater the weight loss and the longer it is sustained, the greater the benefits that can be obtained.

5. **Describe the routine clinical assessment of the individual with overweight or obesity**
   Because of the long-term adverse health consequences of excess body weight, discussions about weight loss and its positive impact on an individual's health should be addressed routinely and continuously. BMI should be assessed at each clinic visit to screen for overweight and obesity, and weight gain and weight loss should be tracked over time. Starting a conversation early about weight goals allows for earlier intervention. Once BMI is $\geq$25 kg/m^2, screening for and discussions about weight-related comorbidities should be routine. Routine and symptom-based screening in people with obesity includes evaluation for T2DM, CVD, hyperlipidemia, hypertension, nonalcoholic fatty liver disease, sleep apnea, osteoarthritis, and depression.

6. **What strategies are available for weight loss?**
   Weight-loss strategies include dietary caloric restriction, physical activity, behavioral therapy, pharmacologic therapy, and metabolic surgery. Asking about motives, barriers, food availability, access to exercise equipment, and cultural circumstances can help the provider further guide a person toward an appropriate strategy. Goal setting allows people to make objective, measurable changes in eating, exercise, and related behaviors. Accountability and self-monitoring must be encouraged. If the individual cannot maintain self-monitoring and >5% weight loss, a high-intensity program of $\geq$16 sessions in 6 months should be recommended.

7. **Is the individual taking medications that tend to cause weight gain?**
Drug-induced weight gain is a common and preventable cause of overweight and obesity. Therefore a thorough assessment of previous medications (that may have resulted in weight gain) and current prescription medications is paramount during all clinic visits when weight management is the focus of care. Medications that are weight neutral or are associated with weight loss should be chosen whenever it is feasible to do so. Medications often associated with weight gain include antipsychotics, antidepressants, glucocorticoids, injectable progestins, anticonvulsants, gabapentin, and possibly sedating antihistamines and anticholinergics.

8. **What antidiabetes medications are associated with weight gain?**
The classes of antidiabetes medications with the most potential to promote weight gain are insulin, insulin secretagogues, and thiazolidinediones. Although these medications are often needed to control hyperglycemia, medications that are weight neutral or associated with weight loss are preferable for people with obesity and T2DM whenever possible. In those requiring insulin therapy, consideration should be given to the addition of insulin-sparing medications, such as metformin, pramlintide, glucagon-like peptide-1 (GLP-1) receptor agonists (RAs), and sodium–glucose cotransporter 2 (SGLT-2) inhibitors.

9. **Why do people often gain weight after initiating antidiabetes medications such as insulin?**
People can gain as much as 10 kg in a short period (3–6 months) after initiating treatment with insulin, sulfonylureas, other insulin secretagogues like meglitinides, and thiazolidinediones. Mechanisms that may result in weight gain after insulin initiation include the conservation of calories when glucose is lowered below the renal threshold, inhibition of protein catabolism, and increased carbohydrate intake to avoid hypoglycemia.

10. **What antidiabetes medications are weight neutral or associated with weight loss?**
Treatments that are weight neutral are dipeptidyl peptidase-4 (DPP-4) inhibitors, alpha-glucosidase inhibitors, colesevelam, and bromocriptine. Medications that may lead to weight loss are metformin, pramlintide, GLP-1 RAs, and SGLT-2 inhibitors. GLP-1 RAs are being approved at higher doses (e.g., dulaglutide) that have been found to result in greater weight loss at 52 weeks.

11. **How do GLP-1 RAs and SGLT-2 inhibitors help with weight loss?**
GLP-1 RAs are the antidiabetes medication class with the potential to promote the greatest weight loss. GLP-1 is an endogenous gut hormone that slows gastric emptying and acts on the central nervous system to suppress appetite; GLP-1 RAs bind to GLP-1 receptors and produce similar effects. For some people, this reduces food-seeking behaviors. Although higher GLP-1 RA doses provide superior hemoglobin A1c lowering and weight loss, side effects may limit their tolerability. GLP-1 RA therapy should be initiated at the lowest dose, with subsequent dose increments as tolerated. SGLT-2 inhibitors reversibly block the reabsorption of filtered glucose from the renal tubular lumen, thereby preventing excessive glucose from returning to the circulatory system. This mechanism is understood to reduce weight by osmotic diuresis and loss of calories through the urine without an effect on appetite.

12. **What dietary approaches are recommended by the American Diabetes Association (ADA) for people with type 2 diabetes?**
The ADA does not recommend a single diet or pattern of eating. However, certain dietary choices should be promoted to people with T2DM, such as increasing intake of nonstarchy vegetables, reducing added sugars and refined grains, and choosing whole foods over highly processed foods. Registered dieticians can help assess a person's overall nutritional status and help formulate a sustainable diet plan. Dietary approaches that may prove beneficial for many people with T2DM and obesity are Mediterranean-style, vegetarian or plant-based, and low-carbohydrate diets. The best available evidence supports that reducing carbohydrate intake improves blood glucose levels in individuals with diabetes. Low-carbohydrate and very low-carbohydrate eating patterns are not recommended for pregnant or lactating women, those with or at risk of disordered eating, and those with renal disease. Additional caution with a low-carbohydrate diet should also be taken by those on SGLT-2 inhibitors because of the potential risk of triggering euglycemic ketoacidosis.

13. **How much of a calorie deficit is needed for weight loss?**
Research has not delineated the optimal percentage of calories from proteins, fats, and carbohydrates for people with diabetes. Meaningful weight reduction can be achieved with lifestyle programs that maintain an energy deficit of 500 to 750 kcal/day. For the general population, this is a target intake of around 1200–1500 kcal/day for women and 1500–1800 kcal/day for men, adjusted for the individual's baseline body weight. Weight loss of just 3% to 5% of body weight can have significant health benefits. People should strive to achieve a healthy, sustainable weight that is deemed safe. Programs that promote more significant energy deficits should be monitored with a healthcare professional's support when possible.

14. **What does the ADA recommend regarding the use of weight-loss medications in people with type 2 diabetes?**
Antiobesity medications are useful in combination with diet, physical activity, and behavioral counseling to achieve energy deficits for certain individuals with T2DM and a BMI of $\geq$27 kg/m². If weight loss of at least 5% body weight is not achieved in the first 3 to 4 months (minimum trial period), the medication should be stopped, and another weight-loss medication or a different treatment approach should be considered. The clinician and individual will need to weigh the risks versus benefits of starting, continuing, or stopping antiobesity medications. Importantly, antiobesity drugs are used as an adjunct to lifestyle modification; people who are provided regular behavioral support are more likely to have better weight-loss outcomes.

15. **What antiobesity medications are available and approved by the U.S. Food and Drug Administration (FDA) for long-term use?**
   - Orlistat (Xenical, Alli)
   - Phentermine plus topiramate ER (Qsymia)
   - Naltrexone plus bupropion SR (Contrave)
   - Liraglutide 3.0 mg (Saxenda)—approved for people who do not have diabetes

16. **Discuss phentermine and its role in weight management**
Phentermine is the most frequently prescribed weight-loss medication in the United States. It is FDA approved to be taken only for 3 months at a time; however, it is often used off-label in a continuous fashion. Usual doses of phentermine range from 15 to 37.5 mg/day. An 8-mg formulation has more recently become available, to be taken 3 times daily before meals. Phentermine is a sympathomimetic amine and anorectic agent that works by reducing appetite. Average weight loss typically is 5% to 6% of body weight and is dose dependent. Some of the typical side effects reported are tachycardia, tremors, restlessness, overstimulation, headache, hypertension, and difficulty sleeping. Phentermine should not be used in people with uncontrolled hypertension or pulmonary hypertension. Blood pressure should be monitored closely in those who take this medication. In low-risk individuals, phentermine has been used for more than 12 months with an observed weight loss of 7.4%.

17. **Explain the expected weight loss, side effects, and costs associated with antiobesity medications**
See Table 26.1.

18. **What is the typical course of weight loss for someone on a weight-loss medication?**
It is expected that most weight loss will occur in the first 3 to 4 months while on an antiobesity medication, and results during that time frame are the only predictor of future success on the drug. It is suggested that people taking weight loss medications be seen by their provider monthly for the first 3 months to assess efficacy and safety and at least every 3 to 6 months thereafter. If <5% of total body weight is lost in the first 3 to 4 months, the medication should be stopped. Pharmacotherapy for weight loss works only while the medication is being taken. It is highly probable that a person will regain the weight lost once the medication is stopped, which is why long-term use for weight-loss maintenance should be encouraged and discussed early. In clinical trials, orlistat, naltrexone/bupropion SR, liraglutide 3.0 mg, and phentermine/topiramate ER resulted in $\geq$5% weight loss in 21%, 35%, 36%, and 41% to 49% of trial participants, respectively. Phentermine/topiramate ER use was most likely to result in $\geq$10% weight loss, with 30% to 40% of people reaching that goal in trials.

19. **Explain the use of orlistat for weight management**
Orlistat is a reversible inhibitor of gastrointestinal lipases. At the prescription strength of 120 mg 3 times a day with meals, it reduces the absorption of dietary fat by approximately 30% by inhibiting the enzymes responsible for fat digestion. Orlistat is not advised for those with chronic malabsorption syndromes or cholestasis. The average weight loss reported is about 5% to 8%. This medication may be preferred in people with mood disorders, heart disease, or poorly controlled hypertension. A 60-mg form is available over the counter; the lower dose reduces dietary fat absorption by 25%. This strength is less effective than the prescription strength, resulting in weight loss of roughly 2% to 4%. Reported adverse events for orlistat (incidence of $\geq$5% and twice that of placebo) are fatty/oily stools, flatus with discharge, fecal urgency, and fecal incontinence. People using orlistat should be advised to take a daily multivitamin containing fat-soluble vitamins.

20. **Explain the use of phentermine plus topiramate extended-release (PHEN/TPM) for weight management**
In clinical trials, subjects taking PHEN/TPM had a mean weight loss of 8% to 10% body weight. The recommended dose is phentermine 7.5 mg plus topiramate ER 46 mg once daily. A higher dosage of phentermine 15 mg plus topiramate ER 92 mg is also available for those who do not lose $\geq$ 5% in the first 3 months on the initial dose. The quick-release phentermine starts working immediately, reducing appetite. The extended-release topiramate releases throughout the day, promoting satiety. PHEN/TPM stimulates the neurotransmitter

Table 26.1 Antiobesity Medications

AGENT	MECHANISM OF ACTION	TYPICAL MAINTENANCE DOSE	AVERAGE PRICE FOR 30-DAY SUPPLY[a]	WEIGHT LOSS[b]	KEY POINTS
Phentermine	Sympathomimetic amineanorectic	8–37.5 mg daily	$39 ($4)	5%–6%	Approved for short-term use, monitor BP
Orlistat	Lipase inhibitor	60 mg TID (OTC); 120 mg TID (Rx)	OTC (Alli): ~$60; Rx (Xenical): $765 ($700)	2%–4%, 5%–8%	A lower dose available OTC, GI side effects
Naltrexone/ bupropion ER	Opioid antagonist/ antidepressant combination	16 mg/180 mg BID	$339 ($285)	5%	Intermediate in effectiveness and side effects (nausea/ vomiting)
Liraglutide 3.0 mg	GLP-1 receptor agonist	3.0 mg daily	$1500 ($1300)	6%	Intermediate effectiveness and side effects, ?CVD benefit, very high cost
Phentermine/ topiramate ER	Sympathomimetic amine anorectic/ antiepileptic combination	7.5–15 mg/ 46–92 mg daily	$232 ($192)	8%–10%	Most effective, intermediate side effects

BP, blood pressure; *CVD*, cardiovascular disease; *ER*, extended release; *GI*, gastrointestinal; *GLP-1*, glucagon-like peptide-1; *OTC*, over the counter; *Rx*, prescription.
[a]Average retail price (discounted price) as listed on GoodRx the week of October 16, 2020
[b]One-year efficacy, difference versus placebo ($P < 0.05$ for all).
From Drugs@FDA. <http://www.accessdata.fda.gov/Scripts/cder/DrugsatFDA/>; and U.S. Food and Drug Administration. Safety alerts for human medical products. <https://www.fda.gov/safety/medwatch-fda-safety-information-and-adverse-event-reporting-program/medical-product-safety-information>

gamma-aminobutyric acid (GABA), which may also suppress appetite and enhance satiety. PHEN/TPM cannot be used during pregnancy or when planning pregnancy because fetuses exposed to topiramate during the first trimester are at increased risk of cleft lip with or without cleft palate. Females of reproductive age should be on contraceptives, should have a negative pregnancy test before starting the medication, and should report monthly pregnancy test results after initiation (as required by the Risk Evaluation and Mitigation Strategy [REMS] program for this medication). The medication cannot be used in people with glaucoma, hyperthyroidism, or a history of kidney stones. Weaning off this medication is recommended when the decision is made to discontinue it. The most common reported drug side effect is paresthesias. This medication also has the potential to cause cognitive and mood-related adverse effects.

21. **Discuss the use of naltrexone plus bupropion sustained-release for weight management**
    Bupropion is a dopamine and norepinephrine reuptake inhibitor that stimulates proopiomelanocortin (POMC) neurons. When bupropion is combined with naltrexone (an opioid antagonist), it helps regulate feelings of pleasure when eating to control cravings. In the hypothalamus, these medications work synergistically to reduce hunger. In the COR-1 study, 62% of people taking naltrexone plus bupropion achieved ≥5% total body weight loss versus 23% of those taking placebo. This medication has a 4-week titration with a final dose of 16 mg naltrexone plus 180 mg bupropion twice daily. The most common side effect is nausea (32%), which tends to improve with time, followed by constipation, headache, and vomiting. The medication should not be used in people with uncontrolled hypertension, angle-closure glaucoma, seizure disorders, anorexia or bulimia, drug or alcohol withdrawal, or the use of monoamine oxidase inhibitors or chronic opioids. This medication has the potential for mood-related adverse effects. It should not be taken with high-fat meals because this increases bupropion and naltrexone absorption, resulting in lowering of the seizure threshold.

22. **Explain the use of liraglutide 3.0 mg for weight management**

    The first FDA-approved GLP-1 RA for weight management is liraglutide 3.0 mg. It is delivered via an injection pen once daily. GLP-1 is a native gut hormone released in response to food and acts as a regulator of hunger in the hypothalamus. Participants in a 1-year study lost an average of 6% of total body weight. Gastrointestinal side effects, such as nausea and constipation, are the most commonly reported. There is also an increased risk of pancreatitis. This medication should be avoided if the individual has a personal or family history of medullary thyroid cancer and/or multiple endocrine neoplasia type 2. Liraglutide 3.0 mg is not indicated for treating T2DM or for use with insulin.

23. **What is the role of metabolic surgery in the management of people with type 2 diabetes?**

    Individuals should be considered for weight-loss surgery if they do not achieve durable weight loss and improved obesity-related comorbidities (including hyperglycemia) with nonsurgical methods. Metabolic surgery should be recommended as a choice to treat T2DM in optimal surgical candidates with a BMI of $\geq$40 kg/m^2 (BMI $\geq$ 37.5 kg/m^2 in some Asians) and considered in those with a BMI of 35.0 to 39.9 kg/m^2 (32.5–37.4 kg/m^2 in some Asians). Surgery can also be suggested as an option for people with a BMI of 30.0 to 34.9 kg/m^2 (27.5–32.4 kg/m^2 in some Asians). When considering surgery for weight loss, the individual should be evaluated for comorbid psychological conditions and other mental health issues that may interfere with postsurgical outcomes.

24. **How effective is metabolic surgery for the treatment of type 2 diabetes?**

    A considerable amount of evidence from randomized controlled trials (RCTs; nonblinded) shows that metabolic surgery achieves superior blood glucose control and reduces CVD risk in people with T2DM and obesity compared with several lifestyle and medical therapies. Sleeve gastrectomy (SG) and Roux-en-Y gastric bypass (RYGB) are now the most commonly performed types of metabolic surgery. RYGB tends to result in more significant weight loss and T2DM remission but higher rates of major short-term complications than SG. The RCTs have reported T2DM remission during postoperative follow-up from 1 to 5 years in 30% to 63% of people following RYGB. The average diabetes-free period after RYGB is 8.3 years.

25. **What other weight-management therapies are emerging or under development for people with type 2 diabetes?**

    The FDA has approved several minimally invasive medical devices, such as gastric balloons, for short-term weight loss in people with obesity. Drawbacks are high out-of-pocket costs, low insurance coverage, and insufficient data in people with T2DM. Medical devices for weight loss are not considered the standard of care for obesity management in individuals with T2DM. Tirzepatide, now in clinical trials, is a dual GLP-1 RA and glucose-dependent insulinotropic polypeptide (GIP) receptor agonist. This drug is designed to promote more significant weight loss and hemoglobin A1c lowering than a GLP-1 RA alone but is not FDA approved at this time. A large international CVD outcome trial evaluating semaglutide in people with obesity is also under way.

KEY POINTS

1. The majority of people with type 2 diabetes also have comorbid obesity, and various management options exist to simultaneously improve both of these conditions.
2. Antihyperglycemic agents may result in weight gain, weight loss, or weight stability. Discussions with individuals about the impact of different agents on their weight during the treatment of diabetes are of paramount importance.
3. Several antiobesity medications are FDA approved for long-term use and often produce 5% to 10% weight loss when used as an adjunct to lifestyle modification.
4. Bariatric surgery is the treatment modality that is most effective at producing long-term weight loss and type 2 diabetes remission.

BIBLIOGRAPHY

1. Apovian CM, Aronne LJ, Bessesen DH, et al. Pharmacological management of obesity: an endocrine Society clinical practice guideline. *J Clin Endocrinol Metab.* 2015;100(2):342–362.
2. American Diabetes Association 8. Obesity management for the treatment of type 2 diabetes: Standards of Medical Care in Diabetes-2019. *Diabetes Care.* 2019;42(Suppl 1):S81–S89.
3. Arterburn D, Wellman R, Emiliano A, et al. PCORnet bariatric study collaborative. comparative effectiveness and safety of bariatric procedures for weight loss: A PCORnet cohort study. *Ann Intern Med.* 2018 Dec 4;169(11):741–750.
4. Centers for Disease Control and Prevention *National Diabetes Statistics Report, 2020.* Atlanta, GA: Centers for Disease Control and Prevention, U.S. Dept of Health and Human Services; 2020. Available at: https://www.cdc.gov/diabetes/data/statistics-report/index.html.
5. Domecq JP, Prutsky G, Leppin A, et al. Clinical review: drugs commonly associated with weight change: a systematic review and meta-analysis. *J Clin Endocrinol Metab.* 2015 Feb;100(2):363–370.
6. Hales CM, Carroll MD, Fryar CD, Ogden CL. *Prevalence of obesity and severe obesity among adults: United States, 2017–2018. NCHS Data Brief, no 360.* Hyattsville, MD: National Center for Health Statistics; 2020.
7. Khera R, Murad MH, Chandar AK, et al. Association of pharmacological treatments for obesity with weight loss and adverse events: a systematic review and meta-analysis. *JAMA.* 2016 Jun 14;315(22):2424–2434.
8. Lewis KH, Fischer H, Ard J, et al. Safety and effectiveness of longer-term phentermine use: clinical outcomes from an electronic health record cohort. *Obesity (Silver Spring).* 2019;27(4):591–602.

CHAPTER 27

IDENTIFYING AND OVERCOMING BARRIERS TO ACHIEVING GLUCOSE CONTROL

Sara Wettergreen, PharmD, BCACP, and Jennifer M. Trujillo, PharmD, BCPS, FCCP, CDCES, BC-ADM

1. **What are the main barriers to achieving glucose control?**
   Despite major advances in the treatment of diabetes, including an abundance of new medications and technologies, there has been no measurable improvement in glycemic control in the last two decades. Clinical and therapeutic inertia are at the root of the problem. *Clinical inertia* is defined as the lack of adherence to guideline recommendations when appropriate to do so. *Therapeutic inertia* is defined as failure to advance therapy or de-intensify therapy when appropriate to do so. Drivers of clinical and/or therapeutic inertia are complex and often divided into three categories: provider related, patient related, and health-system related.

   Provider-related barriers to achieving glucose control include insufficient time or support staff to manage diabetes effectively, lack of knowledge or confidence in applying guidelines, lack of training or experience with newer medications or technologies, overestimation of quality of care, and the use of soft excuses to avoid intensifying therapy. System-related barriers include insufficient time or resources devoted to implementing effective diabetes care initiatives, lack of team-based care, lack of decision support tools and workflow models, lack of patient outreach, and the disconnect between what is recommended in the guidelines and what is reimbursed in practice. Patient-related barriers include concerns regarding medication side effects, fear of hypoglycemia and weight gain, cost constraints, regimen complexity, the burden of self-management, nonadherence, and lack of appropriate education and training, in addition to social determinants of health (SDOH), including access to care and the psychosocial factors of depression and health literacy.

2. **What can you do to overcome therapeutic inertia?**
   Assess your entire population of patients with diabetes using the electronic health record. Identify how many have a glycosylated hemoglobin (A1c) above goal with no recent visit or therapy change and how many have never had diabetes education. This information can help you evaluate therapy delays in your practice. Also, engage with your patients in real time. For example, point-of-care A1c testing allows you to make treatment decisions during a visit rather than after. Schedule "diabetes only" visits, and remind patients to bring glucometers, logbooks, and medication lists with them. Screen for barriers such as diabetes distress, depression, low health literacy, and SDOH. Collaborate with patients to set individualized A1c goals, and adjust the therapy plan when the goal is not met. Schedule follow-up appointments based on the patient's A1c level, and aim for more frequent visits for patients not at goal. Lastly, refer patients for diabetes education whenever possible.

3. **What factors are associated with nonadherence?**
   Adherence has a significant impact on the effectiveness of a treatment plan and includes adherence to medications and diabetes self-management behaviors. Medication adherence becomes a greater challenge with more complex medication regimens and polypharmacy.

   Factors contributing to nonadherence include patient demographics, beliefs about medications, and regimen-related challenges. Demographics associated with medication nonadherence include low health literacy and low income level, and individuals with these characteristics may need additional adherence support.

   Beliefs about the medication regimen can influence medication adherence. This includes general beliefs about medications or beliefs about a patient's specific medications. For example, the perceived efficacy of a regimen can affect medication adherence. Beliefs about medications can be positively influenced by a strong patient–provider relationship and education about the medication regimen.

   Regimen-related factors also influence medication adherence in diabetes, including tolerability, cost concerns, and the complexity of the treatment regimen. Nonadherence with injectable therapies may be a result of fear of needles, pain with administration, the amount of time needed to inject, and concerns for hypoglycemia or weight gain.

4. **How can you screen for nonadherence?**

In routine interactions with patients, asking about adherence in an open-ended, nonjudgmental way can identify medication nonadherence. For example, you may ask, "How many times did you miss a dose of your medication in the last week?" You can also assess medication adherence through a review of refill history, if available. The refill history will not confirm that the patient is taking the medication as prescribed; however, this may give some insight into the patient's medication habits.

5. **What are methods to overcome nonadherence?**

Patients face unique barriers to adherence; thus, there is no single solution to overcome nonadherence.

The five *E*s is a helpful tool that providers can use to assist patients in overcoming medication nonadherence.

1. *Entry:* Help patients to access medications by overcoming insurance-coverage and cost-related barriers.
2. *Explain:* Explain the purpose and potential benefits of medications, and make efforts to simplify the medication regimen whenever possible.
3. *Engage:* Use shared decision making to engage patients in care decisions.
4. *Empower:* Empower patients to self-manage diabetes because this can improve adherence to both medications and behavioral modifications.
5. *Encourage:* Anticipate setbacks, and encourage patients to overcome them.

Even when patients are motivated to take their medications regularly, imperfect adherence is expected. Simple and inexpensive strategies to help with adherence include using a pillbox and storing medications in an easily accessible area as a reminder to take them. Alarm reminders, such as a mobile phone alarm or a traditional alarm clock, are helpful for more simple medication regimens. Mobile apps with reminders are helpful for those with more complex medication regimens, such as MyMedSchedule and PillManager.

6. **How does the patient–provider relationship affect adherence? What communication strategies can support adherence?**

Only about one-third of patients report positive experiences with their diabetes care provider. The provider's communication style can affect the patient–provider relationship and, ultimately, a patient's adherence to a treatment plan.

Clear communication ensures patients know what to expect from their treatment plan and allows patients the opportunity to ask questions. When patients feel the provider's communication is rushed, this results in greater diabetes distress and poor adherence to medication and self-management behaviors. Contrastingly, communication that displays compassion and optimism can positively affect coping abilities.

Simple efforts to enhance empathy within an encounter are explained by the acronym EMPATHY:

- Eye contact: Make meaningful eye contact.
- Muscles of facial expression: A relaxed expression can ease the patient.
- Posture: Get to the patient's eye level and lean in slightly; show openness (e.g., arms uncrossed).
- Affect: Assess the patient's affective state. Consider reflecting your assessment for confirmation. For example, "It sounds like you are hesitant to start taking insulin for your diabetes."
- Tone of voice: Speak in a calm, reassuring tone.
- Hearing the whole patient: Actively listen, and show nonverbal cues of acknowledgment.
- Your response: Use reflective responses to show you are listening.

Although these approaches to communication are important, so is engaging patients in their care. The shared decision-making method is a partnership between the provider and patient, where the provider shares and discussions options and allows patients to choose their plan of care. Engaging patients in their care through shared decision making can improve adherence to a treatment plan.

7. **How can the healthcare team enhance patients' motivation to improve their diabetes?**

Even when patients know exactly what to do to improve control of their diabetes and have the tools to do so, low motivation can prevent successful implementation of the care plan. Communication strategies can help empower patients to make behavioral modifications and to encourage patients to overcome any barriers that arise.

Multiple communication strategies can support patients in making behavioral changes; two examples include empowerment-based communication and motivational interviewing. In empowerment-based communication, the clinician helps the patient to explore and self-identify areas to change through a five-step protocol: explore the problem, clarify feelings and their meaning, create a plan, commit to the plan, and evaluate results.

Contrastingly, motivational interviewing is clinician driven, where a provider directs questions to drive ambivalence toward the direction of change. In this model, providers are encouraged to roll with resistance to change. Providers should look for cues of change talk and focus on these as drivers toward change.

Both of these communication strategies take skill and practice. Additional training is useful for mastering empowerment-based communication and motivational interviewing in practice.

8. **How do SDOH affect glucose control?**

SDOH are the conditions in the environments where people are born, live, learn, work, play, and worship that affect a wide range of health, functioning, and quality-of-life outcomes. SDOH are grouped into five domains: economic stability, education access and quality, healthcare access and quality, neighborhood and built environment, and social and community context. Each of these factors can negatively affect glucose control. Most obviously, financial stress can result in an inability to afford medications and supplies, food insecurity, and the need to limit medical appointments, all of which can lead to poor glucose control. In a study using data from the National Health Interview Survey, one-half of adults with diabetes reported financial stress, and one-fifth reported food insecurity. Food insecurity is directly associated with poor glucose control when patients stretch their budget by purchasing inexpensive, carbohydrate-rich processed foods or when they binge eat after going without food. Furthermore, hypoglycemia can occur when meals are erratic. In addition to the affordability of healthy foods, you should also consider your patient's access to healthy foods, especially for those patients with limited transportation. The U.S. Department of Agriculture (USDA) identifies and maps food deserts throughout the country in which healthy and affordable foods are not available within a 1-mile radius in urban centers or a 10-mile radius in rural areas. Low-income patients may also suffer from housing insecurity or homelessness, which can result in lost or stolen medications and supplies or inappropriate medication-storage conditions. Patients with diabetes and unstable housing are at a much higher risk of diabetes-related emergency department visits or hospitalizations. Language barriers and health literacy are other determinants that affect glucose control. Patients who do not speak English or speak English as their second language face many challenges in navigating the healthcare system, communicating with healthcare providers, and self-managing diabetes.

9. **How do you identify or screen for SDOH?**

SDOH are often unrecognized or underappreciated but have a large impact on successful diabetes management. Screening for SDOH will depend on your practice setting and patient population. System-based mechanisms may help overcome structural barriers and more systematically identify SDOH that should be addressed. Validated screening tools for some SDOH, including food insecurity, homelessness, and limited literacy, can identify overlooked issues and prompt appropriate treatment considerations. Providers working in a low-income community or a federally qualified health center should place greater emphasis on the thorough screening of all patients. Higher rates of food insecurity exist within low-income homes, in single-parent homes, and in all ethnicities besides Caucasian. To screen for food insecurity, the following questions can be asked:
1. "Within the past 12 months, were you worried that food would run out before you got money to buy more?"
2. "Within the past 12 months, did you feel the food you bought did not last and there was no money to buy more?"
   To screen for homelessness, the following questions can be asked:
1. "In the past 2 months, have you been living in stable housing that you own, rent, or stay in as part of a household?"
2. "Are you worried that in the next 2 months, you may not have stable housing that you own, rent, or stay in as part of a household?"

10. **How do you identify or screen for limited health literacy?**

One of the most widely used screening tools for identifying limited health literacy skills is the Newest Vital Sign (NVS), which is available at https://www.pfizer.com/health/literacy/public-policy-researchers/nvs-toolkit. To administer the NVS, the patient is given a nutrition label from a container of ice cream and asked six questions about the label. Correct responses require the ability to interpret text and perform basic math calculations. A score of 0 to 1 is a strong predictor of limited health literacy, a score of 2 to 3 indicates a possibility of limited health literacy, and a score of 4 to 6 almost always indicates adequate health literacy. The assessment takes 2 to 3 minutes to complete.

11. **What are methods to overcome SDOH barriers to glucose control?**

You should consider community-level, system-level, and patient-level solutions to reduce SDOH barriers to glucose control. At the patient level, simply identifying SDOH and considering those factors when making treatment decisions is crucial. You can aim to reduce language barriers by using picture infographics, using a language translation line, and involving the patient's home support system, when available. For those with food insecurity, you can seek local resources that may help patients more regularly obtain nutritious food. System-level structures should be in place to screen for SDOH and support patients who require assistance through a coordinated process with primary care, behavioral health, and social services. In some cases, healthcare facilities can partner with community groups that aid in access to resources. Be sure to have a list of resources available or a care coordinator for your patients when needed.

12. **What are tips to overcome cost-related barriers to accessing medications?**

Cost-related challenges are common in patients with diabetes. In a survey of adults with diabetes in the United States, about half of participants reported financial stress related to managing diabetes, with contributing factors being high out-of-pocket costs for medications and provider visits, in addition to food insecurity.

The Association of Diabetes Care and Education Specialists (ADCES) has helpful access and affordability resources on its website. These include insulin and noninsulin diabetes medication cost-savings resources. ADCES also has a tip sheet to help patients afford their medications. Some of the key takeaways for cost savings include the following:

- Maximize coverage from insurance benefits:
  - Assist Medicare-eligible patients with enrolling in Medicare Part D, and be aware of the potential to reach a coverage gap. Medicare also has a financial assistance program called Extra Help for those who qualify.
  - Depending on the insurance plan, patients may have copay savings when filling prescriptions for a 90-day supply compared with a 30-day supply. Use the pharmacies preferred by the insurance plan.
  - Select medications that are preferred on the patient's insurance formulary.
- Use additional noninsurance resources: These resources can be used for those with insurance and are particularly helpful for the uninsured or underinsured. Many databases are available online that help patients and providers identify eligibility for patient-assistance programs, including Partnership for Prescription Assistance, RxAssist, and Needy Meds. In addition to manufacturer copay cards, other coupons and discounts may be available from sources such as GoodRx.com, RxPharmacyCoupons.com, and Rebates.com.
- Generic Medication Use: When cost and coverage are limited, the use of lower-cost generic medications may be the only option. Consider checking prices between different pharmacies to find the lowest-cost option available, such as on GoodRx.com.

13. **What strategies are helpful when communicating with patients who have lower health literacy?**
When explaining the use of a medication and providing education about diabetes self-management behaviors, it is important to communicate at a level appropriate for the patient's health literacy. The Agency for Healthcare Research and Quality (AHRQ) provides recommendations for communicating with patients of lower health literacy through both verbal and written methods.

When verbally communicating with patients, you should display a warm demeanor, make appropriate eye contact, and actively listen to the patient. Avoid the use of medical terminology, and speak slowly to ensure understanding. Repeat key messages. Use simple pictures and visual aids, when available.

When teaching manual activities, such as the administration technique for an injectable medication, demonstrate the process to the patient first, allowing for questions and patient participation. After answering questions, use the teach-back method to ensure patient understanding. This method confirms the patient understands a process or information by asking the patient to repeat or demonstrate back what was taught. The use of the teach-back method might sound like, for example, "To make sure that I explained this information correctly, can you show me the process you would use to inject your insulin?"

It is also important to ensure written patient education materials are at an appropriate health literacy level. You should discuss written materials with patients within a visit whenever possible. Consider circling or highlighting the most important items that the patient should focus on within the written materials. Provide a method for patients to ask follow-up questions after the visit.

14. **How do psychosocial factors affect glucose control?**
Psychosocial factors that affect glucose control include environmental, social, behavioral, and emotional factors. More specifically, you will want to consider the patient's socioeconomic and cultural context of diabetes self-management; their knowledge and beliefs about diabetes and its treatment; their behavioral skills, including coping, self-control, and self-regulation; their mental health; and their cognitive function. Psychosocial and social problems can impair the individual's ability to carry out diabetes self-management tasks and could negatively affect glucose control.

15. **How do you identify and screen for psychosocial barriers to glucose control?**
The American Diabetes Association Standards of Medical Care recommend that psychosocial screening should include attitudes about diabetes, expectations for medical management and outcomes, affect or mood, diabetes-related quality of life, available resources, and psychiatric history. In addition, patients should be assessed for symptoms of diabetes distress, depression, anxiety, disordered eating, and cognitive capacities using standardized and validated screening tools. A description of these tools is available in Chapter 2. Providers can start with informal verbal inquiries about changes in mood over the last 2 weeks and new or different barriers to treatment or self-management, such as feeling overwhelmed or stressed by having diabetes.

16. **What are methods to overcome psychosocial barriers to glucose control?**
Psychosocial care should be integrated within a collaborative, patient-centered approach. Your patients' perceptions about their own self-efficacy to manage their diabetes are directly related to outcomes. Decision-making education and skill-building programs have demonstrated improvement in glucose control. Routine monitoring and screening will help guide you to appropriate and timely referrals to ensure the patient is thoroughly managed. Collaborative care and a whole-team approach can ensure that your patient is well supported by a variety

of healthcare professionals. In the case of patients who face barriers related to SDOH or psychosocial factors, you should emphasize the importance of follow-up appointments. Consistent contact with the care team will allow patients to feel empowered to take charge of their own healthcare.

KEY POINTS

1. There are many potential barriers to achieving glucose control, with the root of the problem stemming from clinical and therapeutic inertia.
2. The healthcare team should engage with patients through shared decision making, communicate at an appropriate level for the patient's health literacy, and express empathy and compassion for patients.
3. The impact of SDOH and psychosocial factors on glycemic control can be significant, yet these barriers are often underappreciated. Providers should routinely screen patients for SDOH and psychosocial barriers using validated screening questions or tools.
4. Patients may struggle to overcome their individual barriers to achieving glucose control. Acknowledge these challenges and connect patients with resources to help as they seek to overcome these barriers.

BIBLIOGRAPHY

American Diabetes Association. Getting to goal: Overcoming therapeutic inertia in diabetes care. Available at: http://www.professional. diabetes.org/sites/professional.diabetes.org/files/media/overcoming_therapeutic_inertia_factsheet_final.pdf. Accessed October 4, 2020.
American Diabetes Association. Summary of proceedings of the American Diabetes Association Summit "Overcoming therapeutic inertia: Accelerating diabetes care for life." Available at: http://www.professional.diabetes.org/sites/professional.diabetes.org/files/media/ ada_therapeutic/inertia/interior/final.pdf. Accessed October 4, 2020.
American Diabetes Association. 1. Improving care and promoting health in populations: Standards of medical care in diabetes – 2021. *Diabetes Care.* 2021;44(Suppl 1):S7–S14.
American Diabetes Association. 5. Facilitating behavior change and well-being to improve health outcomes: Standards of medical care in diabetes – 2021. *Diabetes Care.* 2021;44(Suppl 1):S53–S72.
Association of Diabetes Care and Education Specialists. Access and affordability resources. Available at: https://www.diabeteseducator. org/living-with-diabetes/Tools-and-Resources/affordability-resources. Accessed September 12, 2020.
Brega AG, Barnard J, Mabachi NM, Weiss BD, DeWalt DA, Brach C, Cifuentes M, Albright K, West DR. AHRQ Health Literacy Universal Precautions Toolkit, Second Edition. (Prepared by Colorado Health Outcomes Program, University of Colorado Anschutz Medical Campus under Contract No. HHSA290200710008, TO#10.) AHRQ Publication No. 15-0023-EF. Rockville, MD. Agency for Healthcare Research and Quality. January 2015.
Cramer JA, Roy A, Burrell A, et al. Medication Compliance and Persistence: Terminology and Definitions. *Value in Health.* 2008;11(1):44–47.
Fisher L, Polonsky WH, Hessler D, Potter MB. A practical framework for encouraging and supporting positive behaviour change in diabetes. *Diabet Med.* 2017;34(12):1658–1666. https://doi.org/10.1111/dme.13414.
Gabbay RA, Kendall D, Beebe C, et al. Addressing therapeutic inertia in 2020 and beyond: A 3-year initiative of the American Diabetes Association. *Clinical Diabetes.* 2020;Aug. https://doi.org/10.2337/cd20-0053.
Healthy People 2030, U.S. Department of Health and Human Services, Office of Disease Prevention and Health Promotion. Available at: https://health.gov/healthypeople/objectives-and-data/social-determinants-health. Accessed October 4, 2020.
Khunti S, Khunti K, Seidu S. Therapeutic inertia in type 2 diabetes: prevalence, causes, consequences and methods to overcome inertia. *Ther Adv Endocrinol Metab.* 2019 May 3. https://doi.org/10.1177/2042018819844694.
Linetzky B, Jiang D, Funnell MM, Curtis BH, Polonsky WH. Exploring the role of the patient-physician relationship on insulin adherence and clinical outcomes in type 2 diabetes: Insights from the MOSAIc study. *J Diabetes.* 2017;9(6):596–605. https://doi.org/10.1111/1753-0407.12443.
Litterbach E, Holmes-Truscott E, Pouwer F, Speight J, Hendrieckx C. 'I wish my health professionals understood that it's not just all about your HbA1c!'. Qualitative responses from the second Diabetes MILES - Australia (MILES-2) study. *Diabet Med.* 2020;37(6): 971–981. https://doi.org/10.1111/dme.14199.
Patel MR, Piette JD, Resnicow K, Kowalski-Dobson T, Heisler M. Social determinants of health, cost-related nonadherence, and cost-reducing behaviors among adults with diabetes: Findings from the national health interview survey. *Medical Care.* 2016;54:796–803.
Polonsky WH, Henry RR. Poor medication adherence in type 2 diabetes: recognizing the scope of the problem and its key contributors. *Patient Prefer Adherence.* 2016;10:1299–1307. Published 2016 Jul 22. https://doi.org/10.2147/PPA.S106821.
Riess H, Kraft-Todd G. E.M.P.A.T.H.Y.: a tool to enhance nonverbal communication between clinicians and their patients. *Acad Med.* 2014;89(8):1108–1112. https://doi.org/10.1097/ACM.0000000000000287.
Swe K, Reddy SSK. Improving Adherence in Type 2 Diabetes. *Clin Geriatr Med.* 2020;36(3):477–489. https://doi.org/10.1016/j. cger.2020.04.007.
Young-Hyman D, de Groot M, Hill-Briggs F, et al. Psychosocial care for people with diabetes: a position statement of the American Diabetes Association. *Diabetes Care.* 2016;39:2126–2140.

CHAPTER 28

DIABETES IN AFRICA

Abdurezak Ahmed Abdela, MD, and Helen Yifter Bitew, MD

1. **How prevalent is diabetes in Africa?**

   Low- and middle-income countries carry the major burden of diabetes worldwide. Eighty percent of people with diabetes live in these countries. The International Diabetes Federation (IDF) Africa region has more than 19.4 million people with diabetes (prevalence of 3.9%), and this number will increase 143% by 2045. However, considering that North Africa is not an IDF Africa region, the actual number of people with diabetes in the African continent is much higher than the number just reported. In addition, 60% of diabetes in Africa is undiagnosed, making this the highest percentage of undiagnosed people with diabetes in the world. There is a significant prevalence variation across different regions and countries within Africa, ranging from 0.8% in Benin to 14.2% in Seychelles. The top four countries with the highest number of people with diabetes, according to the recent IDF report, are South Africa (4.6 million), Nigeria (2.7 million), Democratic Republic of Congo (DRC; 1.8 million), and Ethiopia (1.7 million). The four most populous sub-Saharan African countries (Nigeria, Ethiopia, DRC, South Africa) have varying diabetes prevalence rates of 3.0%, 3.2%, 4.8%, and 12.8%, respectively, among adults 20 to 79 years old.

   Among risk factors, a high prevalence of HIV and combined antiretroviral therapy (cART) may contribute to the increased diabetes prevalence in sub-Saharan Africa as a result of ongoing inflammation and inherent mechanisms of cART despite achieving undetectable HIV viral levels. Moreover, because patients with diabetes are more prone to tuberculosis (TB), the next epidemic of TB cases in the region may be related to the increasing prevalence of diabetes.

   In the African region, an estimated 25,800 children and adolescents under the age of 20 years are living with type 1 diabetes; this is believed to be an underestimate.

2. **What are the peculiarities seen among Africans with type 1 diabetes?**

   Although it is difficult to make generalizations about an entire continent and its people, a few peculiarities can be observed among Africans. Some studies suggest that the frequency of antibody positivity in type 1 diabetes is lower than that reported in American or European populations (7%–44% vs. 80%–97%). One hypothesis for low antibody positivity with type 1 diabetes in Africa is the existence of malnutrition-related or malnutrition-modified diabetes (MRDM) as a cause of insulin-requiring diabetes. Some epidemiologic issues include later average age of onset (by about a decade), male predominance, and poor socioeconomic status correlated with higher risk.

3. **What is MRDM?**

   Although MRDM is not listed in the current classification of diabetes, it is common in parts of sub-Saharan Africa and Asia. MRDM was listed as a type 1 diabetes subtype in the World Health Organization (WHO) 1985 classification but was later removed, citing insufficient evidence. The two forms of MRDM are fibrocalcific pancreatic diabetes (FCPD) and protein-deficient pancreatic diabetes (PDPD), also known as *Jamaica* or *J-type*. The insulin requirements of patients with MRDM are reported to be higher than those in patients with typical type 1 diabetes. African patients' insulin requirements tend to be less than those of Indian or Jamaican patients.

4. **What are the features of MRDM in Africa?**

   The features suggestive of MRDM are onset before 30 years of age, body mass index < 19 kg/m^2, absence of ketosis on insulin withdrawal, poor socioeconomic status, history of childhood malnutrition, and insulin requirements > 2 units/kg/day (suggesting insulin resistance). FCPD is diagnosed if, in addition to the items just listed, the person has a history of recurrent abdominal pain from an early age, pancreatic calculi on plain abdominal x-rays, and/or typical changes on ultrasonogram of the pancreas, in the absence of alcoholism, gallstones, or hyperparathyroidism.

5. **Discuss ketosis-prone type 2 diabetes**

   Some people with phenotypic type 2 diabetes present with acute symptoms of severe hyperglycemia with ketosis. This presentation has been described among Africans and African Americans. It is characterized by a strong family history of type 2 diabetes, young adult age, male gender (men 3× > women), rare islet autoimmunity, and high human papilloma virus-8 prevalence. Although insulin is required for the short-term control of diabetes, unlike classic type 2 diabetes, people with ketosis-prone type 2 diabetes can achieve full remission with no need for continuing medical treatment. However, recurrence is possible.

6. **How is a hyperglycemic crisis diagnosed and treated in resource-limited settings?**
   The diagnosis of diabetic ketoacidosis (DKA) is made based on clinical presentation, blood glucose levels, and urine ketones. Serum ketones, arterial blood gas analysis, and serum electrolytes are not readily available. Most setups use hourly regular insulin injections because of a lack of infusers and insulin analogs. This leads to increased complications. Missed doses of regular insulin result in longer times to clear ketones. The long turn-around time to get results from laboratories adds further difficulty in following the DKA protocol. It is also problematic to confirm DKA resolution, which usually results in earlier discontinuation of hourly insulin and hyperglycemic relapses.

7. **How prevalent is gestational diabetes in Africa?**
   There are few studies done in Africa; only 11% of the 54 African countries have prevalence data on gestational diabetes mellitus (GDM). Prevalence reports from one systematic review range from 0% in Tanzania to 13.9% in urban Nigeria. This difference could be attributable to the use of different diagnostic criteria. Many sub-Saharan countries do not have screening and treatment protocols for GDM. In contrast to the standard practice of using insulin, oral agents (metformin and glyburide) are used to treat GDM without increasing reported fetal or maternal complications. Oral agents are preferred because they are relatively inexpensive, less invasive, and require minimal self-monitoring of blood glucose (SMBG).

8. **What is the most common cause of hospital admission for people with type 2 diabetes in Africa?**
   Diabetic foot disease (ulcer and/or gangrene) is the leading cause of hospital admission for people in Africa with type 2 diabetes. Neuropathy is not reported to be the most common cause of foot ulcer; instead, the reported cause for the majority of foot ulcers is "unidentified." Improperly fitting shoes and blunt trauma contribute to one-third of cases. Foot ulcers result in significant morbidity and mortality, accounting for nearly 50% of amputations and more than 20% of hospital mortality.

9. **How is diabetes care organized in Africa, and what are the care gaps?**
   The rate of undiagnosed diabetes in Africa is high. Patients often present late, increasing the likelihood of chronic complications. In many African countries, care is integrated with other services in primary care. However, most centers fail to meet the IDF criteria for resource-limited settings. Care gaps include an insufficient number of healthcare professionals; patient overload; lack of access to diabetes education, basic laboratory testing, and SMBG; and unavailability and affordability of oral and injectable medications.

10. **What options are there to manage diabetes in areas of the world where there are few endocrinologists/diabetologists?**
    A task-shifting/task-sharing approach is increasingly being used in the management of chronic illnesses in areas with few specialized human resources for health. A similar approach is used in the management of diabetes in Africa. Dedicated nurses, health officers/medical officers, general practitioners, and internists are trained to provide comprehensive noncommunicable disease (NCD) care. The fact that task sharing requires continuous support and mentorship from specialists has shaped the role of the endocrinologist in Africa.

11. **What cultural backgrounds must be considered for people with diabetes in Africa?**
    Africa is home to various indigenous tribes with diverse cultural practices and belief systems. Religious belief, fatalism, and cultural (mis)conceptions are used to explain disease causation. Illness is generally perceived to be an acute process. The distinction between illness and disease is blurred at best. Consequently, chronic disease processes like diabetes are poorly understood by patients and communities at large.

12. **How do cultural beliefs and practices affect diabetes care in Africa?**
    Cultural beliefs and practices, which include supernatural, natural, and social explanations, affect health-seeking behavior, acceptability, counseling, adherence to treatment, and outcomes. These factors warrant an understanding of the cultural explanatory models of diabetes that are critical to the design of culturally sensitive and effective interventions in the prevention and treatment of diabetes.

13. **How does diabetes in Africa fit into the Universal Health Coverage (UHC) model of WHO health prioritization?**
    The WHO UHC model, which integrates a person-centric approach that involves all public health functions (prevention to rehabilitation) with equity considerations across the life span, is designed to create opportunities for delivering optimal diabetes care for all populations. However, there must be an investment in building resilient health systems across Africa that are equipped with the necessary workforce and infrastructure to meet and exceed the dire need resulting from NCDs.

14. What are the challenges of implementing standard comprehensive care interventions in Africa?

The lack of cost-effectiveness studies in the region makes proper prioritization of care very difficult. As a result, most countries rely on standard recommendations for treatment. However, weakly financed health systems with a lack of trained personnel and technologies present a huge hindrance to the implementation of standard recommendations. For this reason, countries are encouraged to adopt the limited care recommendations by the IDF, that is, care that seeks to achieve the major objectives of diabetes management, to meet their respective needs.

15. What is the prevalence of acute and chronic complications of diabetes in Africa?

Prevalence data for diabetes complications in sub-Saharan Africa are scarce. Most regional evidence comes from a single center in one country and mostly from older studies. Attributed to decreased awareness among health workers and the community at large, and health system factors, DKA has been reported to have a high incidence, ranging from 7% to 80% in newly diagnosed patients and 25% to 90% in children who have already been diagnosed with diabetes. Because of the lack of adequate diabetes education and SMBG, severe hypoglycemia was in the 25% to 55% range. Many cases of DKA are underreported or misdiagnosed. Recognized as a form of ketosis-prone atypical diabetes (KPDM), DKA is encountered in a higher proportion of African patients with type 2 diabetes, contrary to the global trend; a 2000 report revealed a prevalence of 34%. A recent study in Nigeria reported the incidence of DKA to be 40%, hyperosmolar hyperglycemic state (HHS) to be 3.6%, and mixed forms (DKA + HHS) to be 50.9% among the various hyperglycemic emergencies.

Vascular complications develop sooner after a diabetes diagnosis in sub-Saharan African patients because of delayed diabetes diagnosis. Microvascular complications appear to be higher than in high-income countries; the most common are retinopathy (7%–63%), neuropathy (27%–66%), microalbuminuria (10%–83%), nephropathy (32%–57%), and cataracts (9%–16%). Diabetes-related cardiovascular disease (CVD) complications are reported to be lower than in high-income countries but are clearly on the rise. Among people with type 2 diabetes, 5% to 8% may have CVD, and up to 50% may have echocardiographic abnormalities, including cardiomyopathy. Nearly 15% of people with a stroke have diabetes, and up to 5% of those with diabetes present with cerebrovascular accidents at diagnosis. Peripheral vascular disease prevalence varies across sites from 4% to 28%. Amputations are frequent outcomes in people with diabetic foot ulcers in sub-Saharan Africa. Around a third of amputations have been associated with neuro-ischemic lesions, progressive infection, or both.

In sub-Saharan Africa in 2014, 76.4% of deaths attributed to diabetes occurred in people <60 years of age. This was mainly attributable to late diagnosis and poorer diabetes care in resource-limited settings. The older estimates of diabetes-related mortality of 1.8% in the region need to be interpreted with caution because there is inadequate recording of causes of death despite the high prevalence of diabetes and the inability of many health systems to properly treat diabetes and its complications. A recent IDF report has revealed 6.8% of all-cause mortality in the region to be attributed to diabetes, with the highest percentage (9.1%) of all-cause mortality resulting from diabetes occurring in the age group of 30 to 39 years.

KEY POINTS

1. According to the IDF, the African region will have the highest increase in diabetes among all the continents by 2045.
2. Peculiarities of type 1 diabetes in the African setting include lower antibody positivity, later average age of onset, male predominance, and poor socioeconomic status being correlated with higher risk.
3. Malnutrition-related and ketosis-prone diabetes are peculiar phenotypes of diabetes in Africa.
4. Chronic complications of DM tend to occur earlier and in younger age groups, related to delayed diagnosis and poorer diabetes control.

BIBLIOGRAPHY

1. International Diabetes Federation. *IDF Diabetes Atlas*, 9th ed. Brussels, Belgium
2. Gill GV, Mbanya JC, Ramaiya KL, Tesfaye S. A sub-Saharan African perspective of diabetes. *Diabetologia*. 2009;52:8–16.
3. Chattopadhyay Partha Sarathi, Gupta Sanjib Kumar, Chattopadhyay Rita, Kundu Prabir Kumar, Chakraborti Rabindranath, Chattopadh Martha Diabetes. Malnutrition-Related Diabetes Mellitus (MRDM), Not Diabetes-Related Malnutrition A report on genuine MRDM. *Diabetes Care*. February 1995;18(2).
4. Alemu S, Dessie A, Seid E, Bard E, Lee PT, Trimble ER, Phillips DIW, Parry EHO. Insulin-requiring diabetes in rural Ethiopia: should we reopen the case for malnutrition-related diabetes? *Diabetologia*. 2009;52:1842–1845. https://doi.org/10.1007/s00125-009-1433-3.
5. Abdulkadir J, Mengesha B, Welde Gabriel Z, Keen H, Worku Y, Gebre P, Bekele A, Urga K, Taddesse A-S. The clinical and hormonal (C-peptide and glucagon) profile and liability to ketoacidosis during nutritional rehabilitation in Ethiopian patients with malnutrition-related diabetes mellitus. *Diabetologia*. 1990;33:222–2276.
6. Siraj ES, Gupta M, Scherbaum WA, Yifter H, Ahmed A, Kebede T, Reja A, Abdulkadir J. *Islet-cell associated autoantibody in Ethiopian patients with diabetes Journal of Diabetes and Its Complications*. August 2016;30(6):1039–1042.
7. Macaulay S, Dunger DB, Norris SA. Gestational diabetes mellitus in Africa: a systematic review. *PLoSONE*. 2014;9(6):e97871. https://doi.org/10.1371/journal.pone.00978719.
8. Gizaw M, Harries AD, Ade S, Tayler-Smith K, Ali E, Firdu N, Yifter H. Diabetes mellitus in Addis Ababa, Ethiopia: admissions, complications and outcomes in a large referral hospital. *Public Health Action*. 2015;5(1):74–78.
9. Wondwossen A, Reja A, Amare A. Diabetic foot disease in Ethiopian patients: a hospital based study. *Ethiop J Health Dev*. 2011;25(1):17–21.

10. Rifat Atun, Justine I Davies, Edwin A M Gale, et al. Diabetes in sub-Saharan Africa: from clinical care to health policy The Lancet Diabetes & Endocrinology Commission Vol August 5, 2017.
11. Ahmed AM. Cultural aspects of diabetes mellitus in Sudan. *Practical Diabetes Int.* 2003;20(6):226–229.
12. Abdulrehman Munib Said, Woith Wendy, Jenkins Sheryl, Kossman Susan, Louise Gina. *HunterExploring Cultural Influences of Self-Management of Diabetes in CoastalKenya: An Ethnography Global Qualitative Nursing Research.* 2016;3:1–13. https://doi.org/10.1177/2333393616641825.
13. http://www.who.int/news-room/fact-sheets/detail/noncommunicable-diseases
14. INTERNATIONAL DIABETES FEDERATION, 2012 Clinical Guidelines Task Force Global Guideline for Type 2 Diabetes.
15. Pastakia SD, Pekny CR, Manyara SM, Fischer L. Diabetes in sub-Saharan Africa – from policy to practice to progress: targeting the existing gaps for future care for diabetes. *Diabetes Metab Syndr Obes.* 2017;10:247–263. https://doi.org/10.2147/DMSO.S126314.
16. Kengne André Pascal, Amoah Albert GB, Mbanya Jean-Claude. *Cardiovascular Complications of Diabetes Mellitus in Sub-Saharan Africa.* December 6, 2005;112(23):3592–3601. https://doi.org/10.1161/CIRCULATIONAHA.105.544312.
17. Majaliwa ES, Elusiyan BEJ, Adesiyun OO, et al. Type 1 diabetes mellitus in the African population: epidemiology and management challenges. *Acta Biomed.* 2008;79:255–259.
18. Murunga AN, Owira PMO. Diabetic ketoacidosis: an overlooked child killer in sub-Saharan Africa? *Tropical Medicine and International Health.* November 2013;18(11):1357–1364. https://doi.org/10.1111/tmi.12195.
19. Nkpozi MO, Ezeani IU, Korubu IF, Chinenye S, Chapp-Jumbo AU. Outcome of hyperglycemic emergencies in a tertiary hospital, South East, Nigeria. *Sahel Med J.* 2019;22:47–54.

CHAPTER 29

DIABETES DIAGNOSIS AND MANAGEMENT IN NEW ZEALAND

Nic Crook, MD

1. **How is diabetes defined in New Zealand?**
   The definition of diabetes mellitus (DM) and gestational diabetes mellitus (GDM) varies depending on geographic location. In New Zealand (NZ), the threshold for a diagnosis of DM has been set at a hemoglobin A1c of ≥50 mmol/mol (6.7%), fasting glucose of ≥7 mmol/L (126 mg/dL), or 2-hour glucose (on a 75-g oral glucose tolerance test [OGTT]) of ≥11.1 mmol/L (200 mg/dL). GDM is defined by the OGTT, with the diagnosis being made by a fasting glucose of ≥5.5 mmol/L (90 mg/dL) or a 2-hour glucose of ≥9.0 mmol/L (182 mg/dL).

2. **What is the virtual diabetes register?**
   The Virtual Diabetes Register (VDR) contains data about people suspected of having DM, identified through their use of diabetes health services. The VDR uses an algorithm to identify these people by data extracted from hospital inpatient and outpatient records, laboratory tests, and pharmaceutical dispensing data; the VDR is collated annually at the end of March. National and regional DM prevalence estimates are calculated based on the number of people on the VDR as of December 31 of the previous year.

3. **What is the prevalence of diabetes in NZ?**
   The most recent prevalence data (2017) based on VDR and census data gives an overall DM prevalence of 3.76% in NZ. The prevalence in Maori (6.83%) and Pacific people (11.14%) was significantly greater than in NZ people from Europe (2.78%). On December 31, 2019, the VDR reported an estimate of 263,938 people with DM in NZ, representing a 40% increase since 2010. Data on the incidence and prevalence of type 1 DM are not available.

4. **How is diabetes healthcare organized in NZ?**
   The vast majority of healthcare in NZ is publicly funded by the central government and is free of cost at the point of care. Visiting a primary care provider usually attracts a small copayment, but treatment in the emergency department or hospital inpatient and outpatient settings does not. Less than 33% of New Zealanders have private health insurance. Primary care oversees around 80% of the DM care, with secondary and tertiary services predominantly caring for persons with type 1 DM, complex type 2 DM, and GDM/pregestational DM in pregnancy.

5. **Who decides what diabetes pharmaceuticals and medical devices are funded by the NZ public system?**
   PHARMAC is a government body formed in 1993 with the stated aim to "secure for eligible people in need of pharmaceuticals, the best health outcomes that are reasonably achievable from pharmaceutical treatment and from within the amount of funding provided."
   PHARMAC receives a budget allocation from the central government and is charged with assessing the available pharmaceuticals and medical devices and funding those that provide the best outcomes for all groups. Any funded medication is available to all appropriate New Zealanders by prescription with either no prescription fee or a nominal prescription fee of $5 per item.

6. **What sort of technology is available to support NZ people with diabetes?**
   A single capillary blood glucose (BG) monitoring system is funded for all people with DM, except those treated with lifestyle modification with or without metformin alone.
   Flash glucose monitors and continuous glucose monitors are not funded by the public system, but the Freestyle Libre and Dexcom G6 systems are available for private purchase.
   People with type 1 DM who have poor glycemic control or recurrent severe hypoglycemia in spite of an optimized regime of multiple-dose insulin are eligible for a funded insulin pump.

7. **Are there any limitations to access to the latest pharmaceutical diabetes therapies in NZ?**
   Starting February 1, 2021, PHARMAC commenced funding of a single sodium–glucose cotransporter 2 (SGLT-2) inhibitor for selected people who have not achieved their target hemoglobin A1c. Although PHARMAC plans to fund one glucagon-like peptide-1 (GLP-1) agonist later in 2021, there are no currently funded GLP-1 agonists, but they are available via private prescription.
   Degludec, Detemir, and Fiasp insulins are not currently funded by the public system.

8. **Are there any ethnic differences in outcomes for people with diabetes in NZ?**
Data from the VDR show that life expectancy at age 25 (LE_{25}) for Maori people with DM is 8.7 years less than that of non-Maori people with DM. Significant work is being undertaken at national and regional levels to narrow and ultimately eliminate this equity gap.

LE_{25} (YEARS)	NON-VDR	VDR	DIFFERENCE
Maori	53.3	44.6	8.7
Non-Maori	58.6	53.3	5.3

Maori and Pacific Island people bear a significantly greater burden of progression to end-stage renal disease. In a retrospective review of the data from a single District Health Board in North Island New Zealand, the crude incidence of dialysis/transplantation among Maoris with type 1 DM (17.3/1000 person-years) was 11-fold higher than that among NZ Europeans. Although the incidence rate of dialysis/transplantation among Maoris with type 2 DM (4.57/1000 person-years) was much lower than that among those with type 1 DM, it was 41 times higher than the rate among NZ Europeans. Adjusted hazard ratios confirmed this finding, with 46 times the risk of dialysis or transplantation for Maori people with type 2 DM.

9. **Are there any unusual patterns of complications in Maori people with diabetes?**
In a community-based screening setting for families identifying as Maori, among those who screened positive for DM, diabetic retinopathy was present in 1.7% of subjects. By contrast, nephropathy, evidenced by microalbuminuria, was present in 29.6% and overt albuminuria in 7.7%. The reasons for this disproportionate propensity to microvascular damage in the kidneys have not been elucidated, but genetic predisposition, higher smoking rates, and earlier hypertension onset have been postulated as drivers.

KEY POINTS

1. Healthcare in NZ is mostly publicly funded by the central government and is free of cost at the point of care.
2. The overall DM prevalence in NZ is 3.76%, but the prevalence is much higher in Maori (6.83%) and Pacific Island people (11.14%) than in NZ people from Europe (2.78%).
3. The crude incidence of dialysis/transplantation among Maoris with type 1 DM is 11-fold higher than for NZ Europeans and is 41 times higher among Maoris than for NZ Europeans with type 2 DM.
4. Life expectancy at age 25 for Maori people with DM is 8.7 years less than that of non-Maori people with DM.

BIBLIOGRAPHY

1. https://www.nzssd.org
2. https://www.health.govt.nz/system/files/documents/publications/screening-diagnosis-management-of-gestational-diabetes-in-nz-clinical-practive-guideline-dec14-v2.pdf
3. https://www.health.govt.nz/our-work/diseases-and-conditions/diabetes/about-diabetes/virtual-diabetes-register-vdr
4. Pharmac.govt.nz
5. Joshy G, Dunn P, Fisher M, et al. Ethnic differences in the natural progression of nephropathy among diabetes patients in New Zealand: hospital admission rate for renal complications, and incidence of end-stage renal disease and renal death. *Diabetologia*. 2009;52:1474–1478. https://doi.org/10.1007/s00125-009-1380-1.
6. Lim S, Chellumuthi C, Crook N, Rush E, Simmons D. Low prevalence of retinopathy, but high prevalence of nephropathy among Maori with newly diagnosed diabetes—Te Wai o Rona: Diabetes Prevention Strategy. *Diabetes Res Clin Pract*. 2008 May;80(2): 271–274. https://doi.org/10.1016/j.diabres.2007.12.018. Epub 2008 Feb 1. PMID: 18242758.

INDEX

Note: Page numbers followed by *f* indicate figures, *t* tables, *b* boxes.